Color Atlas of Vascular Tumors and Vascular Malformations

Color Atlas of Vascular Tumors and Vascular Malformations

Odile Enjolras, MD
APHP, Consultations des Angiomes, Hôpital Lariboisière, Service de Neuroradiologie; and Hôpital d'Enfants Armand Trousseau, Service de Chirurgie Maxillofaciale et de Chirurgie Plastique (Paris, France)

Michel Wassef, MD
APHP, Hôpital Lariboisière, Service d'Anatomie Pathologique, Université Paris 7 Faculté de Médecine (Paris, France)

René Chapot, MD
Service de Neuroradiologie Hôpital Universitaire Dupuytren (Limoges, France)

CAMBRIDGE
UNIVERSITY PRESS

CAMBRIDGE UNIVERSITY PRESS
Cambridge, New York, Melbourne, Madrid, Cape Town, Singapore, São Paulo

Cambridge University Press
32 Avenue of the Americas, New York, NY 10013-2473, USA

www.cambridge.org
Information on this title: www.cambridge.org/9780521848510

First published 2007

Printed in India by Replika

A catalog record for this publication is available from the British Library.

Library of Congress Cataloging in Publication Data

Enjolras, Odile, 1940–
Color atlas of vascular tumors and vascular malformations / Odile Enjolras, Michel Wassef, René Chapot.
p. ; cm.
Includes bibliographical references and index.
ISBN-13: 978-0-521-84851-0 (hardback)
ISBN-10: 0-521-84851-2 (hardback)
1. Blood-vessels—Tumors—Atlases. 2. Blood-vessels—Abnormalities—Atlases. I. Wassef, Michel, 1949– . II. Chapot, René, 1967– . III. Title.
[DNLM: 1. Vascular Neoplasms—Atlases. 2. Arteriovenous Malformations—Atlases. WG 17 585c 2006]
RC280.B56E55 2006
616.99′413—dc22

2006027036

ISBN 978-0-521-84851-0 hardback

This Atlas is dedicated to our much-loved patients and their families, who trusted us through exceptionally difficult times

Contents

Acknowledgments

Figures were provided by:

- Consultation des Angiomes, Department of Neuroradiology and Department of Pathology, Hôpital Lariboisière, Assistance Publique Hôpitaux de Paris, Faculté de Médecine Denis Diderot, Université Paris 7, France.
- Consultation des Angiomes, Department of Orofacial and Plastic Surgery, Hôpital d'Enfants Armand Trousseau, Assistance Publique Hôpitaux de Paris, Faculté de Médecine Pierre et Marie Curie, Université Paris 6, France.
- Department of Dermatology, Hôpital Tarnier/Cochin, Assistance Publique Hôpitaux de Paris, Faculté de Médecine René Descartes, Université Paris 5, France.

We also thank colleagues who provided illustrations and contributed to patient care:

- Our colleagues from the Multidisciplinary Team for Vascular Anomalies, APHP Lariboisière Hospital at Pr Jean-Jacques Merland – Neuroradiology Department, Université Paris 7, 75010 Paris, France: Dr. Annouk Bisdorff (Interventional Radiologist), Dr. Françoise Lemarchand-Venencie (Dermatologist and Laser Surgeon), Dr. Benoit Faucon (ENT and Plastic Surgeon), Dr. Didier Salvan (ENT and Plastic Surgeon), Dr. Michel Borsik (ENT and Plastic Surgeon), Dr. Dominique Deffrennes (ENT and Plastic Surgeon), Dr. George-Marie Brevière (Cardiologist and Pediatrician), Professsor Ludovic Drouet (Hematologist), Mrs. Maya Malet (Psychologist).
- Our colleagues from the Multidisciplinary Pediatric Vascular Clinics, APHP Armand Trousseau Children's Hospital at Pr Marie Paule Vazquez – Orofacial and Plastic Department, Université Paris 6, INSERM U714, 75012 Paris, France: Dr. Véronique Soupre (Orofacial and Plastic Surgeon), Dr. Jacques Buis (Orofacial and Plastic Surgeon), Dr. Virginie Fayard (Dermatologist and Laser Surgeon), Dr. Arnaud Picard (Orofacial and Plastic Surgeon),

Dr. Frédéric Zazurca (Orofacial and Plastic Surgeon), Dr. Patrick Diner (Orofacial and Plastic Surgeon), Dr. Sonia Ariche-Maman (Radiologist), Mrs. Pascale Gavelle (Psychologist).

In addition we thank:

- Professor John B. Mulliken (Plastic Surgeon, Children's Hospital, Harvard Medical School, Boston, USA); Dr. Patrice Josset (Pathologist, APHP-Armand Trousseau Children's Hospital Paris 75012, France); Dr. Claude Laurian (Vascular Surgeon, Department of Vascular Surgery, Hôpital Saint Joseph, Paris); Dr. E. Mazoyer (Hematologist, Department of Hemobiology, Hôpital Avicenne, APHP Paris, France); Dr. Gilles Roger (ENT and Plastic Surgeon, APHP-Armand Trousseau Children's Hospital, Paris 75012, France); Dr. C. Chiron (Department of Pediatric Neurology, Necker-Enfants Malades Hospital, APHP, Paris); Dr. Didier Bessis (Dermatologist, Saint Eloi Hospital, CHU Montpellier, France); Professor Catherine Adamsbaum (Radiologist, APHP Saint Vincent de Paul Hospital, Paris 75014, France); Dr. M. Pelisse (Dermatologist, Tarnier-Cochin Hospital, APHP Paris, France); Dr. Paul Rieu (Pediatric Surgeon, Department of Pediatric Surgery, St. Radboud Hospital, Nijmegen, The Netherlands); Professor Metin Tovi (Neuroradiologist, Karolinska Institute, Stockholm, Sweden); Professor Maureen Rogers (Pediatric Dermatologist, Westmead Children's Hospital, Sydney, Australia); Dr. Eulalia Baselga (Pediatric Dermatologist, Hospital de la Santa Creu I San Pau, Barcelona, Spain); Professor Susan B. Mallory (Dermatologist, Washington University School of Medicine, St. Louis, USA); Dr. Aicha Salhi (Dermatologist, Ain Nadja Hospital, CHU Alger, Algeria).

Introduction: ISSVA Classification

The International Society for the Study of Vascular Anomalies (ISSVA) was born in 1992 after 16 years of biennial international workshops. Interdisciplinary and international collaboration has been the guiding principle of the ISSVA, with a primary goal of improving our understanding and management of these lesions. This continuing workshop has taken place every two years in various countries around the world.

Multiple nomenclatures for "angiomas" or "vascular birthmarks" have long been an important obstacle to communication amongst the various medical specialists (pediatricians, dermatologists, surgeons, radiologists, angiologists, ophthalmologists, ENT surgeons, pathologists, etc.) involved in the management of these patients (13).

During discussions among members of the workshop it was decided to discard the old terms "angioma" and "birthmark." A very basic classification system was adopted by the ISSVA during its 1996 workshop, to give us a common language.

We now distinguish two main types of vascular anomalies: vascular tumors (the most common type is infantile hemangioma, but other rare vascular tumors occur in children as well as in adults) and vascular malformations (10).

This system is based on the founding biological investigation of Mulliken and Glowacki published in 1982, which provided the groundwork for a proper identification of vascular birthmarks (16). Vascular tumors have been differentiated from vascular malformations based on their clinical appearance, radiological and pathological features (21), and biological behavior. The suffix "oma" (used in the term "angioma") means proliferation of a tumor, and thus the words "angioma," "hemangioma," "lymphangioma" are erroneous when used for vascular malformations (10, 16).

Vascular tumors grow by cellular (mainly endothelial) hyperplasia: the very common infantile hemangioma is in reality a benign vascular tumor. In contrast, vascular malformations have a quiescent endothelium and are considered to be localized defects of vascular morphogenesis, likely caused by dysfunction in pathways regulating embryogenesis and vasculogenesis (Table 1). Vascular tumors

Table 1 Vasculogenesis, angiogenesis. As vasculogenesis begins (day 7 in the mouse embryo), the hemangioblasts, then the angioblast, are in a milieu rich in angiogenic factors (high levels of VEGF) and depleted in angiostatic factors (for instance, low levels of interferon, INF). Then, angiogenesis begins, slightly overlapping with vasculogenesis. Slowly over time, angiogenic factors taper and are accompanied by a parallel rise in angiostatic factors. This change in milieu leads to a slow and gradual decline in the relative amount of angiogenic activity, such that by birth, the angiogenic and angiostatic axis meet and global angiogenesis ends.

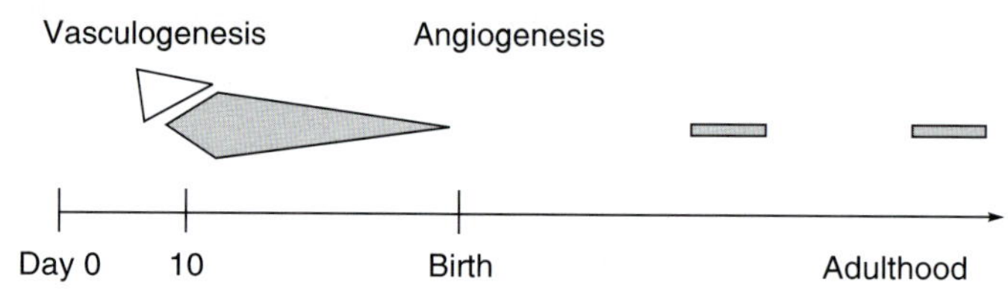

Reproduced with permission from: Chiller KC, Frieden IJ, Arbiser JL. Molecular pathogenesis of vascular anomalies, classification in three categories based upon clinical and biochemical characteristics. *Lymph Res Biol* 2003; **1**: 267–81 (Figure 2).

Table 2 The first "biological" classification of vascular anomalies.

Vascular tumors	*Vascular malformations*
Infantile hemangioma	Slow-flow vascular malformations: • Capillary malformation (CM) • Venous malformation (VM) • Lymphatic malformation (LM) Fast-flow vascular malformations: • Arterial malformation (AM) • Arteriovenous fistula (AVF) • Arteriovenous malformation (AVM)

can regress or persist depending on their type. Vascular malformations never regress, they persist throughout life. Most of them have commensurate growth during childhood, and some worsen over time if not treated (11, 17). Differentiating between vascular tumors and malformations is essential as not only their clinical, radiological and pathologic features and their morbidity, but also their management are quite different.

In addition to separation between vascular tumors and vascular malformations, a subdivision of vascular malformations, based on hemodynamics and on

Table 3 Main differences between the very common vascular tumor, infantile hemangioma, and vascular malformations.

	Infantile hemangioma	*Vascular malformations*
Age of occurrence and course	Infancy and childhood	Everlasting if not treated
Course	Three stages: proliferating, involuting, involuted	Commensurate growth or slow progression
Sex prevalence	3–9 girls/1 boy	1 girl/1 boy
Cellular	Increased endothelial cellular turnover. Increased mastocytes. Thick basement membrane	Normal cellular turnover. Normal number of mastocytes. Normal thin basement membrane
Immunohistochemical expression	Proliferating hemangioma: PCNA +++, VEGF +++, bFGF +++, collagenase IV +++, urokinase ++, TIMP-1 -, mast cells –, LYVE-1/CD31 +++, PROX1 – Involuting hemangioma: PCNA -, VEGF +, bFGF ++, collagenase IV -, urokinase ++, TIMP-1+++, mast cells +++, LYVE-1/CD31 –, PROX1 –	Barely detectable: PCNA, VEGF, bFGF, urokinase Not detectable: collagenase IV Variable staining for TIMP 1
Factors causing flare	None (or unknown)	Trauma, hormonal changes
Pathology	Distinctive aspects of the three phases of the tumor. GLUT1 +	CM, VM, LM, AVM, depending on the type. GLUT1 –
Radiological aspects on MRI	Well-delineated tumor with flow voids	Hypersignal on T2-sequences with VM or LM. Flow voids without parenchymal staining with AVM
Treatment	Spontaneous involution, or pharmacological treatment, or surgery, lasers	Lasers, or surgery and/or embolization/ sclerotherapy depending on the type

VEGF=vascular endothelial growth factor; bFGF=basic fibroblast growth factor; TIMP=tissue inhibitor matrix proteinase; GLUT1=glucose transporter 1; CM=capillary malformation; VM=venous malformation; LM=lymphatic malformation; AVM=arteriovenous malformation; MRI=magnetic resonance imaging.

predominant anomalous channels, was created (10, 11, 21). Vascular malformations are either slow-flow or fast-flow, and they are subcategorized into capillary malformation (CM), venous malformation (VM), lymphatic malformation (LM), and arteriovenous malformation (AVM) (Tables 1–4). This is quite important, since their management, with regard to both diagnosis (Table 5) and treatment (Table 6), will also be quite different depending on their subtype (5–9, 17, 21). Some patients have complex-combined vascular malformations, defined as capillary venous malformation (CVM), capillary lymphatic malformation (CLM), capillary lymphatic venous malformation (CLVM), lymphatic venous malformation (LVM), capillary arteriovenous malformation (C-AVM), or lymphatic arteriovenous malformation (L-AVM). Many of these syndromes are still labeled using eponymous terminology (Table 7).

Since 1982, a number of biological investigations have confirmed obvious differences between vascular tumors and malformations. Markers of cellular proliferation, such as cell nuclear antigen, type IV collagenase, vascular endothelial growth factor (VEGF), and basic fibroblast growth factor (bFGF), are elevated in proliferating hemangiomas, and not in vascular malformations (19). Serum levels

Table 4 Updated ISSVA classification of vascular anomalies.

Vascular tumors

- Infantile hemangiomas
- Congenital hemangiomas (RICH and NICH)
- Tufted angioma (with or without Kasabach–Merritt syndrome)
- Kaposiform hemangioendothelioma (with or without Kasabach–Merritt syndrome)
- Spindle cell hemangioendothelioma
- Other, rare hemangioendotheliomas (epithelioid, composite, retiform, polymorphous, Dabska tumor, lymphangioendotheliomatosis, etc.)
- Dermatologic acquired vascular tumors (pyogenic granuloma, targetoid hemangioma, glomeruloid hemangioma, microvenular hemangioma, etc.)

Vascular malformations

Slow-flow vascular malformations:

- Capillary malformation (CM)
  Port-wine stain
  Telangiectasia
  Angiokeratoma
- Venous malformation (VM)
  Common sporadic VM
  Bean syndrome
  Familial cutaneous and mucosal venous malformation (VMCM)
  Glomuvenous malformation (GVM) (glomangioma)
  Maffucci syndrome
- Lymphatic malformation (LM)

Fast-flow vascular malformations:

- Arterial malformation (AM)
- Arteriovenous fistula (AVF)
- Arteriovenous malformation (AVM)

Complex-combined vascular malformations:

- CVM, CLM, LVM, CLVM, AVM-LM, CM-AVM

C=capillary; V=venous; L=lymphatic; AV=arteriovenous; M=malformation. RICH=rapidly involuting congenital hemangioma; NICH=noninvoluting congenital hemangioma.

Table 5 Diagnostic imaging devices and the various vascular anomalies.

	Infantile hemangioma	*CM*	*VM*	*LM*	*AVM*
Ultrasonography/Doppler	+++	++	++	++	+++
Plain radiographs	–	–	++ (phleboliths, bone)	+/– (bone)	+ (bone)
MRI, MRA, MRV	++	–	+++	+++	++
CT	+	–	+	+	+
Angio-CT scans	–	–	+	–	++
Lymphoscintigraphy	–	–	–	+	–
Biopsy	+	+	+	+	+
Angiography	–	–	+	–	+++

MRI=magnetic resonance imaging; MRA=magnetic resonance angiography; MRV=magnetic resonance venography; CT=computed tomography; CM=capillary malformation; VM=venous malformation; LM=lymphatic malformation; AVM=arteriovenous malformation.

Table 6 Main therapeutic strategies depending on the type of vascular anomaly.

Modality	*Vascular tumors*	*Vascular malformations*
Pharmacological therapies (glucocorticosteroids, interferon alpha 2a or 2b, vincristine, cyclophosphamide, bleomycine, etc.)	+++	+/−
Lasers (FPDL, Nd-YAG, Diode, etc.)	+	CM +++ VM and LM +
Surgical excision/resection	++	++
Direct puncture sclerotherapy	−	VM and LM +++ AVM +
Arterial superselective embolization	+/− (liver hemangiomas, hemangiomas with congestive cardiac failure	AVM +++ VM +/−

FPDL=flashlamp pulsed dye laser; CM=capillary malformation; VM=venous malformation; LM=lymphatic malformation; AVM=arteriovenous malformation.

of VEGF are significantly higher in proliferating hemangiomas than in involuting hemangiomas, vascular malformations, and normal controls (23).

The origin of endothelial cells within the common hemangiomas of infancy has been discussed since it was established that they express GLUT1, merosin, Lewis Y antigen, and $F_{C}\gamma$ receptor II, during the three stages of hemangioma life (proliferating, involuting, and involuted stages) (18). These markers are also present on endothelial cells of placenta microvessels. These proteins are not expressed on endothelial cells of vascular malformations: the placenta-like microvascular phenotype is lacking in all types of vascular malformations (18). As GLUT1 positivity is lost in hemangioma cultures further experiments would determine if hemangioma endothelial cells actually originate from placenta or if both hemangioma endothelial cells and placenta endothelial cells simply share a similarly immature phenotype.

LYVE-1/CD 31 double staining gave positive results in proliferating hemangioma and not in involuting hemangioma, while PROX-1 was negative in both phases of hemangioma, and Dadras et al. concluded that these infantile tumors are arrested in an early developmental vascular differentiation state (8) (Table 3). New, mainly immunohistological, data let us update and complete the ISSVA classification (Table 4).

In roughly half of cases a hemangioma regresses to result in normal-appearing skin; however, it has long been observed that some involuted hemangiomas develop into a prominent fibro-fatty residuum. According to Bischoff (4) and Yu et al. (22) mesenchymal stem cells with adipogenic potential are present in proliferating hemangioma, and these cells probably contribute to this adipogenesis.

Table 7 Syndromes including slow-flow vascular malformations.

Syndrome	*Type of vascular malformation*	*Other main signs and symptoms*
Klippel–Trenaunay syndrome	CM, VM (varicose veins), LM (lymphedema, lymphatic vesicles)	Progressive overgrowth of the affected extremity, possible GI tract and urinary involvement
Proteus syndrome	CM, LM, VM	Disproportionate asymmetric overgrowth, cerebriform connective tissue nevus
Bannayan–Riley–Ruvalcaba syndrome	CM, VM?	Macrocephaly, developmental delay, GI tract polyposis
Cutis marmorata–macrocephaly syndrome	CM	Ocular anomalies, developmental delay
Cutis marmorata telangiectatica congenita	CM	Hypotrophy of affected limbs
Adams–Oliver syndrome	CM	Transverse limb defects, aplasia cutis of scalp
Rendu–Osler–Weber (hereditary hemorrhagic telangiectasia) syndrome	CM	Visceral AVMs
Ataxia telangiectasia	CM	Ataxia, immune deficiency, malignancies
Bean (blue rubber bleb nevus) syndrome	VM	GI tract lesions with hemorrhages, coagulopathy
Maffucci syndrome	VM	Enchondromas
Gorham–Stout syndrome	LM	Bone resorption

CM=capillary malformation; VM=venous malformation; LM= lymphatic malformation; AVM=arteriovenous malformation.

Various theories concerning the pathogenesis of hemangioma have been developed (3). Some suggest an intrinsic defect of hemangioma endothelial cells (hem ECs): the clonality of hem ECs has been demonstrated and a somatic mutation in a single progenitor cell has been hypothesized as the cause of hemangioma. The intrinsic theory is reinforced by the demonstration of loss of heterozygosity in 5q and by paradoxical response to endostatin of cultured hem ECs (3). Other theories suggest that hemangioma endothelial cells respond to extrinsic defects present in the local environment. These are based on various experiments: release of VEGF from in vitro cultured proliferating hemangioma was found (1), and alteration of expression of interferon-β in the epidermis overlying proliferating hemangioma, but not in the keratinocytes distant to the hemangioma, was demonstrated (2).

A balance between intrinsic and extrinsic factors, and between stimulators and inhibitors of angiogenesis, might account for the rapid growth and slow subsequent involution of infantile hemangiomas (3, 12).

It is currently hypothesized that infantile hemangiomas are primarily the consequence of excess angiogenesis ("hemangiogenesis"), while vascular malformations could be the result of errors in vessel remodeling (6). It has long been unclear whether true angiogenesis occurs in some vascular malformations that exhibit a clear propensity to thicken over the years, or expand, or even multiply. An example can be found with the lifelong increasing number of venous lesions in Bean syndrome (also known as blue rubber bleb nevus syndrome). Another example is the lethal, inexorably expanding, unalleviated course of some visceral thoracic and abdominal microcystic lymphatic malformations. New findings indicate that vascular malformations may also be angiogenesis-dependent disorders: urinary high-molecular-weight matrix metalloproteinases (hMW MMPs) and bFGF levels are elevated not only in vascular tumors but also in some vascular malformations, such as lymphatic or lymphatico-venous malformations and arteriovenous malformations (15). It is noticeable that this urinary increase in bFGF and hMW MMPs parallels the extent and progression of the vascular anomaly in patients with expanding, unremitting vascular malformations, while urinary VEGF levels do not (15).

Fewer data are available concerning the pathogenesis of vascular malformations, compared with what is currently known about infantile hemangioma. The excess of proteolytic enzymes like the hMW MMPs probably parallels the tissue remodeling observed in diffuse and expanding vascular malformations, such as some AVM or some LM, and the work of Marler et al. suggests that drugs targeting bFGF or MMPs might be an adequate therapeutic strategy for these patients (15).

The existence of inherited forms of vascular malformations, although rare, has permitted a new insight into the complex process of vasculogenesis and the molecular pathways physiologically involved in vascular malformations (7). As genetic defects are being identified in various types of vascular malformations (VM, glomuvenous malformation, familial lymphedema, arteriovenous-capillary malformation), the objective is to understand how such gene alterations, and modifications in signaling pathways (Table 8) result in abnormal vascular channels, with changes in embryonic blood or lymphatic vessels remodeling, ending in the familial forms of vascular malformations (3, 6, 20).

Molecular biology may completely change our approach to the classification of the various vascular anomalies (20). However, as we do not know whether the biological mechanisms of the sporadic vascular malformations, the most frequent ones, are similar to those of inherited forms, it is currently highly speculative to propose a shift to a genetic classification.

In addition, current progress in the understanding of the pathogenesis of angiogenesis-dependent vascular anomalies offers novel targets for their treatment. As an example, the knowledge of the enzyme defect in Fabry disease has resulted in enzyme replacement therapy with agalsidase alpha treatment, and this has changed the prognosis of this severe familial vascular disease (14). Future therapies for other types of vascular anomalies should be tailored to their specific defects once they are identified.

Treatments for the various vascular anomalies have become more specifically adapted over the last 30 years. Some treatments appeared to have more risks than benefits and were discarded. This was the case for the various types of ionizing radiation therapy. Therapeutic embolization through the arterial route and

Table 8 Genetics defects elucidated in some familial vascular malformations.

Diagnosis	*Transmission*	*Chromosomal location*	*Gene mutated*
VMCM (familial cutaneous and mucosal venous malformation)	AD	9p21	*Tie2* (TEK domain)
GVM (glomuvenous malformation, glomangioma)	AD	1p21–22	*Glomulin gene*
CM–AVM (capillary malformation–arteriovenous malformation)	AD	5q13.3	*RASA1*
Lymphedema of Milroy	AD	5q34–q35	*VEGFR3*
Lymphedema–distichiasis	AD	16q24	*FOXC2*
Cerebral cavernous malformations	AD	CCM1=7q11.2-q21, CCM2=7p15–p13, CCM3=3q25.2–27	*CCM1:KRIT1*, ligand de Krev/Rap1a
Bannayan–Riley–Ruvalcaba syndrome	AD	10q23	*PTEN*
Ataxia telangiectasia	AR	11q22–23	*ATM*
HHT (Rendu–Osler–Weber syndrome)	AD	HHT1=9q33, HHT2=12q13, HHT3=5q31.5–32	HHT1=ENG (endoglin), HHT2=ALK1(activin receptor-like kinase 1), HHT3=*gene*?

HHT=hereditary hemorrhagic telangiectasia; AD=autosomal dominant; AR=autosomal recessive; VEGFR=vascular endothelial growth factor receptor.

sclerotherapy through direct puncture of the lesion now have clear indications for use. Surgical procedures have been adapted and customized by both plastic and vascular surgeons. The development of laser technology, since the early 1960s, has resulted in major progress in the treatment of capillary malformations, with better clinical results as the devices have been improved. When successful, early laser treatment of port wine stains provides better results than the surgical treatments previously performed, and they allow the children to develop a positive self-image, reducing the subconscious psychological impact of the CM. A great deal of progress has been achieved in the field of vascular anomalies, but much still remains to be accomplished, in particular to improve our knowledge of their pathogenesis and the results of therapy.

References

1 Berard M, Ortega N, Carrier JL, Peyri N, Wassef M, Enjolras O, Drouet L. Plouet J. Vascular endothelial growth factor confers a growth advantage in vitro and in vivo to stromal cells cultured from neonatal hemangiomas. *Am J Pathol* 1997; **150**: 1315–26.

2 Bielenberg DR, Bucana CD, Sanchez R. Progressive growth of infantile cutaneous hemangiomas is directly correlated with hyperplasia and angiogenesis of adjacent

epidermis and inversely correlated with expression of endogenous angiogenesis inhibitor, IFN-beta. *Int J Oncol* 1999; **14**: 401–8.

3 Bischoff J. Monoclonal expansion of endothelial cells in hemangioma: an intrinsic defect with extrinsic consequences? *Trends Cardiovasc Med* 2002; **12**: 220–4.

4 Bischoff J. in: Infantile hemangiomas: current knowledge, future directions. Proceedings of a Research Workshop on Infantile Hemangioma. Bethesda Maryland, April 7–9, 2005. *Pediatr Dermatol* 2005; **22**: 383–406.

5 Burrows PE, Laor T, Paltiel H, Robertson RL. Diagnostic imaging in the evaluation of vascular birthmarks. *Dermatol Clin* 1998; **16**: 455–88.

6 Chiller KG, Frieden IJ, Arbiser JL. Molecular pathogenesis of vascular anomalies. Classification into three categories based upon clinical and biochemical characteristics. *Lymphatic Res and Biol* 2003; **1**: 267–82.

7 Cohen MM. Vasculogenesis, angiogenesis, hemangiomas and vascular malformations. *Am J Med Genet* 2002; **108**: 265–74.

8 Dadras SS, North PE, Bertoncini J, Mihm MC, Detmar M. Infantile hemangiomas are arrested in an early vascular differentiation state. *Mod Pathol* 2004; **17**: 1068–79.

9 Dubois J, Garel L. Imaging and therapeutic approach of hemangiomas and vascular malformations in the pediatric age group. *Pediatr Radiol* 1999; **29**: 879–93.

10 Enjolras O, Mulliken JB. Vascular tumors and vascular malformations (new issues). *Adv Dermatol* 1997; **13**: 375–423.

11 Enjolras O, Riché MC. *Atlas des Hémangiomes et Malformations Vasculaires Superficielles.* Paris: Medsi-McGraw-Hill ; 1990.

12 Folkman J. Fundamental concepts of the angiogenic process. *Curr Mol Med* 2003; **3**: 643–51.

13 Hand JL, Frieden IJ. Vascular birthmarks of infancy: resolving nosologic confusion. *Am J Med Genet* 2002; **108**: 257–64.

14 Hoffmann B, Garciade Lorenzo A, Mehta A, Beck M, Widmer U, Ricci R. FOS European Investigators. Effects of enzyme replacement therapy on pain and health related quality of life in patients with Fabry disease: data from FOS (Fabry Outcome Survey). *J Med Genet* 2005; **42**: 247–52.

15 Marler JJ, Fishman SJ, Kilroy SM, Fang J, Upton J, Mulliken JB, Burrows PE, Zurakowski D, Folkman J, Moses MA. Increased expression of urinary matrix metalloproteinases parallels the extent and activity of vascular anomalies. *Pediatrics* 2005; **116**: 38–45.

16 Mulliken JB, Glowacki J. Hemangiomas and vascular malformations in infants and children: a classification based on endothelial characteristics. *Plast Reconstr Surg* 1982; **69**: 412–22.

17 (Mulliken JB, Young AE, eds.) *Vascular Birthmarks: Hemangiomas, & Malformations.* Philadelphia: WB Saunders, 1988.

18 North PE, Waner M, Mizeracki A, Mrak RE, Nicholas R, Kincannon J, Suen JY, Mihm MC Jr. A unique microvascular phenotype shared by juvenile hemangiomas and human placenta. *Arch Dermatol* 2001; **137**: 559–70.

19 Takahashi K, Mulliken JB, Kozakewich HPW, Rogers RA, Folkman J, Ezekowitz RA. Cellular markers that distinguish the phases of hemangioma during infancy and childhood. *J Clin Invest* 1994; **93**: 2357–64.

20 Vikkula M, Boon LM, Mulliken JB. Molecular genetics of vascular anomalies. *Matrix Biol* 2001; **20**: 327–35.

21 Wassef M, Enjolras O. Les malformations vasculaires superficielles: classification et histopathologie. *Ann Pathol* 1999; **19**: 253–64.

22 Yu Y, Fuhr J, Boye E, Gyorffy S, et al., Mesenchymal stem cells and adipogenesis in hemangioma involution. *Stem Cells* 2006; epub ahead of print.

23 Zhang L, Lin X, Wand W, Zhuang X, Dong J, Qi Z, Hu Q. Circulating level of vascular endothelial growth factor in differentiating hemangioma from vascular malformation patients. *Plast Reconstr Surg* 2005; **116**: 200–4.

PART I

Investigations and Radiological Tools

Various imaging tools are available for the diagnosis of vascular malformations (1–5). Techniques must be adapted to the clinical findings and to the aim of imaging, which may be diagnosis, pre-therapeutic assessment, or follow-up with or without treatment.

Conventional X-Rays

These are usually of little interest and are normal in most situations. Venous malformations may be diagnosed if phleboliths are seen on plain radiographs. Bone distortion is only seen in large malformations with an important soft tissue mass effect. Some diffuse venous malformations in the limbs match up with fragile, thinner, curved bones, and sometimes lytic lesions, and a risk of pathologic fracture. Occasionally, an arteriovenous malformation involves a bone and either the intraosseous nidus, or large draining venous channels, after the nidus, create lytic bony lesions.

Ultrasonography in Combination with Doppler

This scan is frequently used as the primary diagnostic tool (4). It often permits distinction between tumors and malformations. It also allows a vascular malformation to be identified and pinpoints the type of lesion. It shows whether the lesion is cystic or tissular, demonstrates the presence or absence of flow, and thus differentiates between fast-flow and slow-flow malformations. Angioarchitecture and vessel density may be analyzed but reliability is often poor. Peak flow velocities and arterial output may also be measured in AVMs. In a patient with an AVM in the head and neck or in an extremity, comparing the arterial output on the normal side to that on the contralateral vascular abnormal side (e.g. both carotid, or both humeral, or both femoral arterial outputs, depending on the site of the AVM), is indispensable to get an idea of the prognosis, and particularly of possible cardiac failure. These techniques are particularly useful for the noninvasive follow-up of AVMs.

Computed Tomography (CT)

This is of limited interest, even after iodinated contrast injection, only allowing us to decide if a lesion is highly vascularized or not. Precise description and diagnosis of soft tissue lesions remain weak, except in macrocystic lymphatic malformations where the cysts are clearly depicted. The presence of phleboliths may direct us towards a diagnosis of venous malformation as these round calcifications develop on thromboses linked to the slow flow. Bony displacement or alteration can also be seen due to chronic compression in VMs and LMs. Transcranial connections are also identified by CT in head and neck VMs. CT scan angiography, with 3-D reconstruction, however, may superbly map the enlarged vascular channels in an arteriovenous malformation.

Magnetic Resonance Imaging (MRI)

This is the best diagnostic tool, allowing optimal analysis of soft tissue masses and adequate diagnosis, differentiating tissular from cystic lesions, and showing fast and slow circulating vessels. As an example, MRI is indispensable in the diagnosis of peri-ocular hemangioma (3). Venous and lymphatic malformations have a characteristic pattern, being hyperintense on spin echo T2-weighted sequences, and optimally seen on fat suppression sequences. Fat suppression T1-weighted sequences with gadolinium injection show an intense enhancement in infantile hemangioma tumors, whereas the enhancement is variable and progressive on dynamic sequences in venous malformations. Gadolinium contrast injection permits differential diagnosis between VM and LM. LMs can be differentiated from VMs as they show only enhancement at the margins of the cysts, while VMs are usually clearly stained. MRI is not only useful for identification and diagnosis of the lesion, but is also mandatory before treatment to delineate the extent of the lesion and depict the relationship between the vascular malformation and neighboring vessels and nerves. In fast circulating vessels, they will appear as flow voids on most sequences. MR-angiography may then be performed, confirming the diagnosis of fast circulating vessels, but it remains insufficient for precisely depicting the AVM nidus and analyzing the angioarchitecture.

Conventional Vascular Imaging

These techniques are mostly not indicated for the diagnosis of a vascular malformation, except for fast-flow vascular lesions.

Indirect phlebography is usually of little interest and should not be used systematically in VMs as opacification of a venous malformation is inconsistently seen. It is of some interest in some diffuse extremity VMs, before a therapeutic decision is made.

Direct percutaneous phlebography is valuable for depicting a VM and to show the draining pattern. However, it should only be used as a pre-therapeutic step, immediately before sclerotherapy, and not as a diagnostic tool.

Conventional angiography has few indications in slow-flow vascular malformations as it will show a variable blush with a nonspecific pattern. Angiography remains, however, indispensable for the diagnosis and pre-therapeutic assessment of an AVM, the characteristic feature of which is an early venous drainage. Angiography also allows us to analyze the angioarchitecture of the AVM, to precisely identify its location, and to depict the arterial suppliers and draining veins and its relationship to the normal surrounding arteries and veins. Angiography is specially indicated to establish the diagnosis in quiescent AVMs, simulating a capillary malformation, where it may be important not to miss the diagnosis before proposing a treatment that may trigger the growth of a dormant AVM, such as pulsed dye laser treatment (5).

References

1 Burrows PE, Laor T, Paltiel H, Robertson RL. Diagnostic imaging in the evaluation of vascular birthmarks. *Dermatol Clin* 1998; **16**: 455–88.

2 Dubois J, Garel L. Imaging and therapeutic approach of hemangiomas and vascular malformations in the pediatric age group. *Pediatr Radiol* 1999; **29**: 879–93.

3 Millischer-Bellaiche AE, Enjolras O, André Ch, Bursztyn J, Kalifa G, Adamsbaum C. Les hémangiomes palpébraux du nourrisson. *J Radiol* 2004; **85**: 2019–28.
4 Paltiel H J, Burrows P E, Kozakewich H P, Zurakowski D, Mulliken JB. Soft-tissue vascular anomalies: utility of US for diagnosis. *Radiology* 2000; **214**: 747–54.
5 Wu JK, Bisdorff A, Gelbert F, Enjolras O, Burrows PE, Mulliken JB. Auricular arteriovenous malformation: evaluation, management, and outcome. *Plast Reconstr Surg* 2005; **115**: 985–95.

PART II

Vascular Tumors

CHAPTER II.A

Infantile Hemangioma (IH)

Introduction

Infantile hemangioma (IH) is also known as "strawberry mark" and "immature hemangioma;" the other names, "capillary hemangioma" and "cavernous hemangioma," have long caused confusion with vascular malformations. IH is a very frequent benign vascular tumor that grows rapidly in an infant over a period of a few weeks or months after birth (the proliferating phase). Then it slowly and constantly regresses over some years (the involuting phase), to leave nearly normal skin, or skin and shape changes (the involuted phase). This third stage is rarely reached at the age of 1 or 2 years, and is most commonly attained around 5 or 6 years, and sometimes not before 10 years. No such tumor occurs in an adolescent or adult; thus, using the wording "hemangioma" or "capillary hemangioma" for a vascular tumor appearing in an adolescent or an adult is misleading.

IHs affect about 10% of children. Dark-skinned infants have a lower incidence than fair-skinned infants. Transcervical chorionic villus sampling increases the risk of IH in the newborn, but not amniocentesis.

The incidence of hemangioma is increased in premature infants of very low birth weight (under 1000 g) (4). A group of US Pediatric Dermatologists, the Hemangioma Investigator Group, confirmed this finding in a prospective study presented at the NIH-sponsored research workshop held in April 2005 at the Bethesda Campus (41). They also highlighted an increased incidence in cases of high maternal age for a first baby, multiple gestation, placental abnormalities, placenta praevia, or preeclampsia.

Numerous factors inducing postnatal growth of hemangioma and subsequent involution have been documented (9, 41, 99, 95), but the very first event initiating the lesion itself remains unidentified, as the reasons for growth starting soon after birth, and for the shift from proliferation to involution after a few months of proliferation remain unknown (9).

It has been shown that IH has a distinctive placenta-like microvascular phenotype (82) that is stable in vivo and lost in culture.

Two hypotheses currently rely on this finding:

1. the hemangioma could result from a somatic mutation occurring in a regulatory gene in a progenitor endothelial cell ending in an immature placental endothelial phenotype; and
2. it could originate from the clonal expansion of embole of placental endothelial cells (82).

IHs are subcategorized into three groups: superficial, deep, and the "mixed" type which is both superficial and deep. They are single or multiple, or disseminated (the miliary type or disseminated neonatal hemangiomatosis (DNH)). An IH is of variable size: from a small dot to a diffuse plaque-like or bossed tumor covering the face, part of the trunk, or an extremity. Color depends on the dermal extent: a very superficial IH has the brightest red color, a deeply growing IH gives a bluish shade and telangiectasia to the overlying skin, or is situated under normally colored skin.

IH predominantly affects the skin (ubiquitously), the oral and genital mucous membrane, the orbit, the airway, and the parotid. Specific locations, such as the lids, nose or lips, have distinctive aspects and complications. It has been suggested that facial hemangiomas develop in a nonrandom distribution (104). Visceral involvement is uncommon. Muscles are not affected but IH may infiltrate the fascia between muscles (in the literature venous malformations of muscles are too often incorrectly labeled intramuscular hemangiomas). Bones are not affected (the so-called hemangioma of bones in the literature corresponds mainly to bony venous malformation). A very rare facial bony tumor present at birth may mimic IH on pathology, but it is GLUT1 negative (OE, unpublished data). GLUT1 is a highly selective immunohistochemical marker for IH, of major value when the pathological diagnosis is somewhat doubtful (81, 82).

The three phases of an IH, proliferation, spontaneous involution, and involuted, sometimes with sequelae, are of variable duration depending on the patient. In visceral locations they follow the same three-phase course as superficial IH.

A majority of IHs (80 to 90%) are small and not dangerous, and may be left to recede spontaneously. However, location has a crucial role in determining possible risks (26). IHs that are alarming due to size, site, volume, function-threatening location (eyelid and orbit, airway, etc.) or that are life-threatening (massive tumor, ulceration and subsequent infection, visceral location, recurrent hemorrhages, congestive heart failure), will require active therapeutic management.

Infants with DNH are at greater risk of visceral involvement. The liver is the most common location; however, many patients with diffuse liver IH do not have skin lesions or only a few lesions (41). IHs can develop in many other visceral sites: GI tract, pancreas, kidney, lung, heart, meninges, brain, etc. A majority of skin and liver DNHs follow a benign self-limiting course, and are assessed by regular clinical and ultrasonographic follow-up; involution of both superficial and visceral lesions usually begins in the latter part of the first year. On rare occasion in infants they develop in life-threatening visceral locations; liver lesions, when multifocal or diffuse, can create massive hepatomegaly and congestive heart failure, requiring aggressive medical treatment, embolization and even liver transplant (39). Based on 43 reports and four personal cases Metry et al. (72) reported on the association of solitary segmental IH of the skin and visceral IH: among 47 patients with facial IH (79%), or facial IH plus at another location, the liver was the most frequent associated visceral location (43%), followed by the GI tract (34%), brain (34%), mediastinum (19%), and lung (15%), other associations being very rare. In this study liver and GI tract lesions were responsible for the death of one-quarter of these patients.

Individual cases of structural abnormalities (brain, heart, vessels, and sternum) associated with hemangiomas have long been reported. Those occurring in association with cephalic IH have also long been recognized (84, 85). They are now known as PHACE(S) syndrome, an acronym denoting the major features of the syndrome: **P**osterior fossa anomalies, **H**emangioma, **A**rterial intracranial and extracranial anomalies, **C**oarctation of the aortic arch and cardiac defects, **E**ye abnormalities, and **S**ternal malformations or supraombilical raphe (40, 41). Details of the many manifestations of patients with PHACE(S) syndrome (OMIM 606519) reported in the literature (128 cases) can be found in the paper by Metry (73). In the same settings a progressive cerebral vasculopathy with aneurismal and occlusive changes can result in cerebral infarction and neurological sequelae (10, 18). Early stroke has been reported in five newborns with PHACE syndrome (26). They developed progressive vasculopathy, and the brain vascular anomalies and ischemic changes were located ipsilaterally to the facial IH (26). PHACE syndrome was first detected in adulthood in a woman who had an involuted hemangioma of the left forehead, and complained of headaches and neurological deficit: she had complex intracranial arterial anomalies of the left internal carotid artery (Dr. Monique Boukobza, Hôpital Lariboisière, Paris, unpublished data); this case stresses the need for prolonged follow-up when PHACE, as is usual, is detected in infancy. The incidence of this neurocutaneous syndrome is still unknown (41, 71). The structural anomalies may be symptom-free and thus not detected if not specifically screened for. We had 12 patients affected in a group of 175 infants, but the series had a bias: all had severe IH (33); in addition this number might have been an underestimation, as not all infants underwent brain and heart investigations. Developmental defects also happen with lumbosacral and lower extremity IH. Hemangioma in the mid-lumbosacral area requires neuroradiological imaging only if it is associated with one or several other markers of spinal dysraphism; for example, when a dimple, a dermal sinus, a lipoma, a skin tail, a hairy tuft, or a deviated gluteal cleft are associated (50).

IHs always have a female predilection (about 3/1 female/male ratio) but a female preponderance for the most severe cases (9/1) is quite striking (including extensive superficial IH, visceral IH, and IH associated with PHACE(S) syndrome or other developmental defects) (22, 33, 41, 47, 71). IHs occurring in a segmental morphology carry a higher risk of complications (22, 74). The cause of PHACE(S) syndrome is unknown and the female predominance leads to the hypothesis of an X-linked defect surviving by mosaïcism with lethality in males (16, 41). Concerning the association of a vascular tumor, the IH, with structural malformations Bauland et al. hypothesized either developmental field anomalies or single gene defects (9).

Pathology

During the proliferative phase, IHs are made of endothelial cells and pericytes, forming organized capillaries, often with virtual lumen, grouped in lobules with afferent and efferent thicker-walled arteriolar-like vessels. The lesion expresses bFGF, VEGF, IGF2, E-selectin, urokinase and collagenase IV (63, 99, 95). In the involuting phase, the capillary lumen becomes more obvious, the number of vessels progressively decreases, and thickening and lamination of their basement membrane occur associated with apoptosis (42, 58, 93) and secretion of TIMP-1 (99). North et al. showed that IH endothelial cells express several markers also expressed in the placental endothelial cells (erythrocyte type glucose transporter1 (GLUT1), Lewis Y antigen, FcγRII and merosin) or in nervous system endothelial cells (GLUT1 and merosin) (81, 82). This immunophenotype is unique to IH endothelial cells, and not present in vascular malformations; therefore it is of major diagnostic interest (Table 9). GLUT1 is also commonly used in the differential diagnosis of IH and other vascular tumors since GLUT1 is

Table 9 Diagnosis of infantile hemangioma.

Diagnostic methods	*Diagnostic value*
Clinical evaluation: age, appearance, course	Best diagnostic factors in more than 90% of infants
US/color Doppler evaluation	Very effective in skillful hands (but risk of misdiagnosis of AVM)
CT scans with iodinated contrast	Indicates the extent and the vascular nature of the lesion, but is not specific
MRI	Indicates the extent of the tumor; images allow better, more precise diagnosis of hemangioma than CT
Angiography	No longer necessary for diagnosis
Biopsy	Rarely necessary (atypical lesions). If performed, GLUT1 staining is indispensable (100% + in IH).

US = ultrasonography; AVM = arteriovenous malformation; CT = computed tomography; MRI = magnetic resonance imaging; GLUT1 = glucose transporter 1; IH = infantile hemangioma.

positive in 100% of IH endothelial cells and negative in the other infantile vascular tumors, including congenital hemangiomas, tufted angioma, and kaposiform hemangioendothelioma.

Treatment

We must first emphasize the fact that a majority of IH are small lesions, often located in areas covered by clothes, and are left to spontaneously disappear. After regression either normal skin is restored or there are some sequelae, such as telangiectasia, anetoderma, and fibro-fatty residuum. Nothing predicts the occurrence of the fibro-fatty residuum after regression. Interestingly, the presence of mesenchymal stem cells with adipogenic potential in cultures of proliferating IHs has been demonstrated (106). The infants requiring treatment during the proliferating or early involuting phases probably represent 10 to 20% of cases, including pharmacological and early surgical therapies. Among the 1109 infants followed by Akyuz et al. (2) only 4% received oral glucocorticosteroid treatment.

Some authors advise treating small and flat IHs in their early expansion using cryotherapy (cryosurgery) or pulsed dye laser treatments in order to try to stop their early growth. Though long suggested, results of these therapeutic modalities are not yet clearly established and they are difficult to appraise, as nothing helps us to predict the final enlargement and particularly the thickening of a proliferating IH. Contact cryosurgery with new cooling devices limiting the working temperature to −32°C was reported as effective, with few side-effects compared to the use of liquid nitrogen (94). The usefulness of flashlamp pulsed dye laser treatment of IH in the early weeks of life is still controversial (8, 55, 56). Improvement in color can be achieved, but without preventing progression of a deep component of IH, or without appreciable resolution of the existing bulk of tumor (5, 43, 90, 97). Other lasers used for the treatment of IH are Nd-YAG or carbon dioxide lasers; however, there is a higher risk of scarring.

Radiotherapy is no longer recommended because of the risk of malignancies in the long term.

Embolization has limited indications (liver hemangiomas or very large superficial hemangiomas, with cardiac failure, poorly responding to pharmacological treatment).

Oral glucocorticosteroid (GS) treatment is still the first step in the pharmacological treatment of dangerous IHs: for example, large IHs of alarming growth, facial IHs impairing vision, severely skin and shape-altering IHs with a risk of permanent and difficult to restore deformity, airway location often linked to

Table 10 Guidelines for the management of an infant with alarming and dangerous cephalic infantile hemangioma.

Clinical examination (clinical pictures taken)

- Every two weeks during the first 2 or 3 months of life
- Then usually every month during the growth phase and early involuting phase (more if needed)

Ultrasonography and color Doppler

- For deeply growing IH without bright red typical superficial growth (e.g. parotid mass under normal skin)

MRI (of face and brain) (and MRA)

- To detect orbital extension in case of eyelid location or exophthalmos
- To detect deep location of IH (cheek, parotid, hypopharyngeal, airway, neck)
- When brain and cerebrovascular anomalies of PHACE syndrome can be associated (mainly when IH is segmental and located on the forehead, upper eyelid, and centrofacial area)

Cardiac ultrasonographic evaluation

- If cardiac or aortic malformation of PHACE(S) syndrome can be linked (mainly IH of both mandibular areas and midline anterior neck or thorax, with midline supraumbilical congenital raphe, and sternal malformation)
- When a bulky IH with increasing arterial flow may create congestive heart failure
- When the child is receiving long-standing glucocorticosteroid treatment

Laryngeal and tracheal endoscopy

- When airway IH may exist (laryngeal and tracheal IH in association with "beard IH")
- And if any respiratory symptoms is associated with a cephalic IH

Hearing tests

- When both external ears are obstructed by the IH growth
- In some large parotid, ear and neck unilateral IH, even when no external ear involvement, because of possible internal ear IH
- In some infants with PHACE(S) syndrome

Ophthalmological monitoring

- When there is eyelid (upper or lower) and/or orbital IH, putting pressure on the cornea and eyeball, hiding the visual axis, or creating dystopia
- In case of PHACE syndrome

hemangioma in the beard area, and visceral IHs (Table 10) (36). In our experience (31, 33), no more than 30% of infants with life- and function-threatening IH experience a dramatic and persisting response to GS; about 40% undergo stabilization of the tumor growth, with ensuing involution as slow as expected without treatment; 30% are nonresponders and they fail to respond to even increased dosage or adding pulse therapy of GS. Good response was obtained in 36% of patients with severe IH by Akyuz et al. (2), and the response was independent of dosage and pharmacological agent. The quantitative systematic review of the literature by Bennett et al. (10), assessing stabilization and involution coincident with GS use, and IH of variable severity, gives a mean response rate of 84%, with an apparent dose—response relationship, and with rebound in 36%. Prednisone or prednisolone are the GS habitually prescribed (starting dose usually 2–3 mg/kg/day). Betamethasone is also prescribed with a dosage of 0.15 to 0.25 mg/kg/day. There are various regimens for oral GS treatment of IH. We use GS given by the oral route in a single morning dose, with an initial dose maintenance for as long as 8 weeks in most cases. Sometimes an even longer initial period is required. Then slow tapering of the dose is performed over 2 to 3 months, in order to prevent rebound growth of the tumor and to allow adrenal suppression to recover. Careful monitoring of the child is required. Nearly inevitable side-effects of GS include irritability, insomnia, gastric irritation and increased reflux, Cushingoid face with hairiness, and growth suppression. Growth curves normalize after 2 years of age (13). In the literature, hypertension has been underestimated or not assessed at all, even in studies reporting on prolonged and very high daily doses of GS. Hypertension developed more quickly in patients who were given a higher initial dose of GS (13, 46, 100). Other rare complications of GS are: hypertrophic cardiomyopathy (91, 100), cataract, infection (one report of pneumocystis carinii pneumonia (6)), osteoporosis with protracted GS treatment, and prolonged adrenal suppression. Infants with more pronounced growth suppression might be at higher risk of adrenal suppression (41). Careful monitoring of the infant is recommended for the developement of side-effects.

Neurodevelopmental impairment was reported in preterm infants who received early postnatal dexamethasone treatment for lung disease (105); no such adverse effect has been appraised in infants treated for IH; however, this requires precise further evaluation.

Intralesional glucocorticosteroid treatment is sometimes preferred for rapidly growing nodular IH, for example in the cheek, tip of the nose, forehead, or lip. There is a risk of cutaneous atrophy and hypochromia, both transient (21). Periocular injections of corticosteroid in IH, introduced by Kushner in 1982, yield distinctive complications. They carry rare but severe risks, including blindness linked to retrograde flow migration of GS particles in the central retinal artery (probably dependent on high injection pressure), ulceration, lid necrosis, sclerodermiform linear atrophy, hypopigmentation, and perforation of the globe (29, 30, 65, 98, 101). Adrenal suppression was also noticed but not as often as with oral GS treatment. Response rates seem similar to those with oral GS treatment.

Topical corticosteroid has been used, mainly on superficial IH, with as yet unclear results (16, 45).

Failure of GS treatment for alarming, endangering, function- or life-threatening hemangiomas requires alternative therapy.

Interferon alpha 2a or 2b (IFN) was first employed in the early 1990s (37). Daily subcutaneous injection of 3 million units/m^2 is usually prescribed for 6 to 12 months. Results are good, particularly on the bulk of the tumor in our experience, in the vast majority of patients (20, 37, 44, 67,). The main indications have been sight-threatening IH (52) and airway IH (69) as well as any life-threatening IH (26). However, we now limit its prescription because, beside the well-known and reversible side effects (flu-like symptoms, alteration of hematological, liver and thyroid parameters, and possibly seizures or personality changes), a distinctive neurological complication (spastic diplegia) has been reported in these infants (7, 28, 34, 37). Infants receiving IFN must be closely monitored for any neurological change, and the treatment must be stopped if the monthly neurological examination documents some anomalous sign. A meta-analysis confirmed that this unwanted, yet poorly understood effect, occurred only in infants receiving IFN for a vascular tumor: 6.1% of 441 children with hemangioma or another vascular tumor developed either spastic diplegia (SD, 11 cases) or mild motor developmental disturbance (MDD, 18 cases), while none of 2140 children receiving IFN for chronic hepatitis had SD or MDD; the authors advocate prescribing IFN as a last resort and, if possible, in children older than one year (76).

Vincristine (VCR), a vinca-alcaloid, was introduced as an alternative to IFN for dangerous corticoresistant skin and visceral (airway, orbit, liver) IHs. VCR is prescribed once a week, by IV injection, at a dosage of 1 mg/m^2, or lower (0.75mg/m^2) if the infant's body weight is less than 5 kg. In our experience VCR is effective, but the number of necessary injections may vary from 5 to 25. It was particularly rapidly successful as first-line therapy in a newborn affected with multifocal liver IH and congestive heart failure (35). Adams also reported good results in patients with complicated superficial or visceral IH who received VCR because of significant side-effects of their GS treatment inability to diminish GS, or no response to GS (1). Short-term side-effects reported with VCR included constipation and abdominal pain, worsening of esophageal reflux ileus, peripheral neuropathy, alopecia, hematological toxicity; long-term side-effects are very limited.

Intralesional bleomycin treatment has recently been introduced in the treatment of unsafe hemangioma; it looks very effective (89). However, a protocol has not yet been clearly established to avoid the risk of pulmonary fibrosis.

Prospective trials are still needed to define the best first- and second-line pharmacological therapy for dangerous IH.

Surgical treatment has a role during three periods in the life of an IH: surgery in emergency for some complication (for example an impossible-to-stop hemorrhage from an ulceration), early excision during the proliferating phase or at the beginning of the involuting process, and late repair of residual after-effects (101). Early surgery during the proliferating phase is used in some locations (sight-threatening eyelid-deep IH, Cyrano-nose IH), as well as for some "pendulum" IH, for IH distorting an adjacent structure if a cosmetically acceptable surgical scar can be expected, and for some complications (extremely painful ulceration with no propensity to heal with medical care and dressings) (24, 41, 79, 101).

Surgical procedures are chosen to match particular locations, for example laryngeal surgery for airway lesions (103). Airway IH is probably the most frequent visceral IH. In a large review of the outcome of treatments of subglottic hemangioma, including 116 patients from three centers, 77% of those who received GS treatment did not respond adequately; CO2 laser applications gave either good or minimum benefit with a high risk of stenosis; open approach laryngotracheoplasty in a single stage modality was recommended for patients who have a subglottic lesion causing more than 70% subglottic narrowing, those with bilateral or circumferential lesion, and in nonresponders to GS treatment (92). A literature review of 372 infants highlighted the claim that oral GS are poorly effective in symptomatic airway IH, with only one-quarter of patients responding (12).

Late surgical removal of damaged, expanded, lax skin and fibrofatty residuum, and reconstruction of structural consequences of IH take place in the late involuting or involuted phase. For example, a lip IH often results in distortion requiring progressive harmonization of the contour of the mouth (101). Flashlamp pulsed dye laser treatment clears residual telangiectasia. Laser resurfacing may somewhat improve the appearance of irregularly pigmented wrinkled skin of the involuted stage.

Figures

INFANTILE HEMANGIOMA (IH)
Pathology

During the proliferation phase, IHs are made up of densely packed capillaries, often with virtual lumen, grouped in distinct or more confluent lobules.

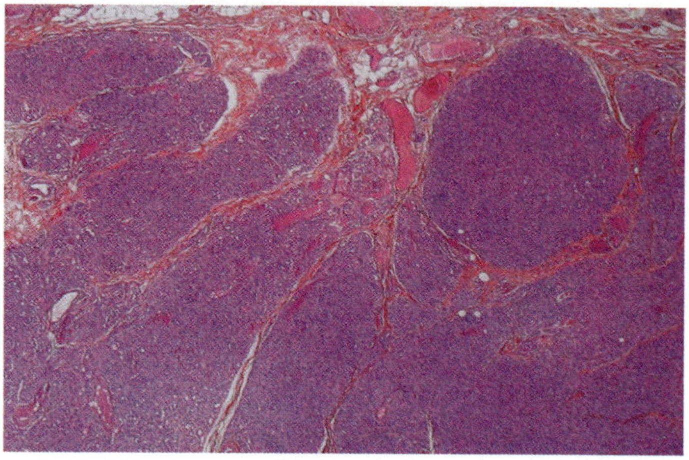

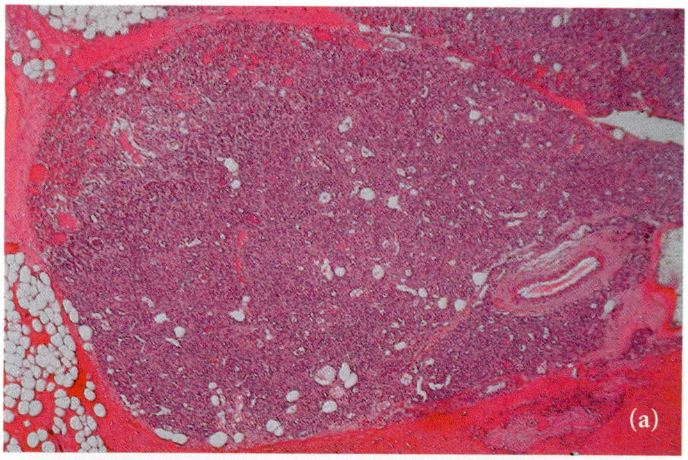

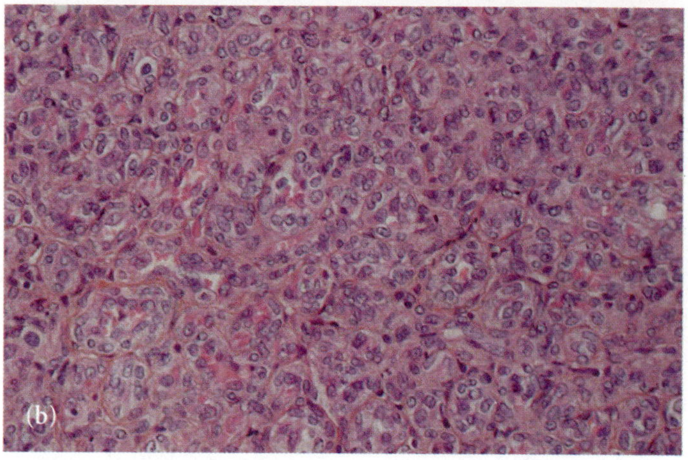

Many of the lobules are associated with afferent and efferent arterial-type vessels with a well-defined muscular media (a). The capillaries are made up of an internal layer of endothelial cells surrounded by a layer of pericytes; some anisocaryosis and mitosis are frequently seen (b).

Pathology

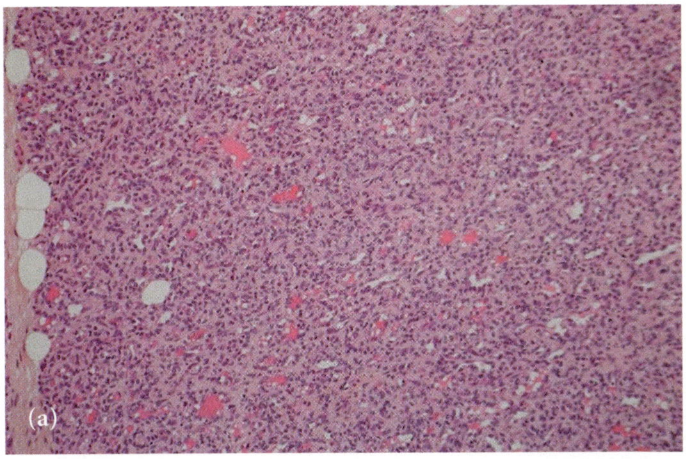

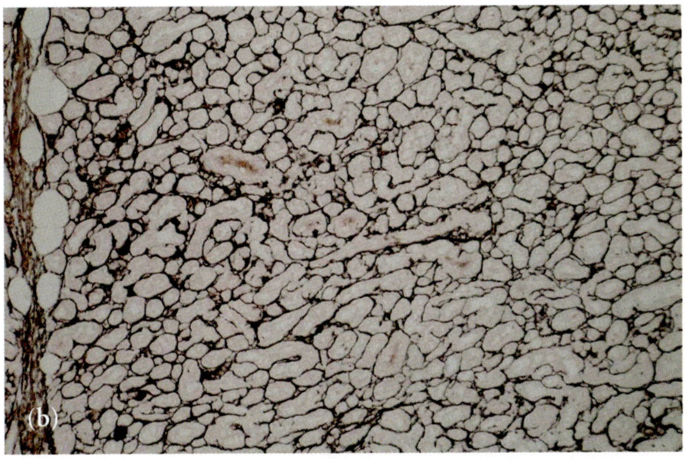

During the proliferation phase, cellular density and the absence of open lumen may obscure the vascular nature of the lesion (a). Reticulin stains highlight the regular vascular architecture of the lesion (b).

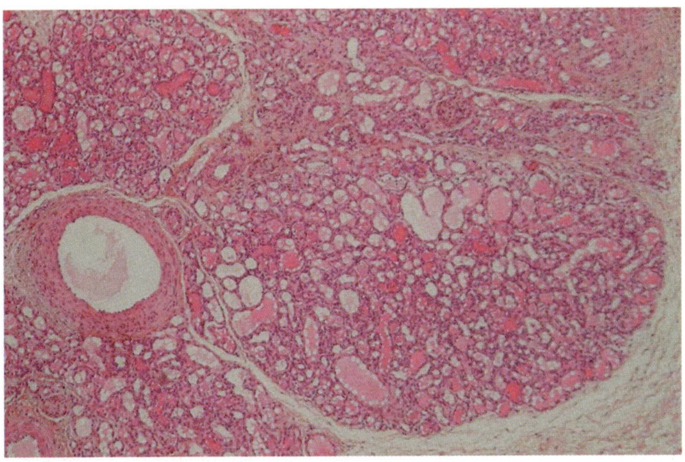

At the end of the proliferation phase, and during the involuting phase, the vascular lumen are open and the vascular nature of the lesion is obvious. Afferent or efferent arteries are still present.

Pathology

At a higher magnification the double layer of endothelial cells and pericytes is more evident.

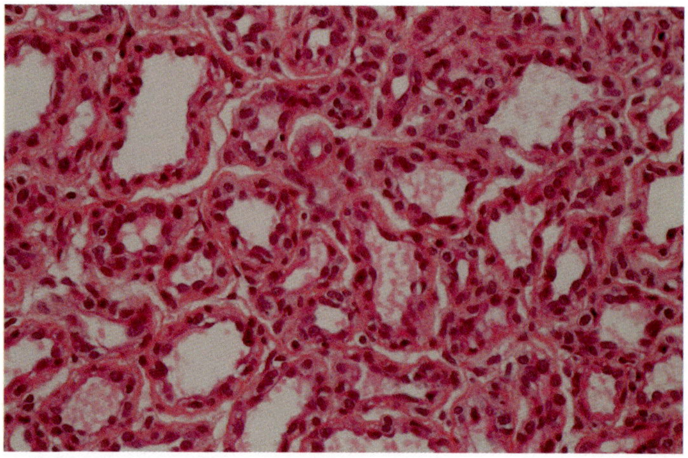

In this figure, the capillary pericytes are colored in brown with an anti-smooth muscle-cell alpha-actin antibody. The endothelial cells show only blue nuclear staining. Mitosis may be seen in both endothelial cells and pericytes.

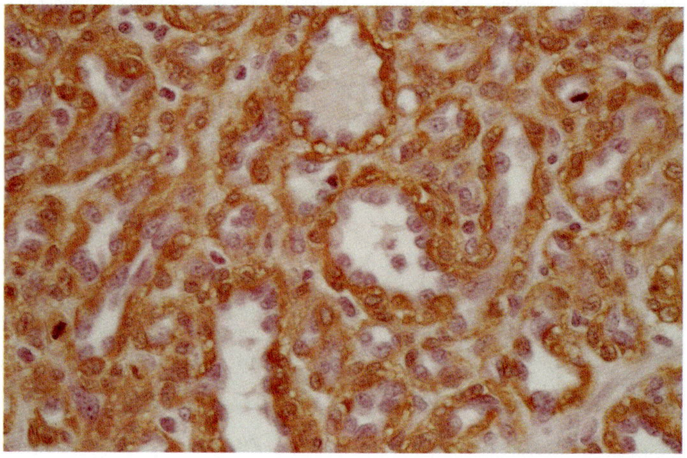

GLUT1, the isoform 1 of a glucose transporter, is a specific immunohistological marker of the endothelial cells of IH. Note that the endothelial cells of the afferent/efferent artery are not stained.

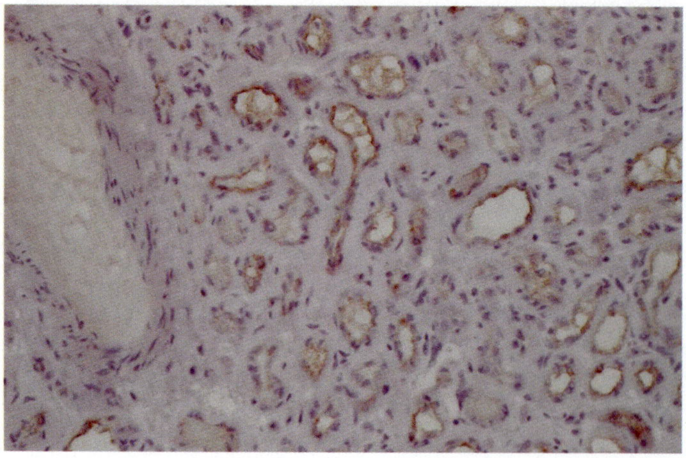

Pathology

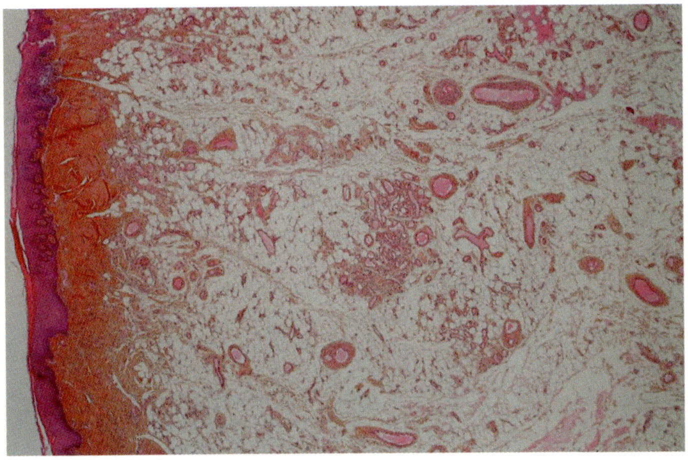

At the involuted phase, the capillaries progressively disappear and are replaced with fibrous or fatty tissue. Some afferent/efferent arteries and small groups of capillaries, reminiscent of the lobular organization may persist.

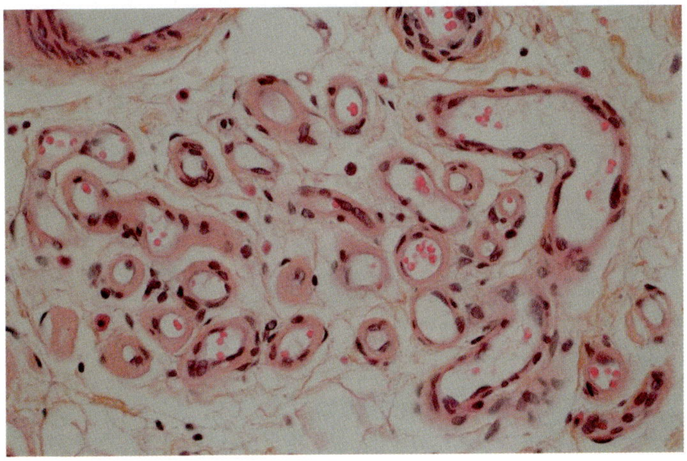

The persisting capillaries often show thickened and hyalinized walls.

Pathology

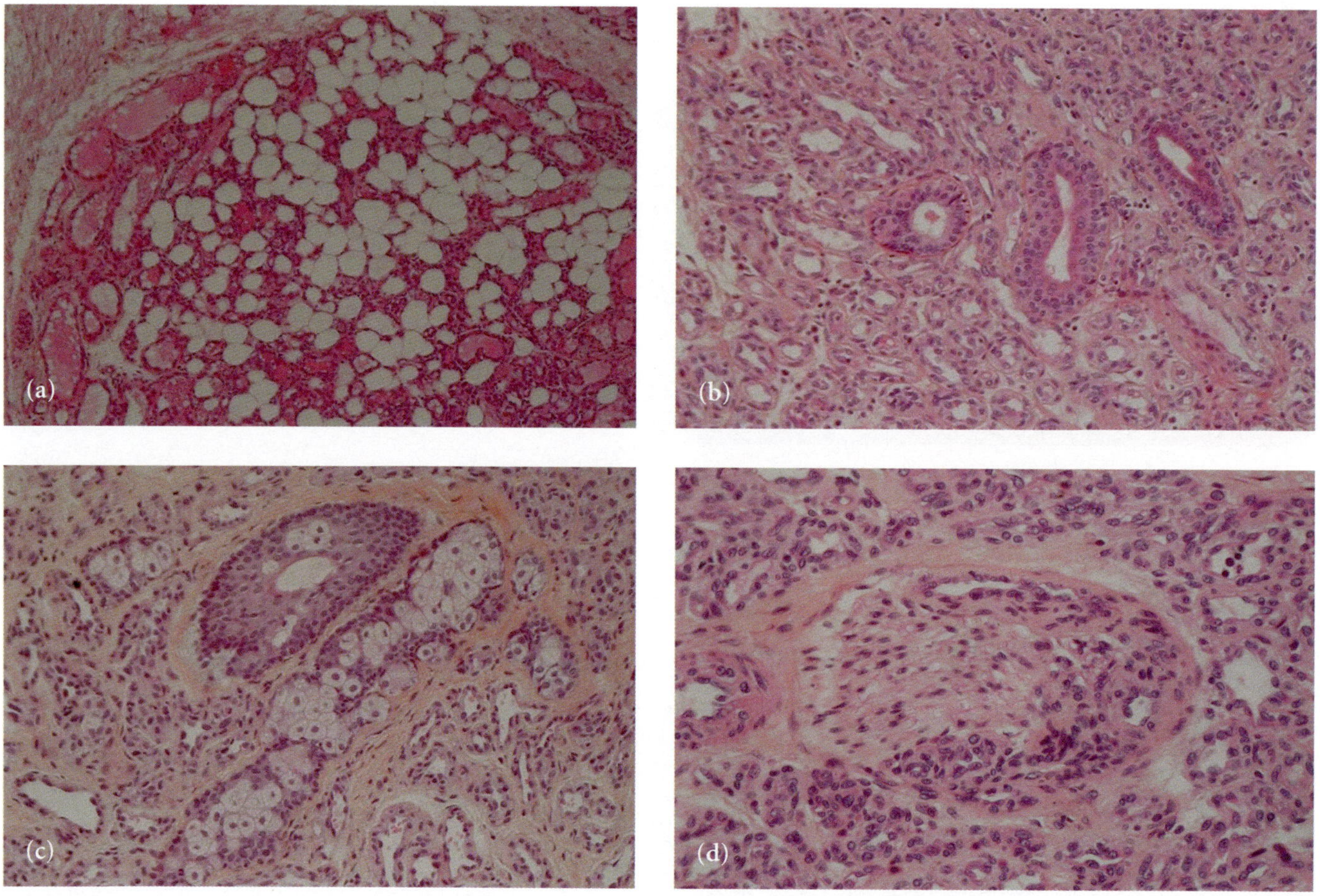

The capillary lobules may enclose normal fat cells (a), sweat glands (b), pilo-sebaceous follicles (c), or minor salivary gland acini. Small nerves may be permeated by the capillary proliferation (d). In an IH, this must not be considered as a sign of malignancy.

Clinical Aspects, Investigations, and Treatment

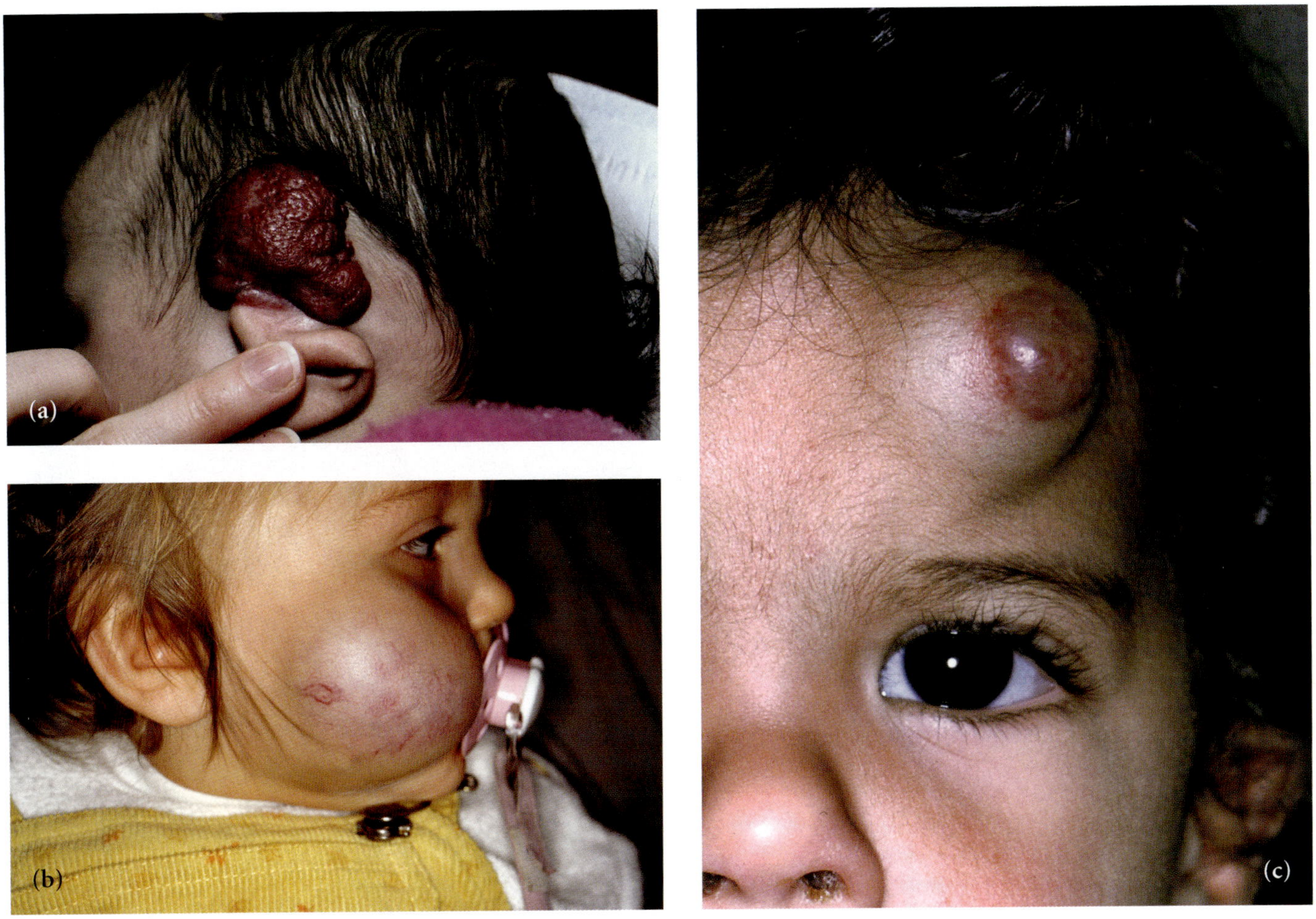

An infantile hemangioma (IH) grows as superficial, crimson red, mammillated tumor, the "strawberry mark" (a); or as a bump under normal or bluish or slightly telangiectatic skin, the subcutaneous "deep hemangioma" (b); or as a deep and superficial mixed hemangioma, with a bluish deeper expansion secondarily developed and growing beyond the red component (c). According to Nakayama (80) who reviewed 1247 patients with IH, subcutaneous hemangiomas make up only 3.1% of cases.

Clinical Aspects, Investigations, and Treatment

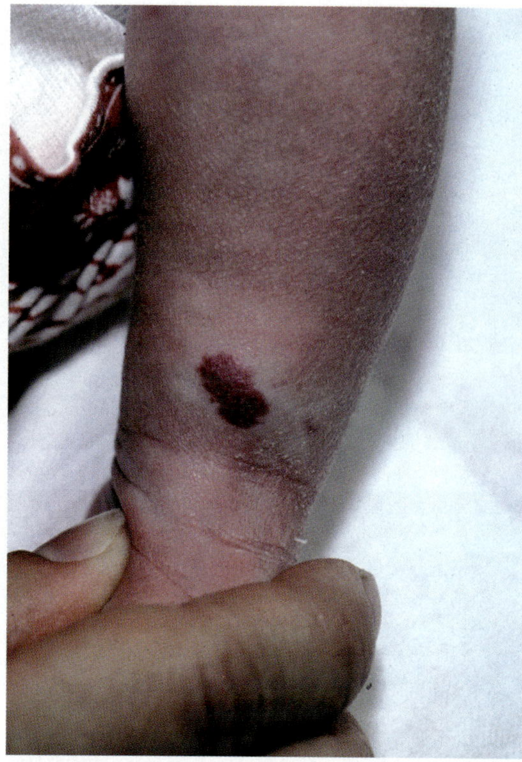

In this newborn's leg the pale "anemic" area of vasoconstriction predicts the growth of a superficial IH, which is just erupting in the center, and announces its future shape.

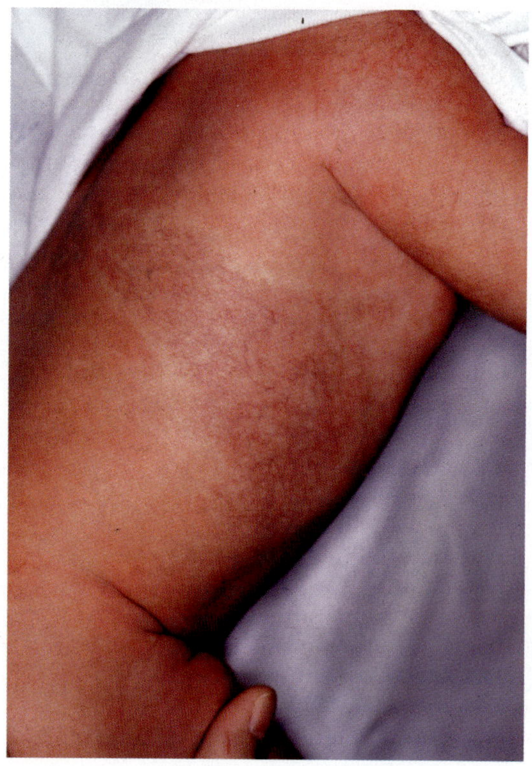

This pink area of skin with linear telangiectasia and a thin white margin of hypothetical vasoconstriction announced the proliferation of an IH. Precursors of hemangioma at birth are either red macular patches, white "anemic" macules, pseudo-bruises, or areas of telangiectasia. All these congenital stains forecast the growth of the IH: a careful neonatal skin inspection detects them in almost half of the newborns who will develop an hemangioma.

Clinical Aspects, Investigations, and Treatment

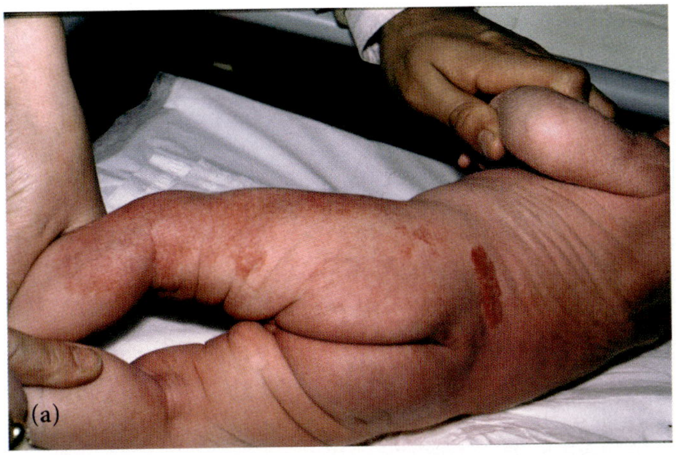

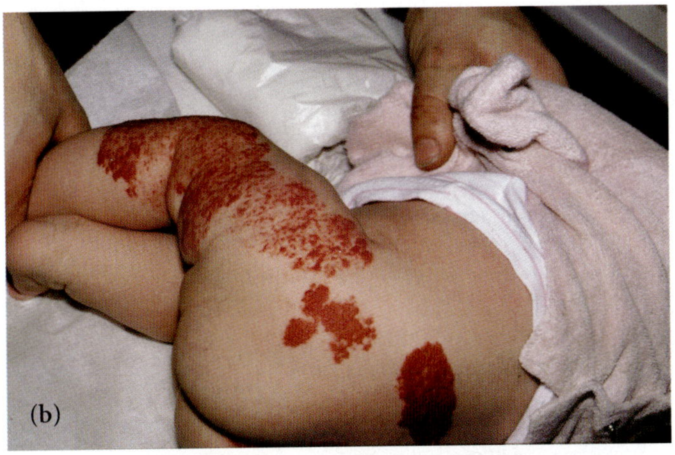

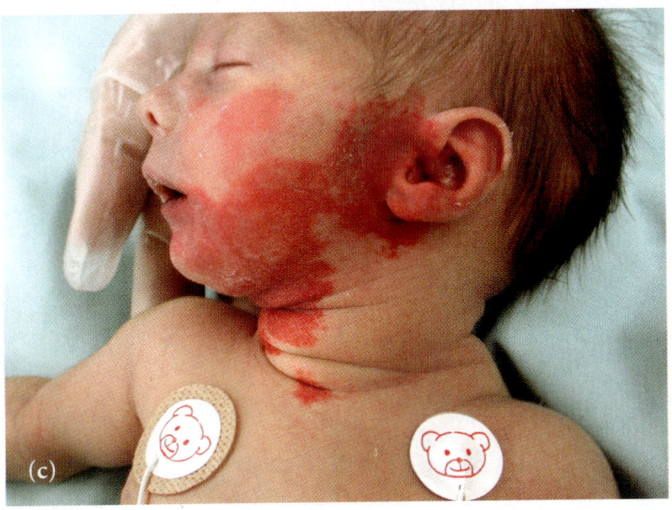

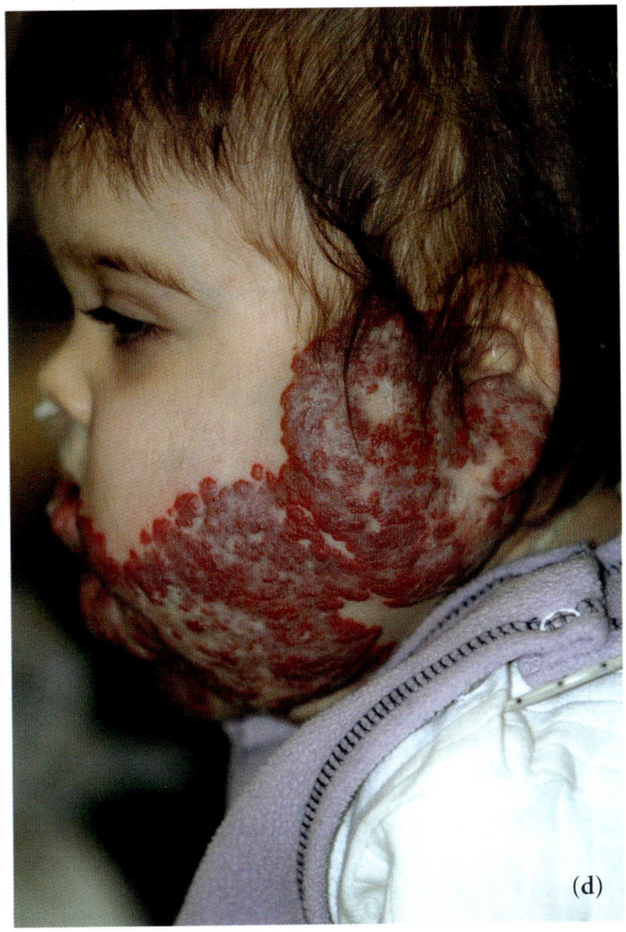

Precursors of IH at birth, like this telangiectatic stain (a) or this red stain mimicking a CM (c), prefigure quite well the size and shape of the upcoming proliferating IH but nothing allows us to predict the final volume of the tumor. In the female infant in (a) the IH remained superficial (b), while in the other (c) who also had early respiratory distress from airway IH, a bulky bilateral mandibular tumor grew (d). Larger lesions often have a longer growth phase of 12 to 24 months.

Clinical Aspects, Investigations, and Treatment

IH of the scalp is commonly found on the anterior fontanel: this does not represent any specific risk and brain imaging is not necessary. Alopecia is common on a scalp IH in its proliferating phase. When hair begins to grow, as seen in this picture, the involuting phase is under way.

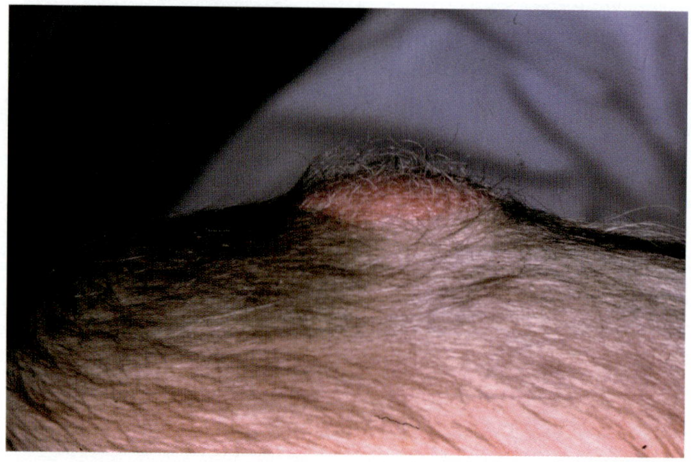

At birth this infant had a large red stain of the forearm and hand. Small papules of IH emerged on top over a few weeks (a). One year later the red stain (precursor) had vanished and the small papules of IH were involuting (b). In this patient the diagnosis of IH is obvious because of the tiny papules apparent on the congenital stain. But in some infants no typical IH develops on the congenital stain ("aborted IH"): the diagnosis may be confused with a CM; however, the precursor of IH is usually more telangiectatic than a CM and spontaneous regression is attained in about a year; laser treatment is not necessary.

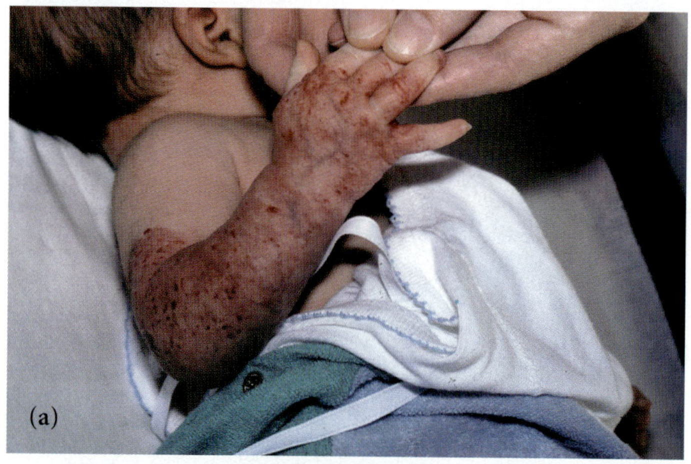

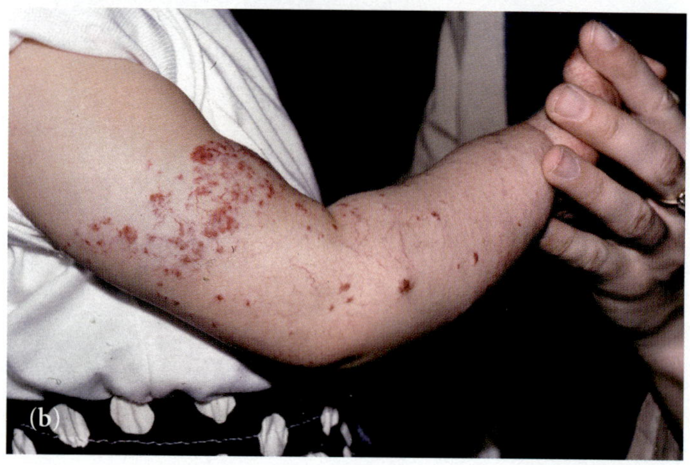

Clinical Aspects, Investigations, and Treatment

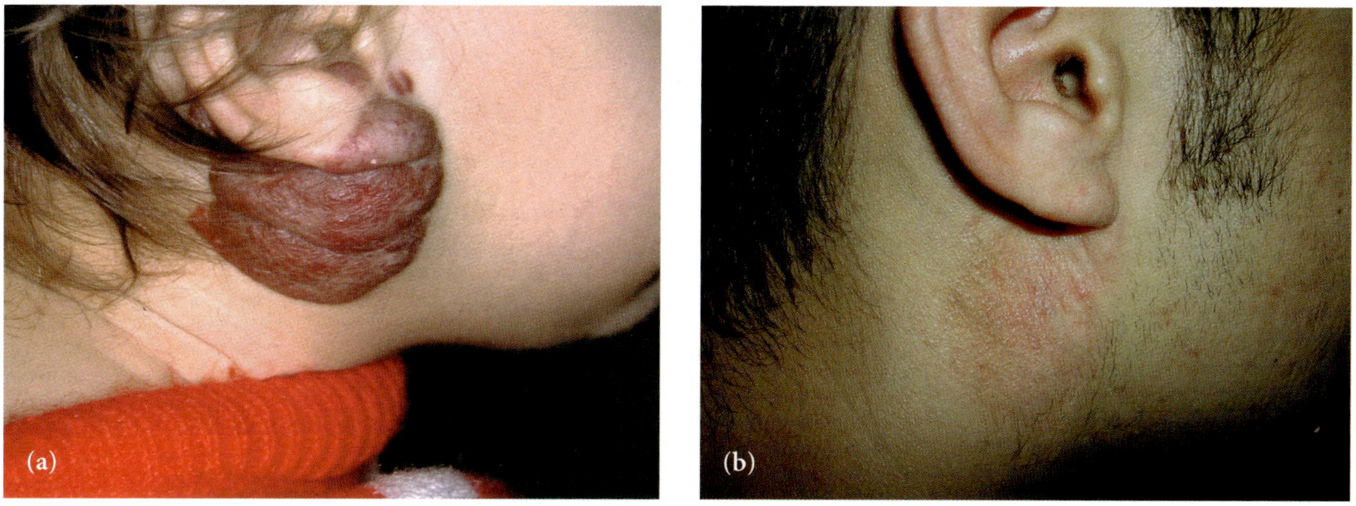

Nothing really predicts the length of the involuting process and the quality of the skin when the involuted stage has been reached: this rather thick superficial IH (a) progressed to practically normal skin (b) after 6 years of spontaneous involution.

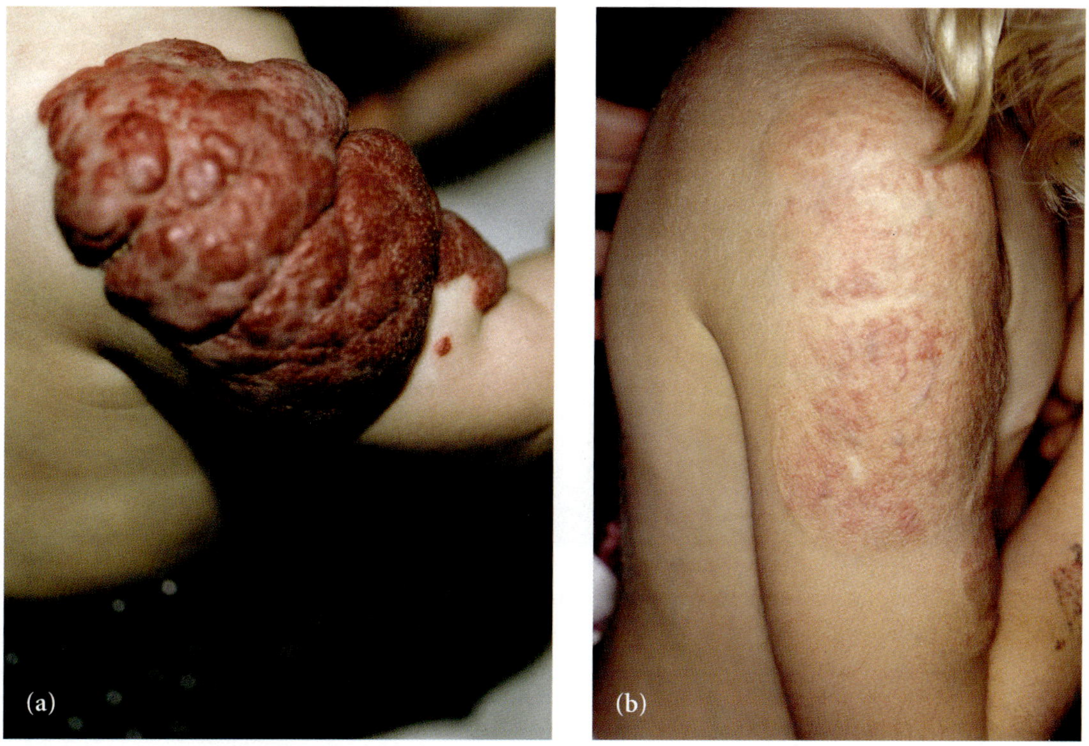

This 5-month-old infant developed this large and thick, deep and superficial IH of the shoulder (a); she had no treatment. The IH regressed relatively rapidly; however, when the girl was 4 years old the area was left with altered, yellowish skin (anetoderma) (b).

Clinical Aspects, Investigations, and Treatment

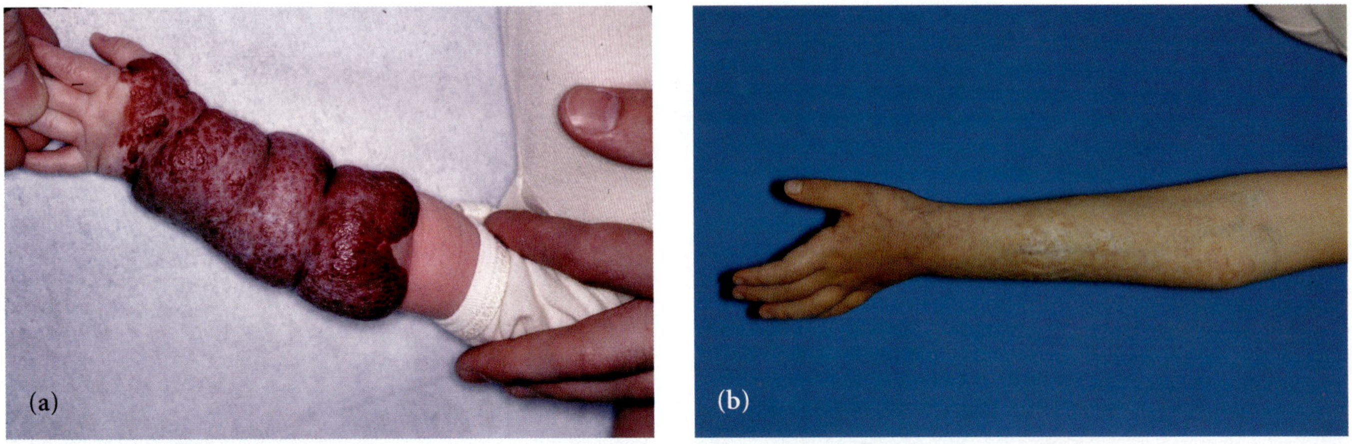

Multiple small painful ulcers arose on this large and thick IH of the hand and forearm during its proliferating phase. It was demonstrated that nerves are most numerous in growing hemangiomas (59): one can hypothesize that these nerves may contribute to the sharp pain suffered by the infant when an ulcerated hemangioma is exposed to air or physical contact. Corticosteroid treatment (CS) and hydrocolloid dressings helped the ulcers healing in this infant. After 1 month of treatment white macules of involution had developed (a) but the lesion was still thick and folded. Four years later the skin folds had fully receded. Multiple scars were noticeable on the forearm, as a consequence of the many ulcers, and some telangiectasia remained on the dorsum of the hand (b).

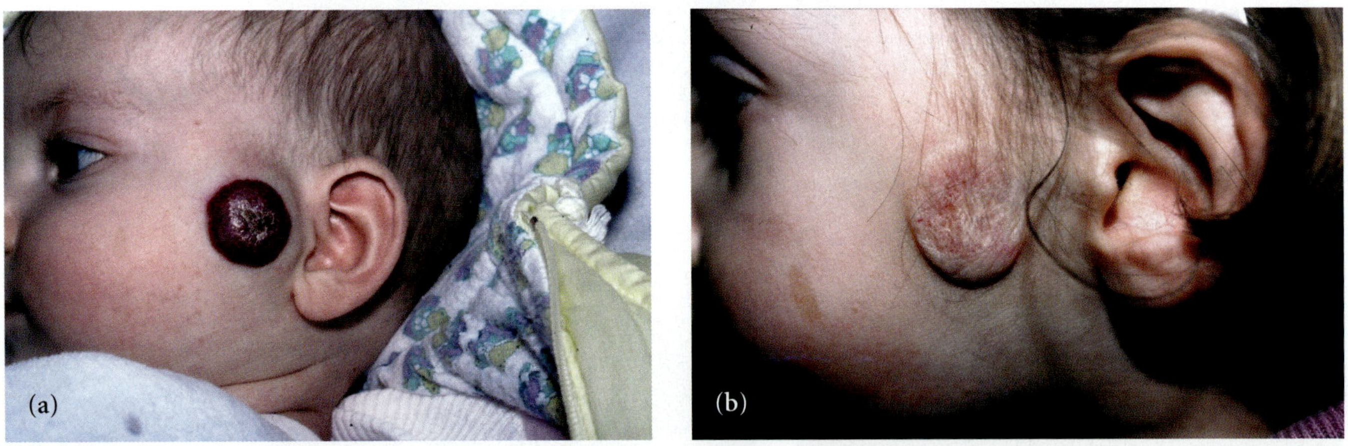

Nothing predicts the occurrence of a fibro-fatty residuum with slack skin after regression of IH. Interestingly, Yu et al. demonstrated the presence of mesenchymal stem cells with adipogenic potential in cultures of proliferating IHs (106).

Clinical Aspects, Investigations, and Treatment

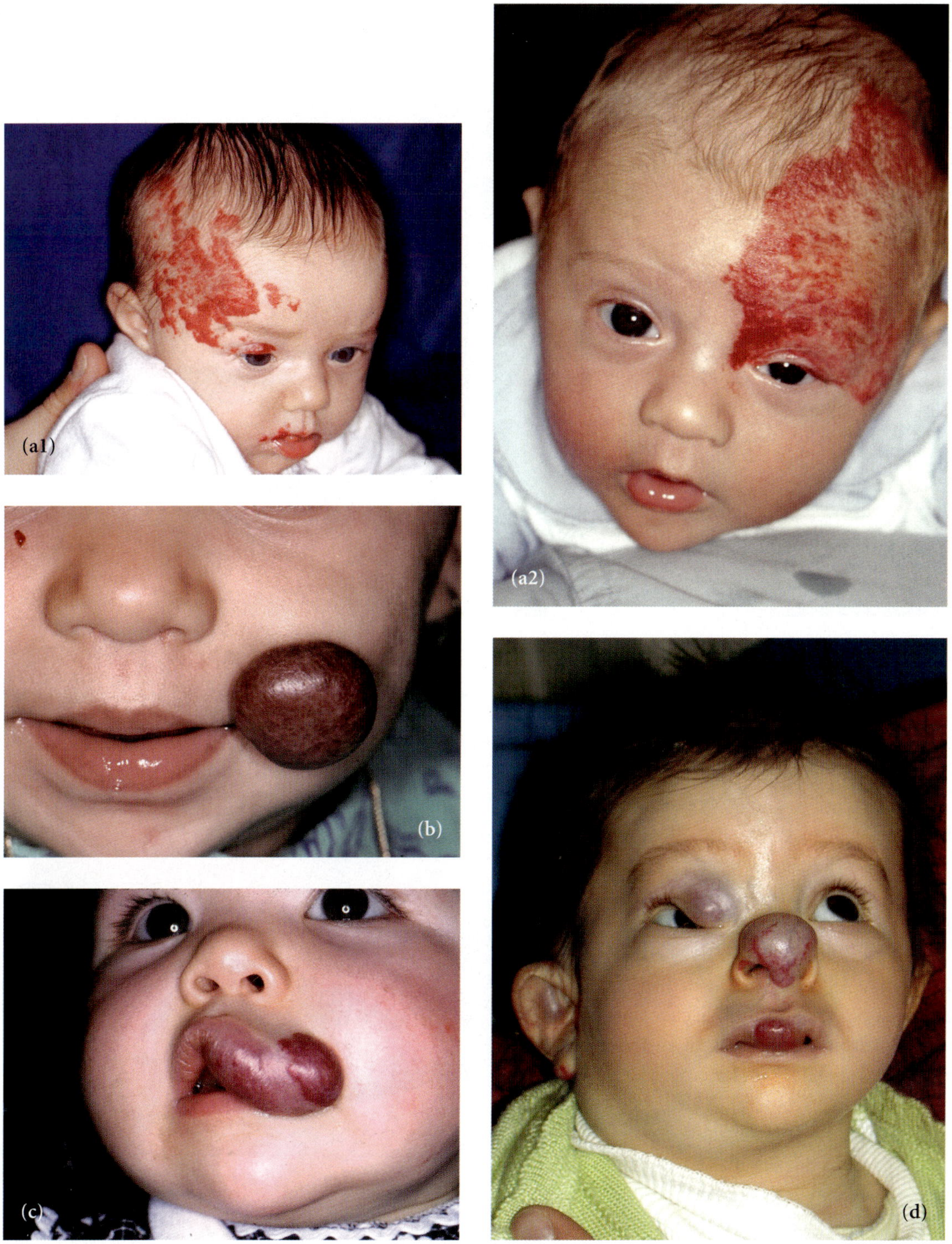

IH in the cephalic area may follow a striking anatomical distribution, reminiscent of the distribution of some facial CM and suggesting some developmental error, and a nonrandom distribution. IHs were classified into four groups: segmental (a1, a2), localized and focal (b), indeterminate (c), and multifocal (d) (22, 104). The girl in (d) had not only multiple facial nodular focal IH but also IH of the ear, scalp, neck, and trunk.

Clinical Aspects, Investigations, and Treatment

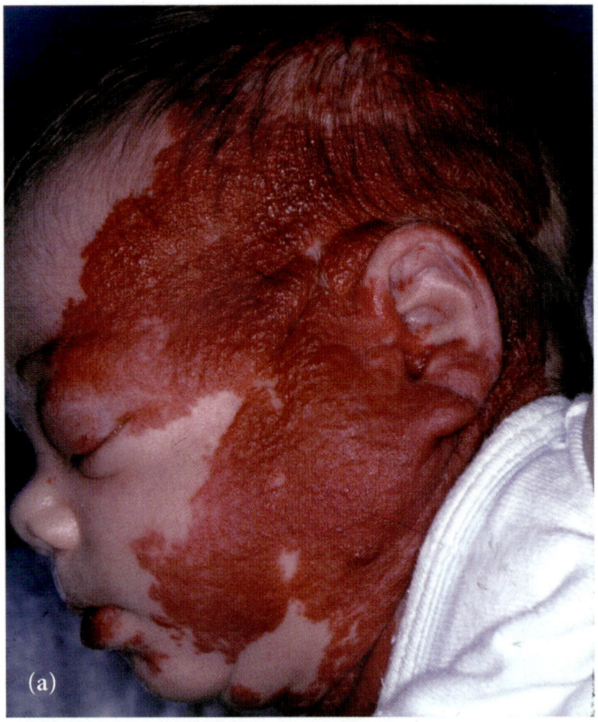

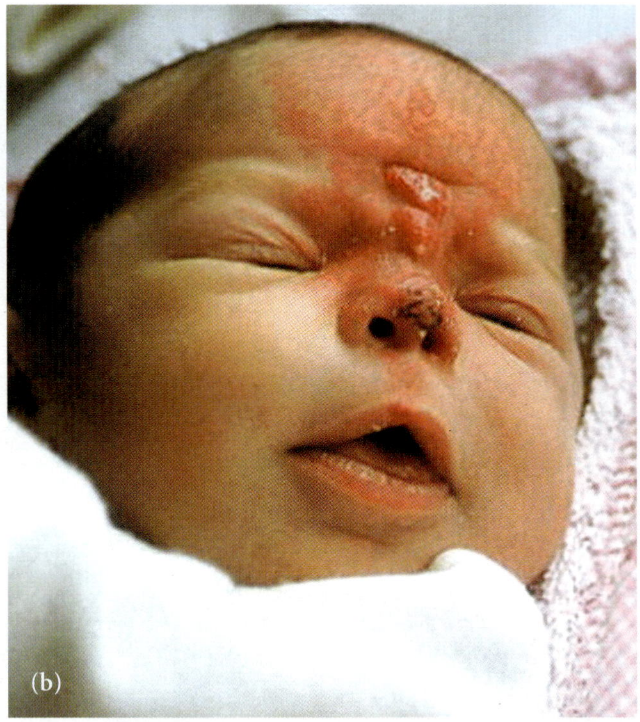

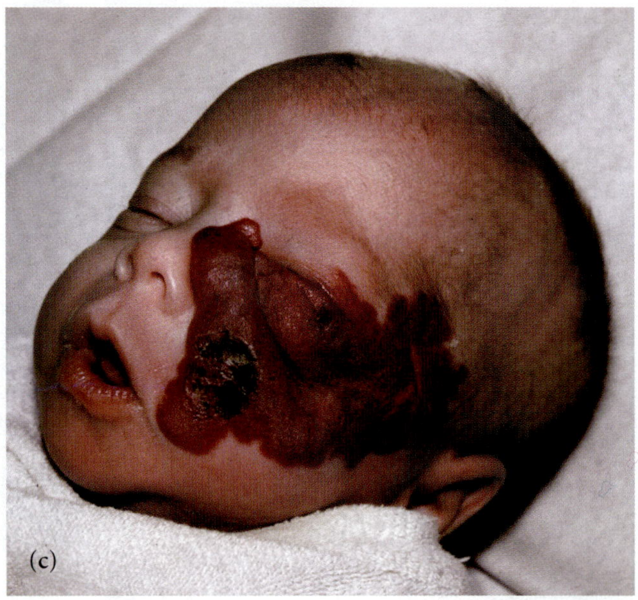

Segmental facial IH may be multiple (b). Haggström et al. classified the large facial hemangiomas into four segments: frontotemporal lateral (S1) (see in a), frontotemporal medial (S4) (b), maxillary (S2) (c) and mandibular (S3) (see in a); some patients have IH encompassing more than one segment (51). According to their image analysis they described S1 as involving the lateral forehead, upper eyelid and part of the temporofrontal scalp; S2 occupies the cheek, sparing the philtrum and preauricular skin; S3 covers the mandibular skin and lower lip; and S4 occupies a sort of centrofacial triangle extending from the forehead to the philtrum. The authors discuss the possible relationship between hemangioma endothelial cells and the distinctive facial cellular environment with neural crest cells derivatives (51). These anatomical segments, of easily recognizable configuration, may reflect specific developmental units. They also allow us to identify a group of infants at greater risk for hemangioma-related complications (ulceration, infection, "worrisome rapid growth," associated visceral IH – not only of the airway and orbit, but also the liver, GI tract and brain IH, etc.) and/or associated structural anomalies (16, 22, 72). Various authors have stressed the fact that most structural anomalies were ipsilateral to the cephalic hemangioma (eye (61), heart (15), brain (26, 84, 85), etc.).

Clinical Aspects, Investigations, and Treatment

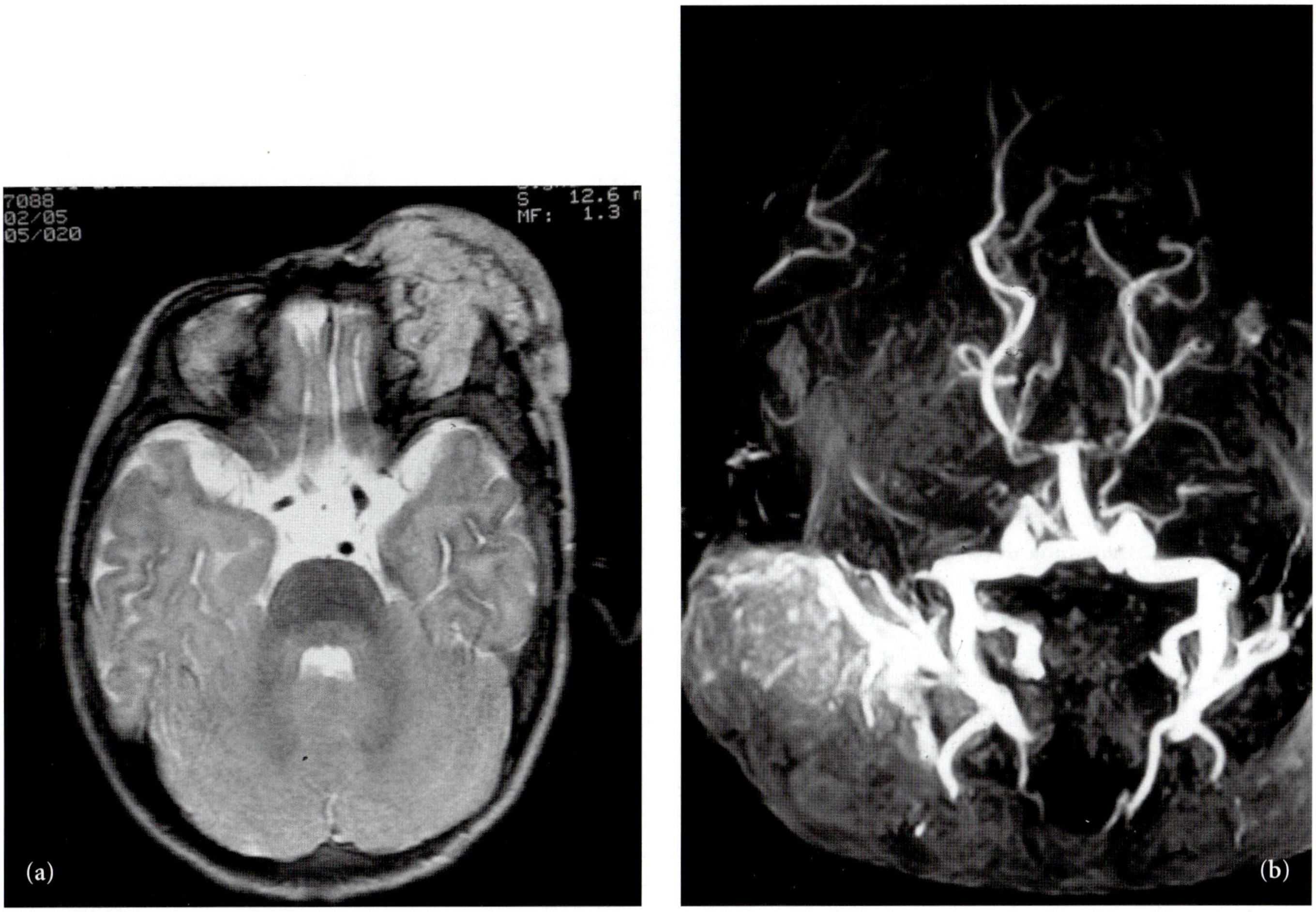

MRI and US/color Doppler are the most useful diagnostic tools for IH (17, 27). On MRI the tumor is isointense on T1 (a), hyperintense on T2 and intensely enhanced after gadolinium injection; flow voids are present within the mass. IH is a fast-flow tumor, as evidenced on the MR angiogram of this parotid IH disclosing the large arterial feeders arising from the external carotid artery (b). Because of the high flow it is sometimes misdiagnosed as AVM by US/color Doppler duplex scan.

Clinical Aspects, Investigations, and Treatment

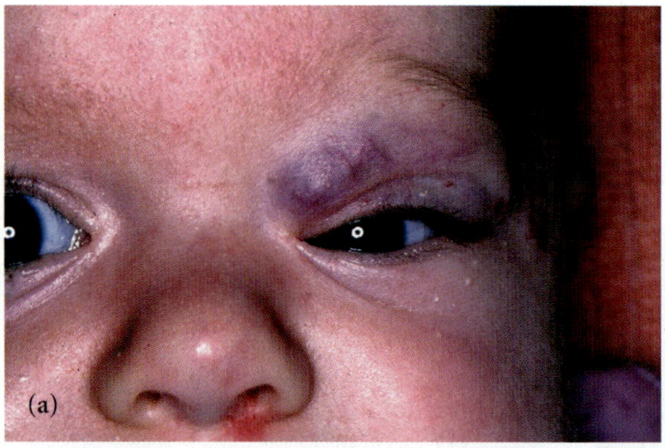
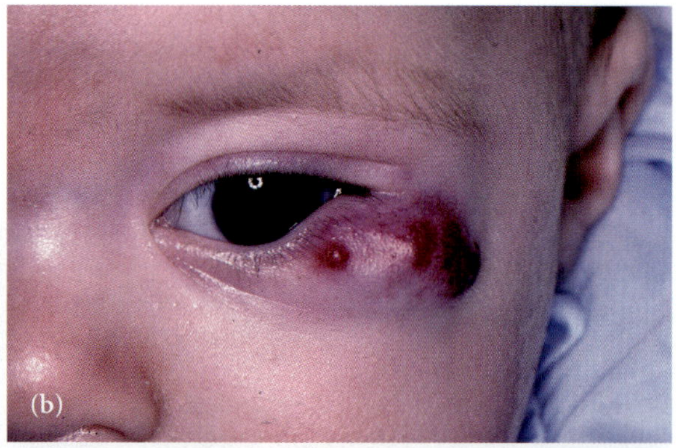

Ophthalmological examination is indispensable: even a small IH of the eyelids with minor incidence on the visual axis may create refractory trouble (mainly astigmatism) as soon as it infringes upon the young developing cornea and applies pressure to the globe (a, b). Dystopia, with displacement of the globe upward or downward requires rapid therapeutic intervention: when the displacement of the globe has not been changed for years (c), irreversible amblyopia is produced. Displacement of the eyeball is always an indicator of orbital extension of IH. There is a strong correlation between a clinically appraised ocular deviation and an intraorbital extension of an eyelid IH; on the other hand there is no correlation between the extent and volume of the eyelid IH and a possible location of IH in the orbit (77) (see also figures on (pages 68–69).

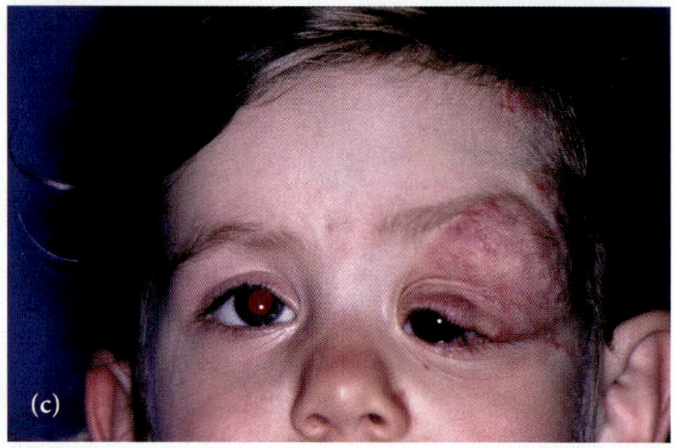

In this child proptosis is the consequence of orbital location of the IH. In addition blockage of the lacrymal duct by compression creates constant tears (epiphora). Radiological imaging is useful to help decide which treatment (pharmacological therapy or early surgery) is the best option. A sight-threatening IH is a therapeutic emergency which can cause amblyopia, ensuing from three mechanisms: deprivation amblyopia secondary to visual deprivation in the first two months of life (eye closed); anisometropic amblyopia linked to a refractive error (mainly astigmatism, or induced myopia, because of the pressure of the IH on the globe and cornea) and strabismic amblyopia as a consequence of extraocular muscle infiltration and dystopia.

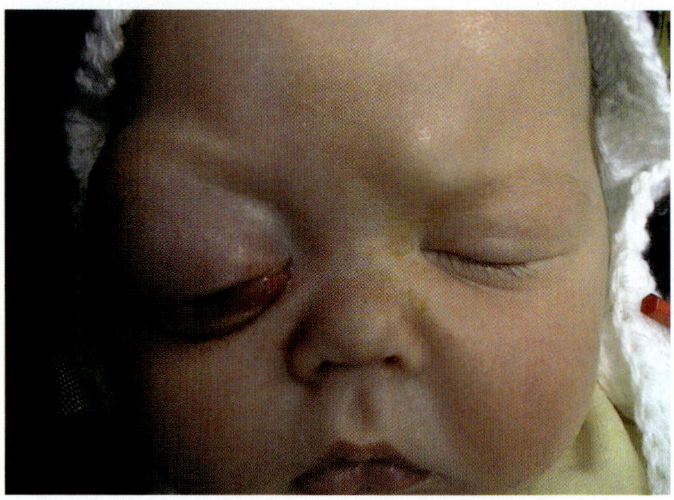

Clinical Aspects, Investigations, and Treatment

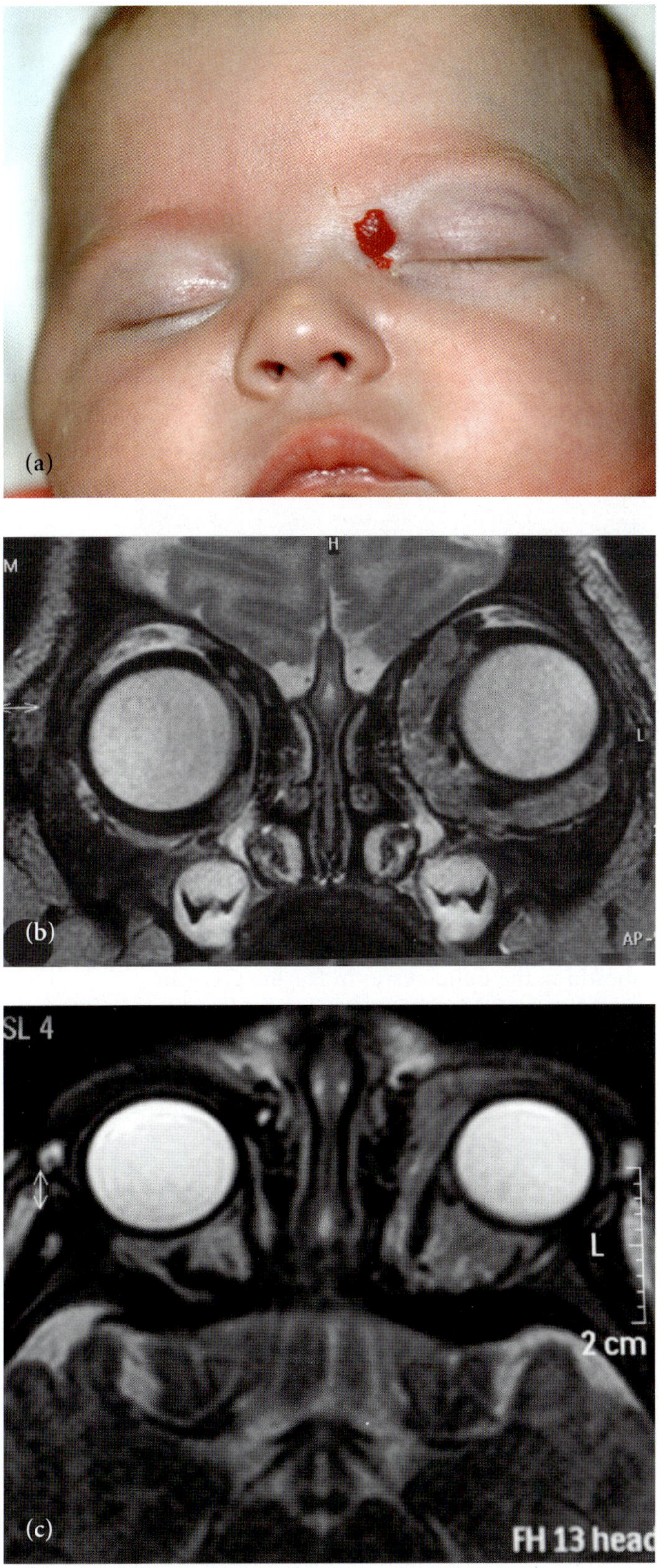

This infant had a small superficial red hemangioma in the internal canthus area and minor exophthalmos of the left eye. (a) MRI, coronal (b) and axial (c) images, showed huge orbital extra- and intraconal involvement; the brain had no associated anomaly. We cannot predict from the size of the eyelid IH if there is, or is not, orbital involvement; the only warning signs are dystopia and exophthalmos. With MRI, T1-sequences and T2-sequences with fat saturation, and images in the three planes (sagittal, axial, and coronal) gave us sufficient information, with no need of gadolinium injection when the diagnosis of IH is clinically sure because there is some red superficial constituent of the tumor (77). We advise to always investigate the brain in parallel with orbital assessment, to check for intracranial symptoms of PHACE syndrome.

Clinical Aspects, Investigations, and Treatment

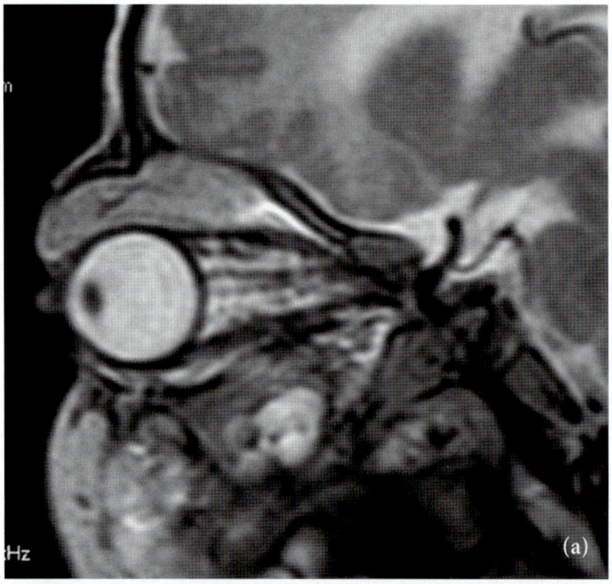

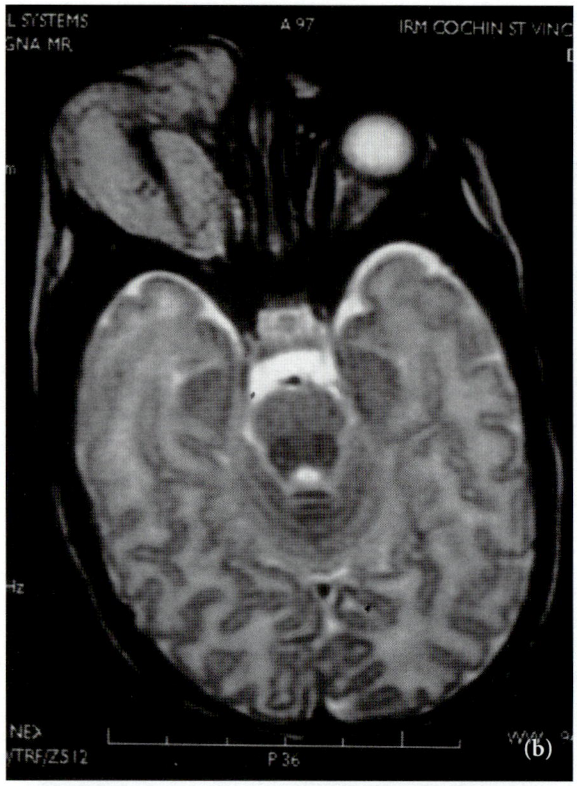

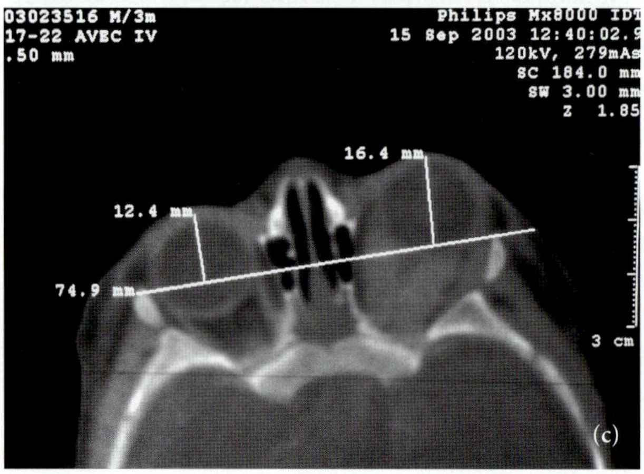

Three cases of IH in the orbit. In (a) the MRI T2 sagittal image reveals an intraorbital extraconal IH, extending along the roof of the orbit. In (b) MRI T2 axial imaging shows the lid and paranasal IH, but also intraconal involvement with the IH encircling and sheathing the optic nerve. In (c) the CT scan with iodinated contrast reveals an intraconal orbital IH embedding the optic nerve and exophthalmos.

Clinical Aspects, Investigations, and Treatment

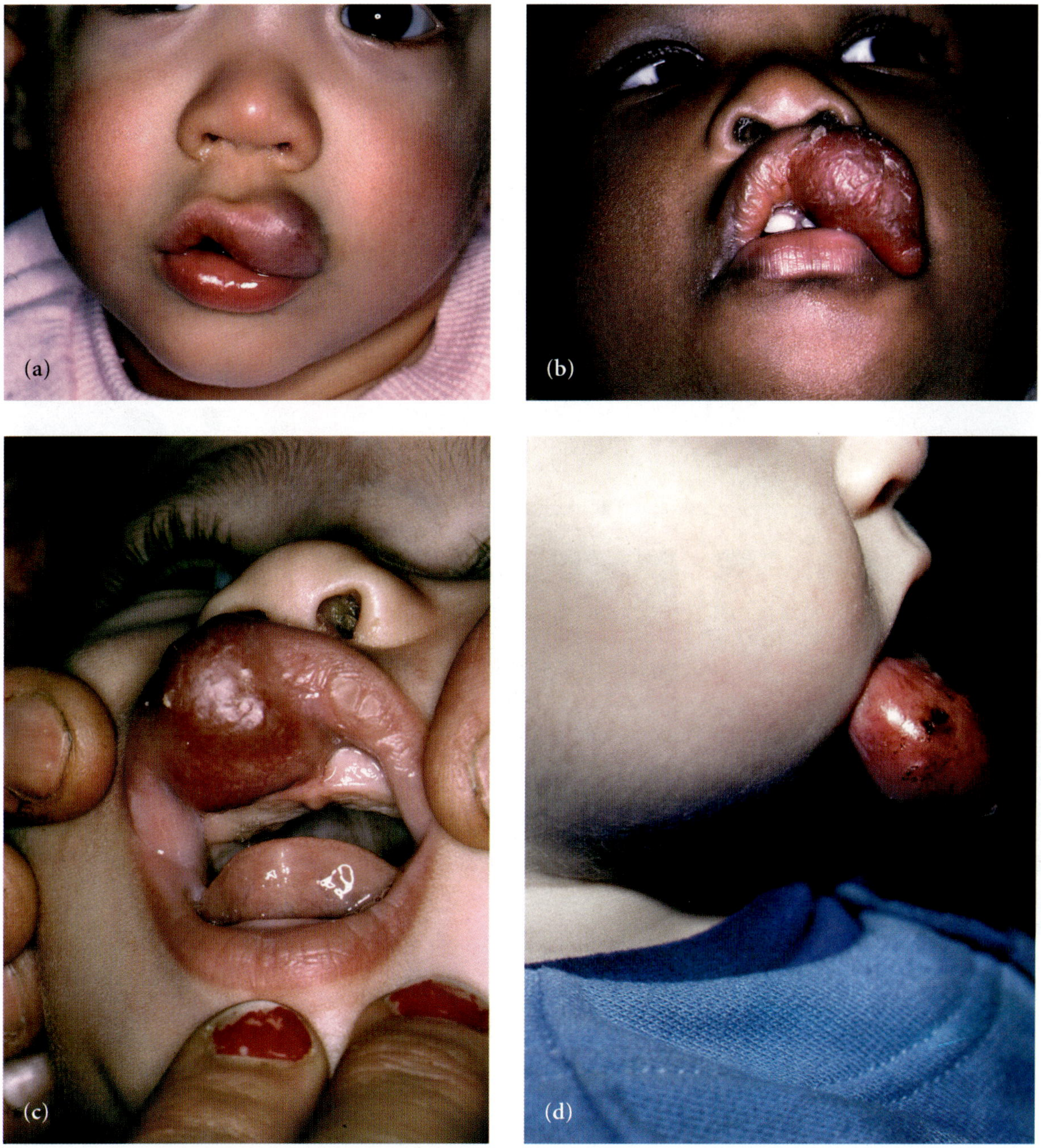

IH commonly affects the lips. Even when localized (a, b) it lastingly expands the thin tissue. The mucosal side of the lip is commonly affected (c) creating some pressure on the maxillary bone. After involution many children are left with some lip discoloration and lip distortion requiring surgical management. A large IH of the lower lip creates severe expansion (d), both because of true proliferation and because of the weight of the lip hanging down. During both the proliferating and involuting phases the lips are dry because the normal close contact is missing; this facilitates cracking, ulceration, pain, and bleeding. Frequent application of vaseline ointment is recommended to maintain some moisture on the lips and soothe the fissures.

Clinical Aspects, Investigations, and Treatment

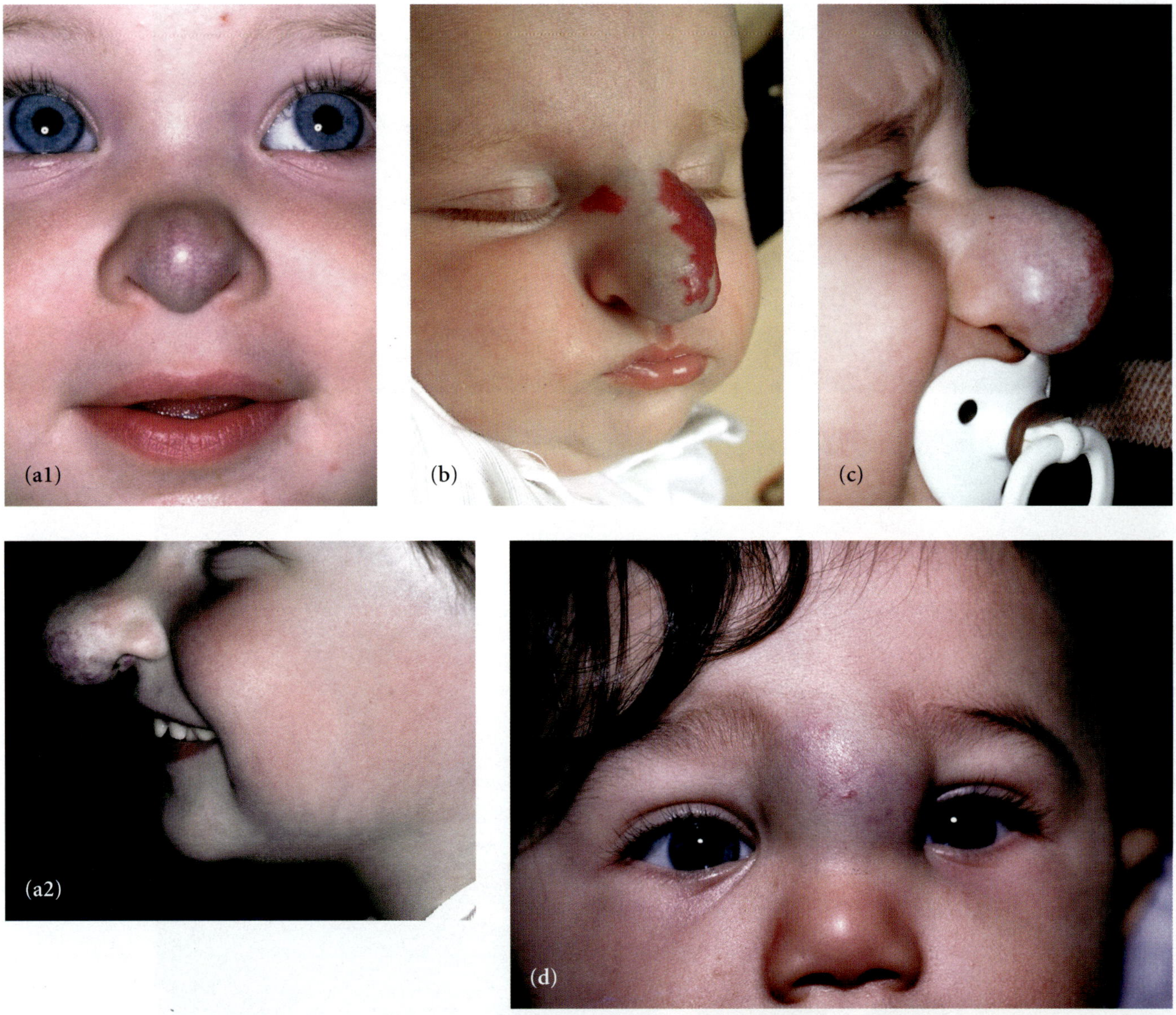

IH of the nose may affect the tip of the nose in a more or less pronounced expansion (the Cyrano nose) (a1, a2), or may involve the full nasal pyramid (b, c), or may be located in the glabellum (d). Early surgical treatment of Cyrano-nose IH is often performed around 2 years of age, to avoid permanent residual deformity (38).

Clinical Aspects, Investigations, and Treatment

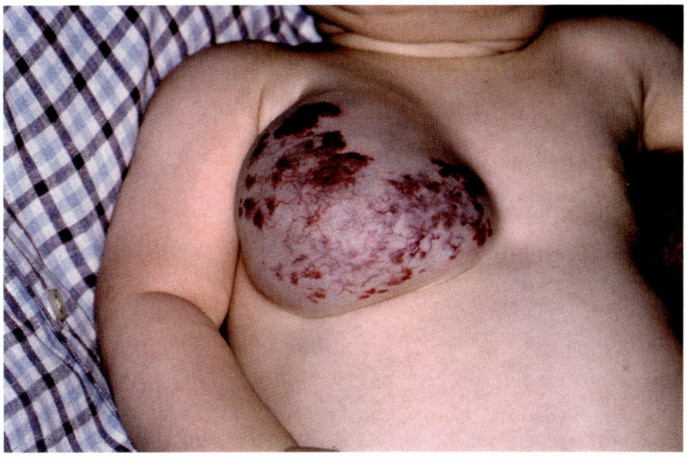

Hemangioma affecting the breast area may be small, or large, as in this girl whose lesion encompasses the mammary bud. In our experience, the risk of developing a small "Amazon" breast at puberty has often been overestimated and the breast may grow normally. If excess skin has been left after involution, we never offer surgical repair before the full growth of the breast, to avoid damage to the fragile arterial feeders of the mammary bud. If necessary, cosmetic repair is considered after pubertal breast growth.

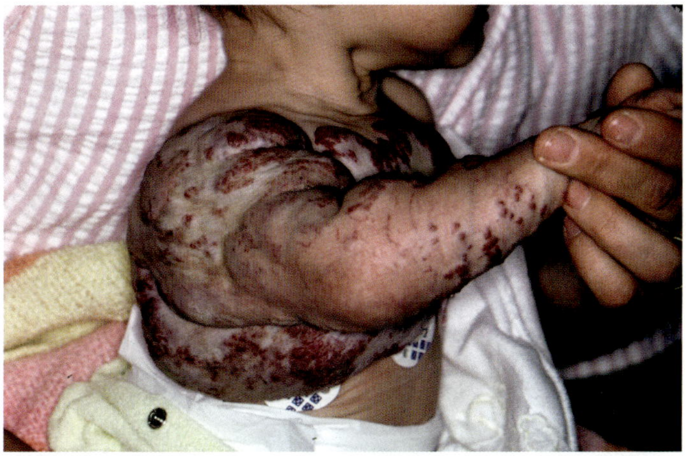

Large thoracic and arm IH may induce congestive heart failure (CHF) due to the high flow through the numerous arterial feeders. Monitoring of cardiac function is recommended. Medical treatment of CHF is necessary, in addition to the pharmacological treatment of the tumor. Occasionally, embolization through the arterial route using particles helps alleviate the cardiac overload.

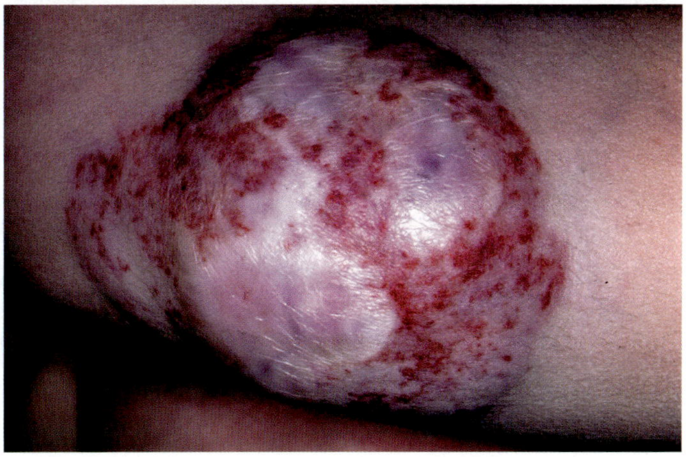

An IH susceptible to ulceration is an IH with a superficial bright red component (deep hemangioma under apparently normal skin usually do not ulcerate) and this can be a side-effect of a local treatment (cryotherapy, lasers). In this infant three ulcers were caused by cryotherapy applied during the proliferating phase. After healing of the necrotic areas the patient developed three bad white scars, while the part of the IH left to spontaneously regress was clearly achieving a better quality of skin.

Clinical Aspects, Investigations, and Treatment

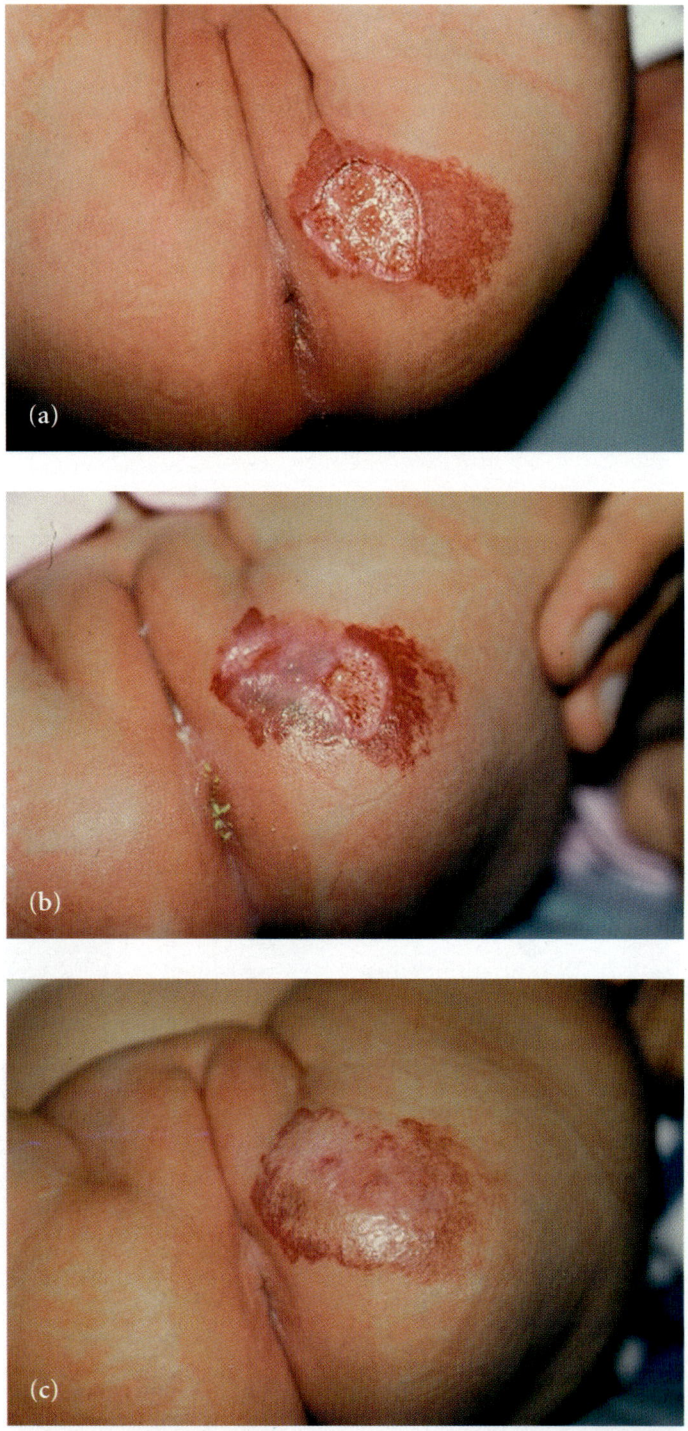

Spontaneous ulceration of hemangioma is quite common in the buttocks. This girl had an ulcerated IH of the left buttock and extreme pain when urine and stools came into contact with it. She had a first procedure of flashlamp pulsed dye laser treatment (a); 20 days later healing was nearly complete (b), a second laser application was made and rapid healing obtained (c) (operator: Dr. Virginie Fayard, Paris, France). Reported benefits of laser treatment for ulcerated hemangioma range from rapid relief of pain, rapid healing, accelerated involution, or no response at all (23). The most common dressings applied to ulcerated IHs are the hydrocolloid dressings, or the hydrocellular dressings in case of important fluid outflow; both protect the wound and reduce pain. Some authors use antimicrobial ointments or zinc oxide paste. Becaplermin gel (Regranex®), a recombinant platelet-derived growth factor used in the cure of diabetic ulcers, has been reported to be effective for severely ulcerated IH not responding to conventional local treatment and systemic therapy (75).

Clinical Aspects, Investigations, and Treatment

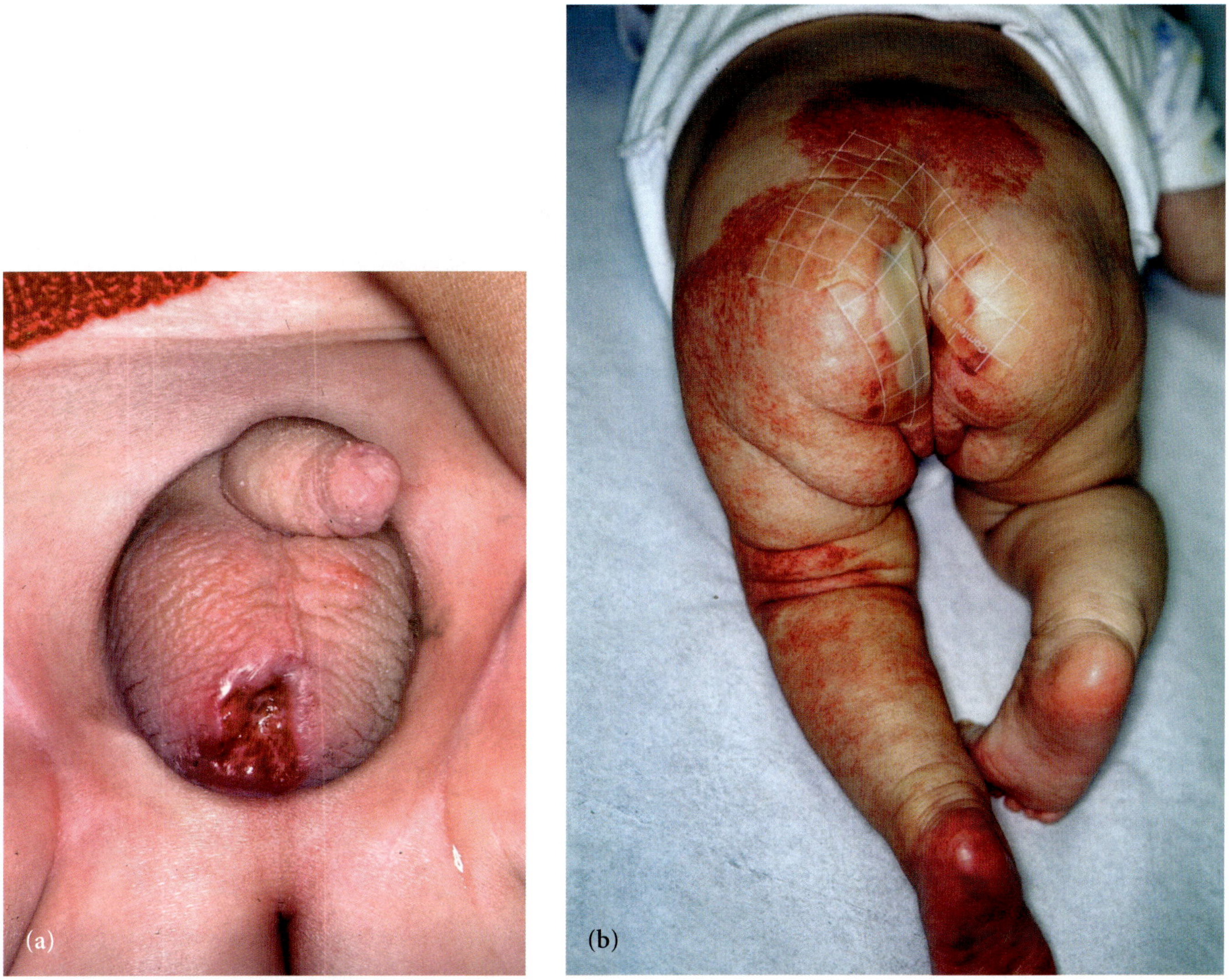

IHs in the perineum and buttocks have a high propensity to ulcerate, in part because of the wet environment and the napkin rubbing the skin. Ulcers are particularly severe in infants with thin and telangiectatic IH of the perineum and leg. Sometimes the IH is barely noticeable at birth before it ulcerates (a). In others it presents in a regional distribution (b). The hydrocolloid dressing (b) helps healing of the ulcer and it alleviates pain.

Clinical Aspects, Investigations, and Treatment

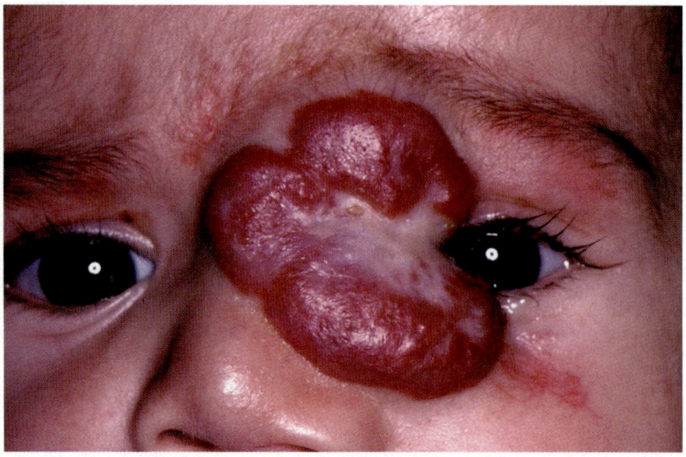

Crust followed by ulceration occurs in the center of the IH, while some minor areas of whitening (involution) are also seen over the whole surface. After healing of the ulcer, at the margin of the tumor, a rim of still-proliferating protruding IH surrounds a white central atrophic scar. It has been suggested that, as in many malignancies, the involution of IH, an apoptotic process (70, 93), starts from the center of the tumor, and that the ulceration is basically an excessively fast vanishing process. In addition, in this infant the internal canthal location of the IH blocked the lacrymal duct creating epiphora.

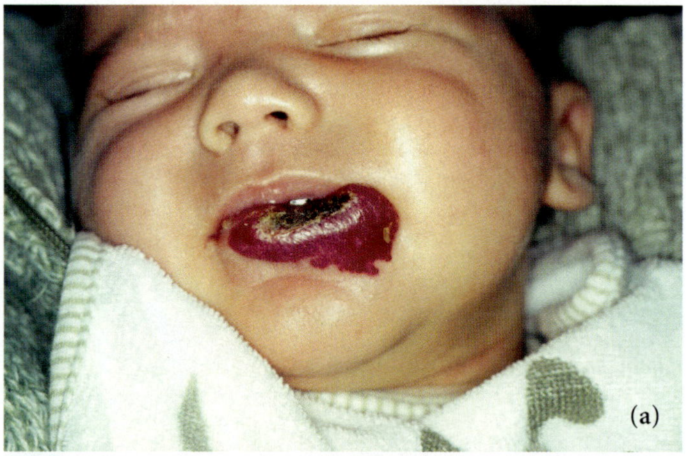

(a)

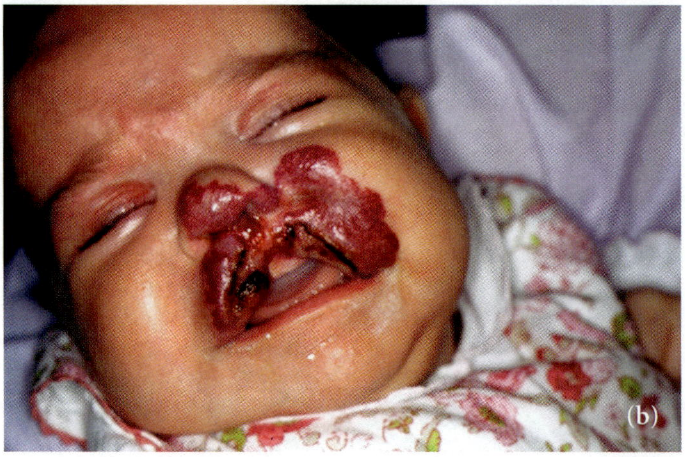

(b)

Ulceration of lower or upper lip IH is another daunting problem: pain may prevent normal feeding, by either breast or bottle sucking, and nourishment of the infant through a nasogastric tube may be required. Crusts (a) can be minimized using vaseline ointment. When a very extensive and painful ulceration is not controlled by pharmacological treatment and flashlamp pulsed dye laser application (b), excision of the necrosis and suturing are considered.

Clinical Aspects, Investigations, and Treatment

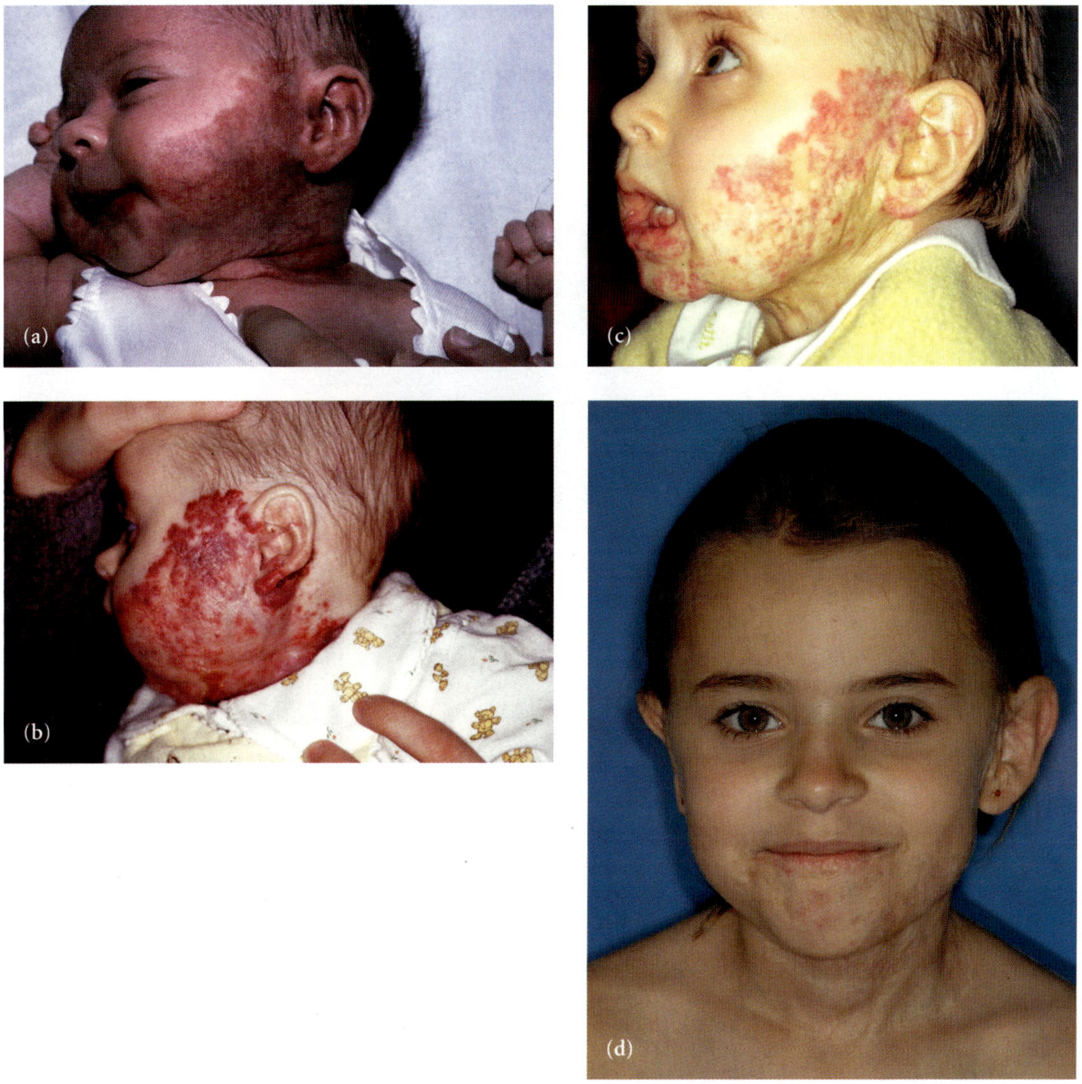

This newborn was transferred to us with a misdiagnosis of CM; the lesion was in fact a precursor of a bilateral mandibular, ear and neck IH (a). "Beard" IH is known to carry a high risk of associated airway IH (36, 83). At that early stage, a pharyngeal and a nonobstructive circumferential laryngeal subglottic IH was observed on fiberoptic laryngoscopy. She received high dosage of glucocorticosteroid (GS), but after 1 month she became tachypneic with a stridor even at rest. At 7 weeks of age she had a single-stage laryngotracheoplasty: open-approach excision of the airway lesion and graft of auricular cartilage for augmentation of the subglottis (operator: Dr. Gilles Roger, Hôpital Armand Trousseau, Paris, France). Respiratory outcome was excellent. Despite ongoing GS treatment, the superficial IH grew to create a bilateral massive parotid tumor with multiple large painful ulcerations in the neck (b). GS were tapered and stopped when she was 3 months old. Then, she received interferon alpha 2b treatment over 10 months, without unwanted side-effects. Healing of the ulcers was obtained after 4 weeks. Rapid shrinkage of the bilateral tumor occurred, resulting in lax skin with widespread scars. The involuted stage was reached at 14 months of age (c) and surgical procedures (four facelift procedures and a neck CO2 laser resurfacing) began at 24 months of age. At 7 years (d) she is a bright happy girl who copes with the residual leucomelanodermic scars on her neck and lower face, undergoing various procedures of laser treatment.

Clinical Aspects, Investigations, and Treatment

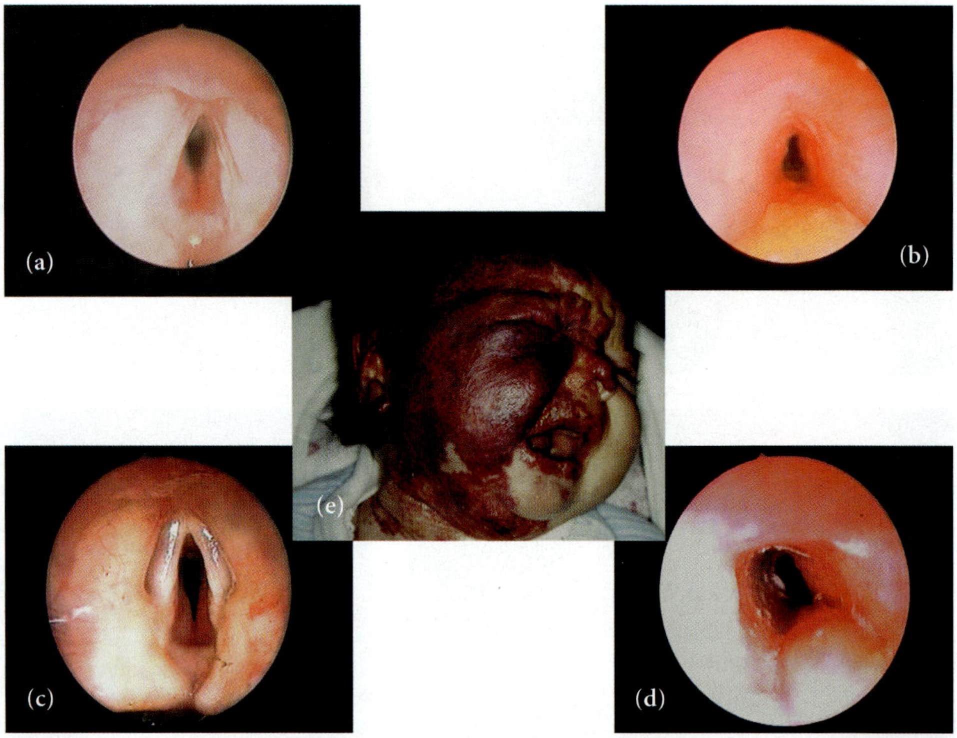

This infant was referred at 2 months of age for dyspnea and a diffuse bright red, plaque-type hemifacial and cervical IH, grown on a congenital pseudo port-wine stain; it closed her right eye and ulcerated her lips and nose margins (columella necrosis). She had been on steroid treatment for 2 weeks (prednisolone 2 mg/kg daily); the dosage was increased to 3 mg/kg daily, without improving her breathing. Brain MRI and hepatic ultrasonography were normal. Laryngotracheal endoscopy (courtesy of Dr. G. Roger, Division of ENT Surgery, Hôpital Armand Trousseau, Paris, France) demonstrated major pharyngo- and laryngotracheal involvement with significant subglottic stenosis (60% estimated) and extension to the right lateral wall of trachea down to the carina (a, b). The main bronchi were disease free. Tracheal involvement was not accessible to surgical treatment. Laser was not an option (because of the risk of stenosis). Vincristine IV weekly injection was then initiated while steroids were tapered and stopped within 3 weeks. Dyspnea progressively disappeared. Serial endoscopies indicated that the implantation of the hemangioma remained identical but the amount and burden of tumor decreased (c, d). After a total of 23 vincristine injections, over 9 months, the facial IH had a reduced volume and was lightening. Scars and telangiectasia, at 3 years of age (f) before any repair and reconstructive procedure.

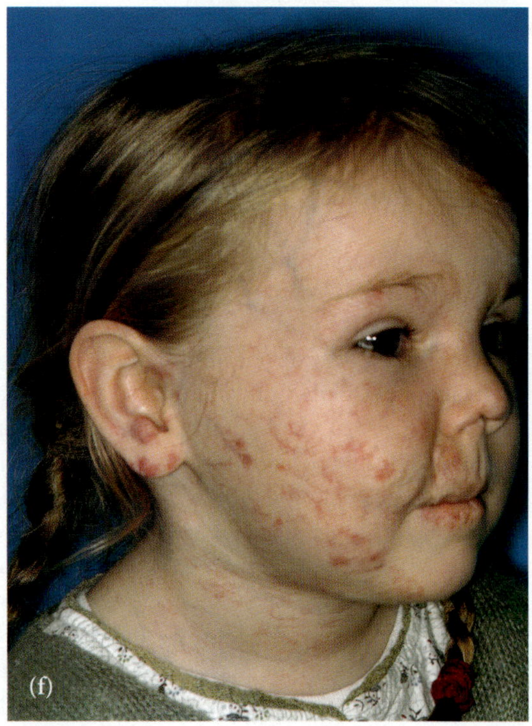

Clinical Aspects, Investigations, and Treatment

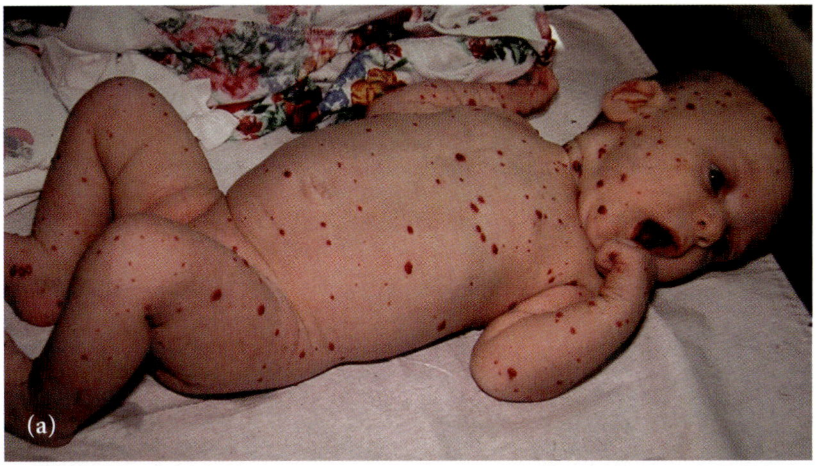
(a)

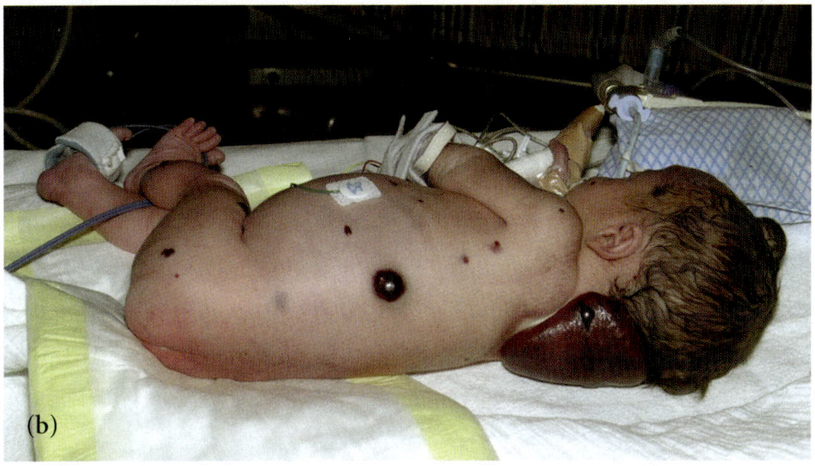
(b)

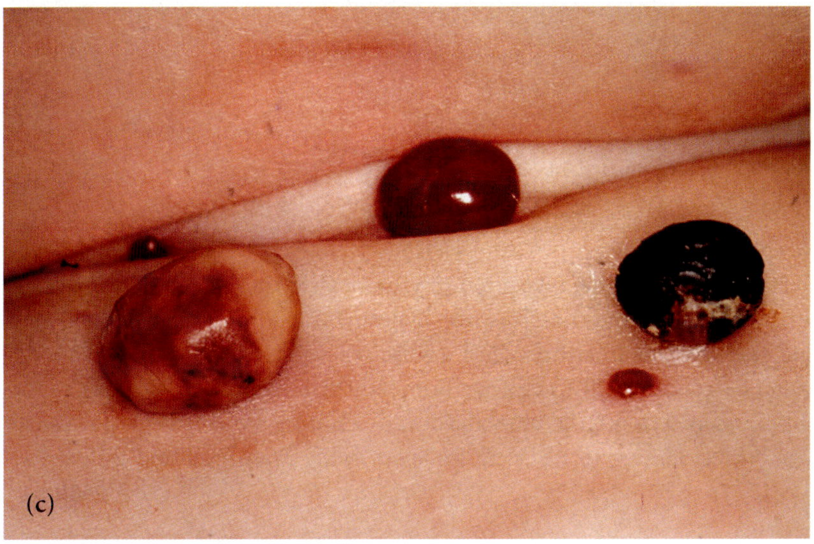
(c)

Multiple miliary-type hemangiomas also known as disseminated neonatal hemangiomatosis (DNH) develop rapidly soon after birth; in a few days or weeks lesions proliferate on the skin and mucous membranes (a, b). They are rare: only 0.4% in a series of 1247 patients had more than 17 lesions (80). Some infants combine small and large superficial lesions and visceral locations at birth or soon after, with either good outcome (a) or an often rapid lethal outcome (b). Rarely, multiple pyogenic-granuloma-like lesions, with aggressive growth and abundant bleeding of the friable lesions arise (96): the boy in (c) was referred to us with significant anemia; blood transfusion was necessary and 12 lesions were excised; IHs continued to proliferate in the skin and liver, and were not stabilized with glucocorticosteroid treatment. Finally vincristine treatment was initiated with significant regression of liver and skin lesions by 1 year of age. Newborns with DNH require careful repeated monitoring because they are at highrisk of developing visceral hemangiomas. The liver is the most common location, followed by the GI tract.

Clinical Aspects, Investigations, and Treatment

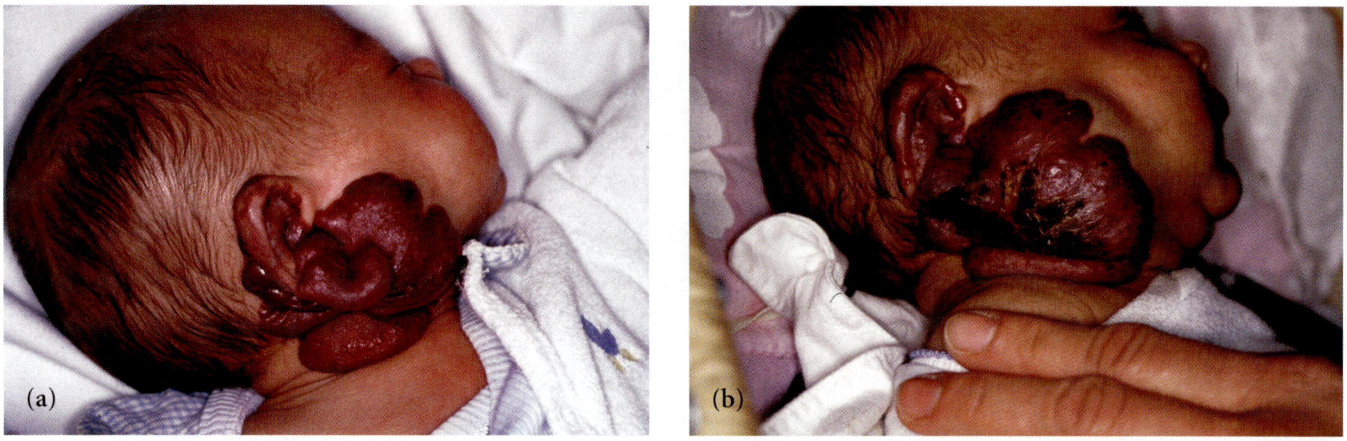

This 4 lb premature girl developed a large IH in the peri-auricular area and ear soon after birth; the color was bright red and the surface shiny, an indication of a risk of spontaneous necrosis (a). One month later, deep IH of the parotid, full involvement of the external ear and a large painful crusted ulceration were present (b). Often, when a parotid hemangioma is unilateral, even if it extends to the external ear, there is no risk of deafness. However, some infants may grow an IH in the inner ear even without having external ear involvement, and thus may develop unilateral deafness.

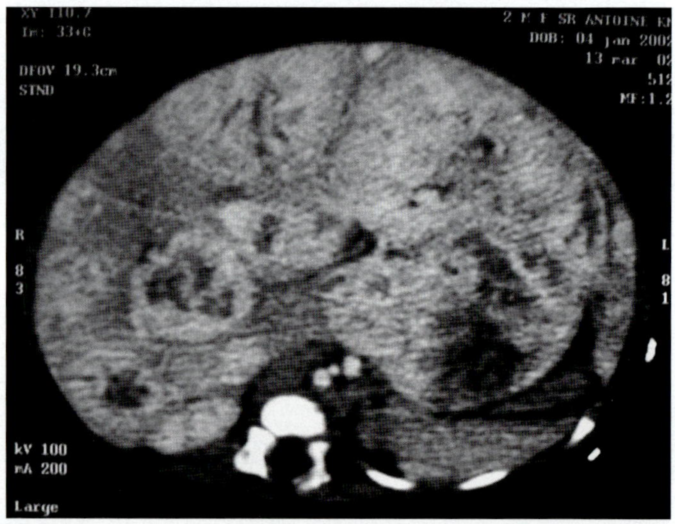

CT with contrast shows multifocal liver IH with centripetal contrast enhancement in a newborn with congestive heart failure. Kassarjian et al. (60) described different imaging (CT and MR) patterns from a selection of 55 patients with liver hemangiomas: focal lesions were present in 22/55, multifocal ones in 33/55; shunts were shown in 17 cases and calcifications in 16. Focal and multifocal IH appear as round, well-defined hypoechoic spherical masses on transverse sonogram. They appear as spherical strongly T2-hyperintense masses on MRI, and with gadolinium injection there is a centripetal enhancement. Some imaging findings are predictive of the clinical course. Massive diffuse hemangiomatosis of the liver is often lethal, being associated with abdominal compartment syndrome, due to vena cava compression, and severe hypothyroidism linked to the secretion of an inactivating selenoenzyme, type 3 iodothyronine deiodinase, by the tumor tissue (39, 57). However, if the liver hemangiomas respond to treatment and regress, the hypothyroidism may improve (62). Focal and multifocal liver IH (a) may wane without the need for treatment. The diffuse type of liver IH (b) is a therapeutic emergency and if there is no response to pharmacological treatment, liver transplant is considered (39). Focal lesions with AV shunting are less common and respond to arterial embolization. According to pathology, focal hemangioma of the liver is usually GLUT1 negative, corresponding to RICH in the liver, while multifocal and diffuse IHs of the liver are GLUT1 positive (41).

Clinical Aspects, Investigations, and Treatment

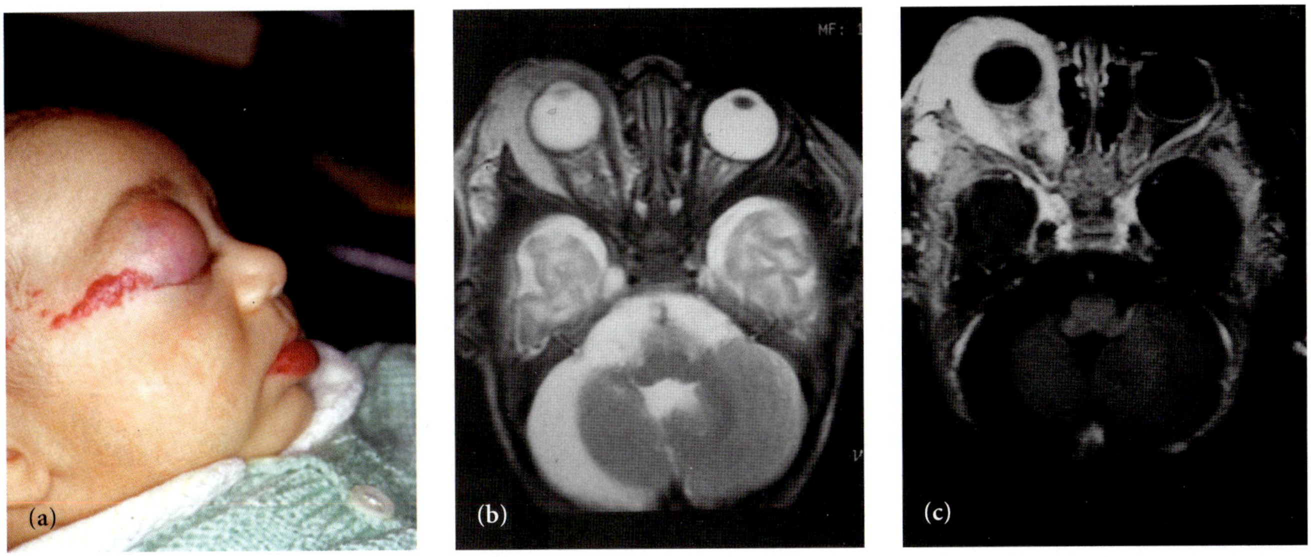

Children at risk of PHACE syndrome should receive neurological, ophthalmological and cardiac assessment (71). This girl had a deep IH of the upper eyelid and minor IH staining of the temporal skin and lower lip (a). MRI showed signs of PHACE syndrome with posterior fossa malformation; hypoplasia of hemi-cerebellum and a complex anomaly of the cerebellar vermis. MRI T2-sequence (b) and T1-sequence with gadolinium injection (c) display eyelid, temporal, and full orbital involvement. Eye abnormalities are an important part of PHACE syndrome. Some ocular abnormalities result from the presence of the periocular hemangioma and they vary from strabismus, refractive error and amblyopia, to proptosis or ptosis. Others correspond to ocular structural defects, such as optic nerve atrophy, coloboma, optic disc excavation or congenital cataract, and these are part of the PHACE syndrome (64).

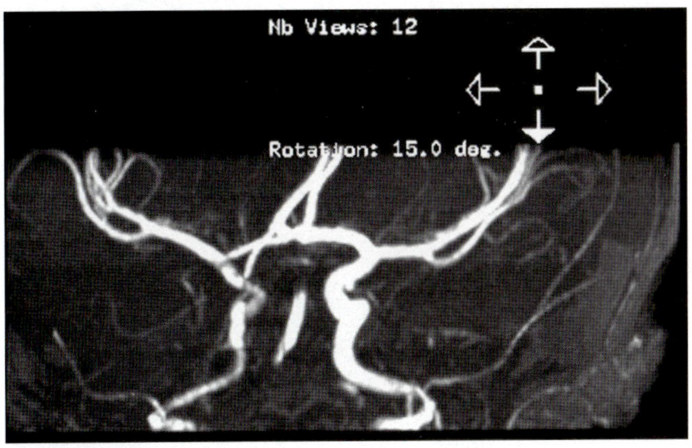

A girl who was developmentally normal at 1 year of age, had a right facial parotid IH, right microtia. PHACE syndrome was diagnosed because of various intracranial arterial anomalies detected on MRI/MRA imaging (courtesy of Dr. I.J. Frieden and Dr. C. Dowd, UCSF, San Francisco, USA). She had a significantly diminished in caliber right internal carotid artery, compared to the left, and fenestration or duplication of the anterior communicating artery. PHACE (OMIM 606519) is an acronym for a neurocutaneous syndrome encompassing the following features: posterior fossa brain malformations, hemangiomas, arterial anomalies, cardiac anomalies, and eye abnormalities. Ventral developmental defects such as sternal cleft or supraombilical raphe may also be present (PHACE(S) syndrome) (40, 41, 85). Diagnosis is made when one or more associated anomalies are present in addition to hemangioma. Most patients do not have all the associated features. Cerebrovascular anomalies consist of persistent embryonic arteries, agenesis or hypoplasia of major arteries and dilatation and tortuosity of others. Patients may be asymptomatic or can have seizures, stroke, developmental delay, and headaches (18, 26, 71, 86).

Clinical Aspects, Investigations, and Treatment

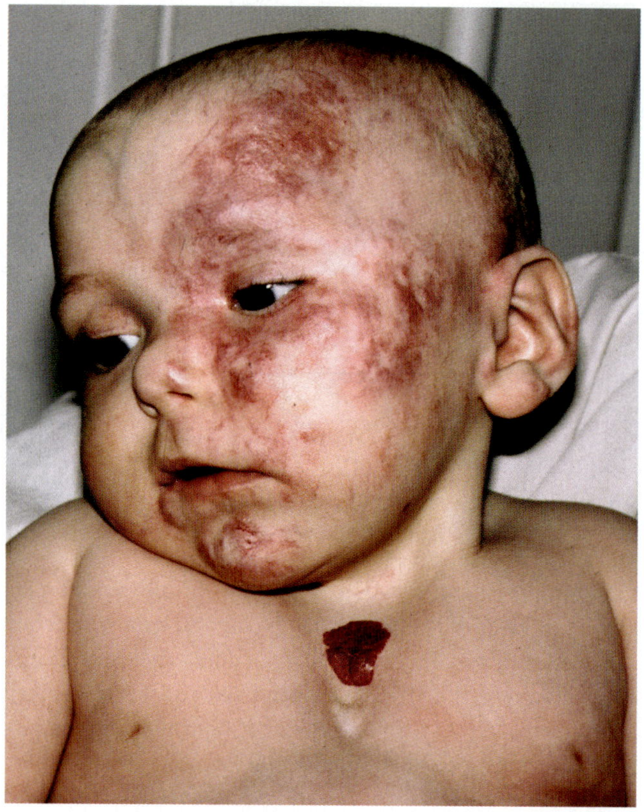

This girl was referred at 6 months for a thin telangiectatic diffuse left hemifacial hemangioma with dilated veins over the forehead and scalp, and a small IH of the mid-thorax. She had total absence of fusion of sternum, creating the large sunken area on the anterior thorax, with heartbeats visible under the skin. Four years later headache and progressive neurological deficit appeared: complex brain arterial anomalies, including hypoplasia of left internal carotid artery and of the proximal left vertebral artery, left intrapetrous fusiform aneurysm, occlusion of right internal carotid artery and Moyamoya-type collateral vessels; a dystrophic left cerebellar hemisphere was also detected (case no.1 reported in: Bhattacharya et al. (11). Intracranial arterial anomalies of PHACE syndrome include dilatation, stenosis, occlusion, tortuosity, aberrant course or origin of arteries, persistent embryonic vessels, fusiform or berry aneurysms (18, 68). Patients experience seizures, stroke, hemiparesis, monoparesis, headaches and developmental delay, or they have normal psychomotor evolution, on long-term follow-up (10, 18, 68, 84, 90). Intracranial vascular alteration may evolve over the years as illustrated in a woman followed over 28 years by Pascual-Castroviejo (86, 87).

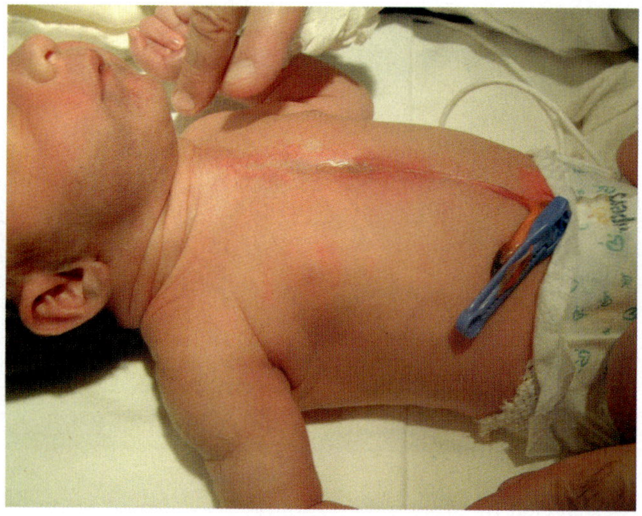

This girl had at birth a supra-umbilical midline raphe, extending from the upper sternum to the umbilicus, and in the cephalic beard area a precursor of IH giving the skin a bluish, pseudo-bruise color (then a thick beard IH and airway involvement expanded, as well as mediatinal IH). This association, first referred to as cavernous hemangioma of face and supraombilical midline raphe (OMIM 140850), is now considered part of PHACE(S) syndrome (OMIM 606519). Sternal fusion defects are rare and most often an isolated finding; the association with supraombilical raphe and craniofacial IH is very rare and has a marked female predilection (54).

Clinical Aspects, Investigations, and Treatment

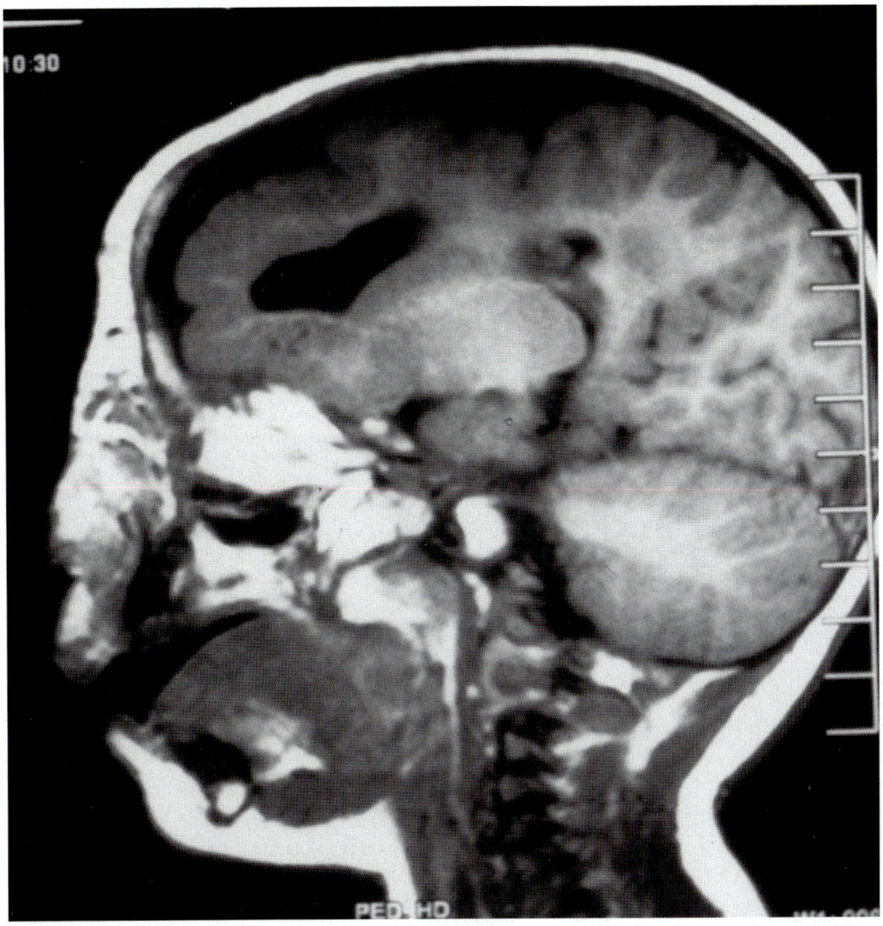

This girl has a different structural developmental anomaly of the brain associated to a rare location of facial hemangioma: a purely centrofacial IH that ulcerated and destroyed the collumella and nostrils. MRI showed frontal lissencephaly. Progressive microcephaly with delay in developmental milestones occurred. Grosso et al. (49) reported another case of complex cortical malformation: a girl with facial hemangioma and a deeply infolding left frontal pachygyric cortex with hypoplasia of the entire left hemisphere.

Clinical Aspects, Investigations, and Treatment

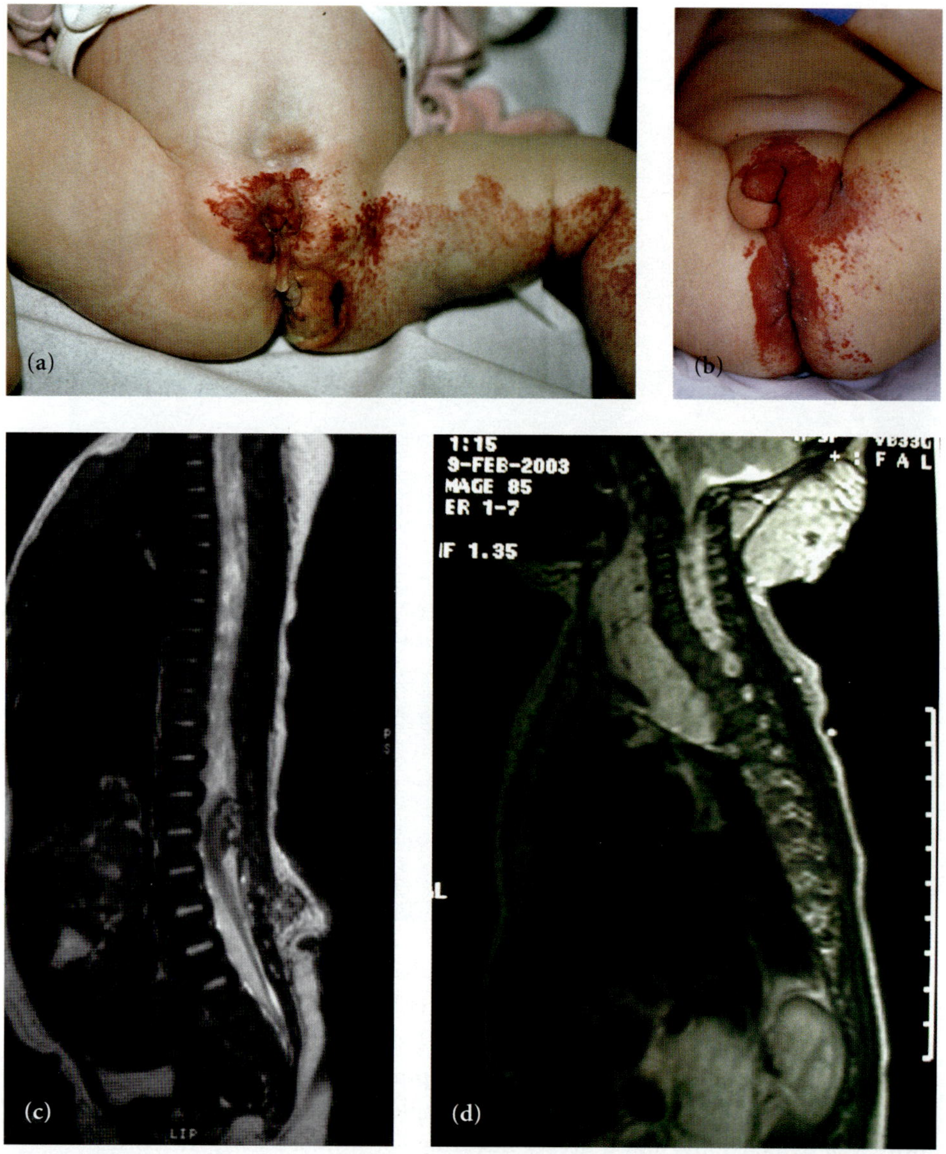

IH of the buttocks, perineum and lower extremity, proliferating in a diffuse regional distribution, are sometimes associated with abnormal genitalia, imperforate anus, and anomalous urinary tract (14). The boy in (b) (courtesy of Dr. Bessis, Saint Eloi Hospital, Montpellier, France) had ambiguous external genitalia. The girl in (a), with perineal ulceration, had incomplete bladder exstrophy and a low position of the navel. Spinal dysraphism, as illustrated by the MRI scan in (c), is present if spinal IH occurs in conjunction with other cutaneous markers of dysraphism (3, 50). The acronym PELVIS was recently created to underline the association of *P*erineal hemangioma, *E*xternal genitalia malformations, *L*ipomyelomeningocele, *V*esicorenal abnormalities, *I*mperforate anus, and *S*kin tag (14a). Some infants have deeply invasive IH without true associated dysraphic anomalies: the infant in (d) remained asymptomatic, although she had developed a deep IH in the nape after birth, and systematic MRI had revealed mediastinal, paraspinal, and intraspinal extension of the IH, a difficult diagnosis as already reported (53).

Clinical Aspects, Investigations, and Treatment

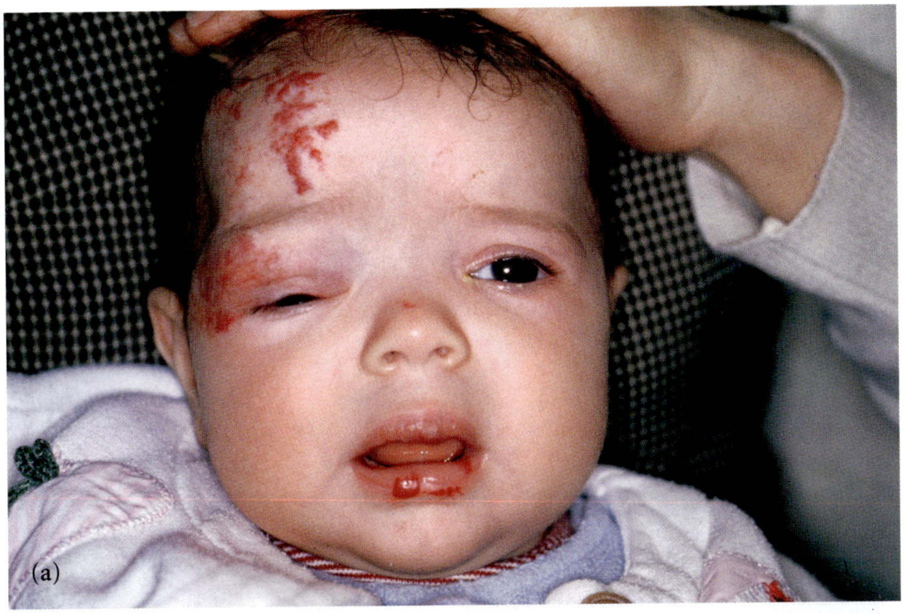

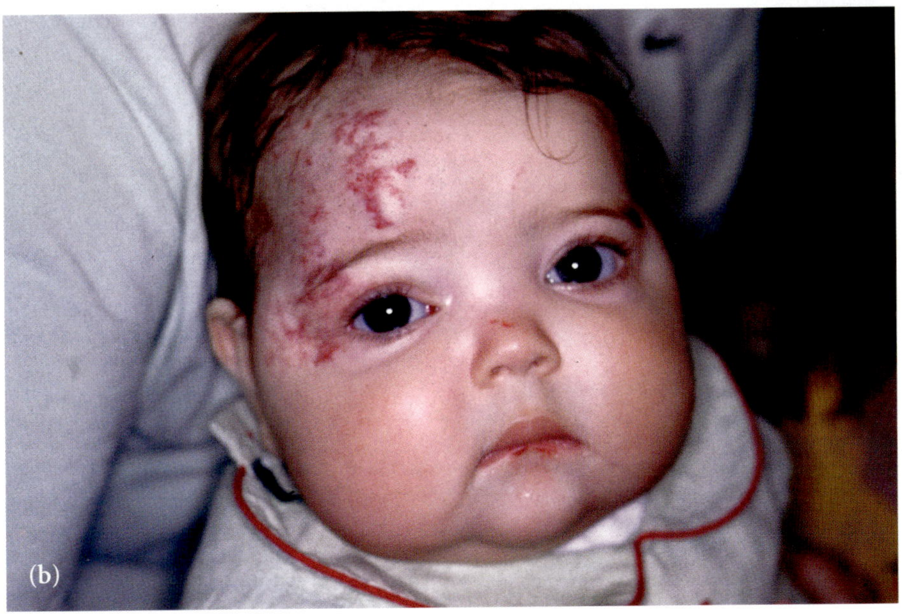

Glucocorticosteroid (GS) treatment remains the first option for dangerous IH. In this girl, the sight-impairing IH (a) involved the upper eyelid as well as the orbit on MRI. There was no PHACE syndrome. The right visual axis was occluded. Oral GS treatment induced rapid cessation of proliferation and reopening of the eye in 1 month (b). She had a total of 4 months of treatment including the tapering phase, with good tolerance. No rebound growth occurred at the end of the treatment. Excellent cosmetic outcome was achieved at the last follow-up when she was 3 years old. However, astigmatism of the right eye required patching and glasses. Infants receiving systemic GS must have close monitoring including frequent blood pressure measurement. Cardiac left ventricular hypertrophy may also be detected by US cardiac evaluation, without any relationship with hypertension. Adrenal suppression seems to correlate with higher daily doses and total dose received.

Clinical Aspects, Investigations, and Treatment

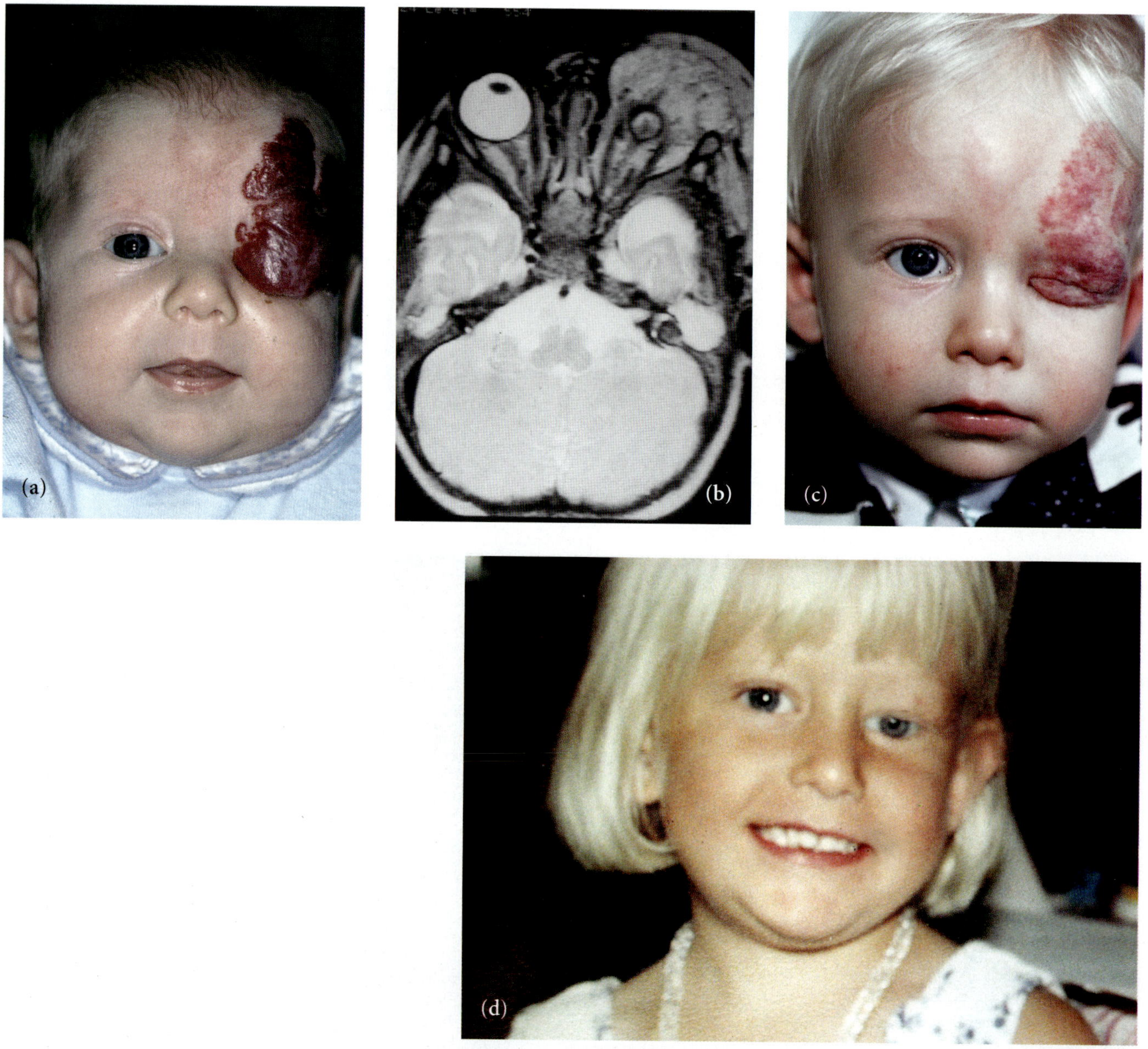

This infant developed an IH soon after birth that completely masked the eye. Because of the risk of deprivation amblyopia, she received corticosteroid treatment during the first weeks of life without any improvement (a). MRI evaluation showed an upper eyelid and orbital intraconal IH and microphthalmos, cataract, and hypoplasia of the optic nerve (b), allowing the diagnosis of PHACE syndrome. No other associated anomaly was present. Structural eye anomalies of PHACE syndrome encompass optic nerve hypoplasia, microphtalmos and cataract (as in this infant), glaucoma, coloboma, morning glory and peripapillary excavation, or optic atrophy (66). It was decided to treat this girl with interferon alpha 2a, 3 million units/m^2 a day for 6 months (lyophilized sterile powder of IFNα 2a). She achieved excellent improvement with no adverse effects, but she still had an apparent ptosis of the eyelid because of the tiny globe (c). However, due to the volume attained by the orbital hemangioma at the end of its proliferating phase, the orbit had reached a correct size. The abnormal eye was enucleated and a prosthetic eye was provided, with excellent cosmetic results (d).

Clinical Aspects, Investigations, and Treatment

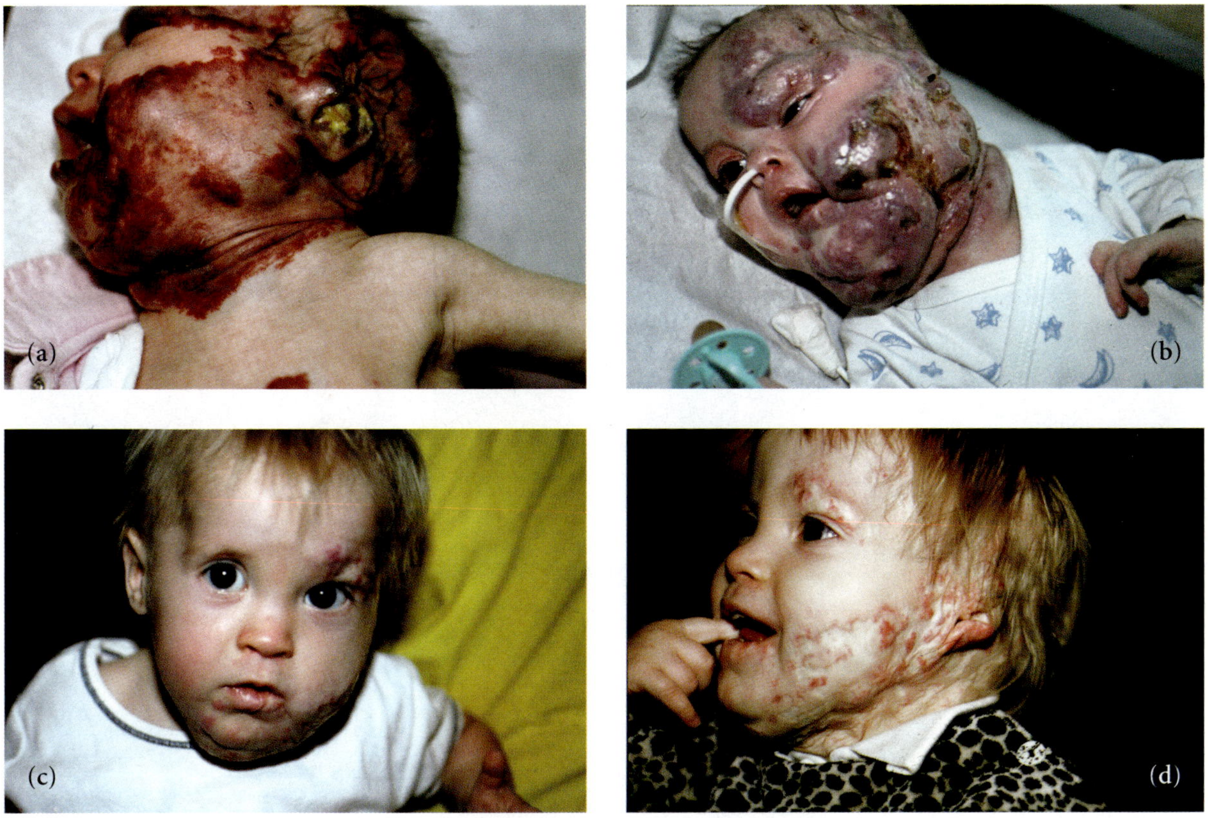

This extensive left hemifacial, scalp, and neck IH with a laryngeal IH was not improved with high-dose glucocorticosteroid (GS) treatment, including megadoses. On the contrary, at 3 months of age necrosis of the lower lip and of the left ear auricle occurred, the IH was still growing, while her general health was deteriorating. No PHACES syndrome was detected. At 7 months of age, only a mild fading of the superficial part of the IH was obtained; but the left eye was partly masked and a parotid mass had developed (b), she was fed through a nasogastric tube, and was enduring extreme pain, not diminished by morphine, from increasing multiple deep ulcerations in the cheek and neck. Interferon alpha 2a (IFN) treatment was then introduced and GS slowly tapered. She had a dramatic response to IFN. After 4 months all ulcers had healed, the eye was wide open and the left parotid mass had shrunk. Eight months later (c) she was in good health, in the late involuting stage of her IH. When 21-months old her IH reached the involuted stage. Diffuse scars were noticeable on the lower part of her left cheek and neck (d), which required further therapeutic procedures, including surgical repair. The scars were much less significant on the forehead and eyelid. Astigmatism of the left eye required orthoptic management.

Clinical Aspects, Investigations, and Treatment

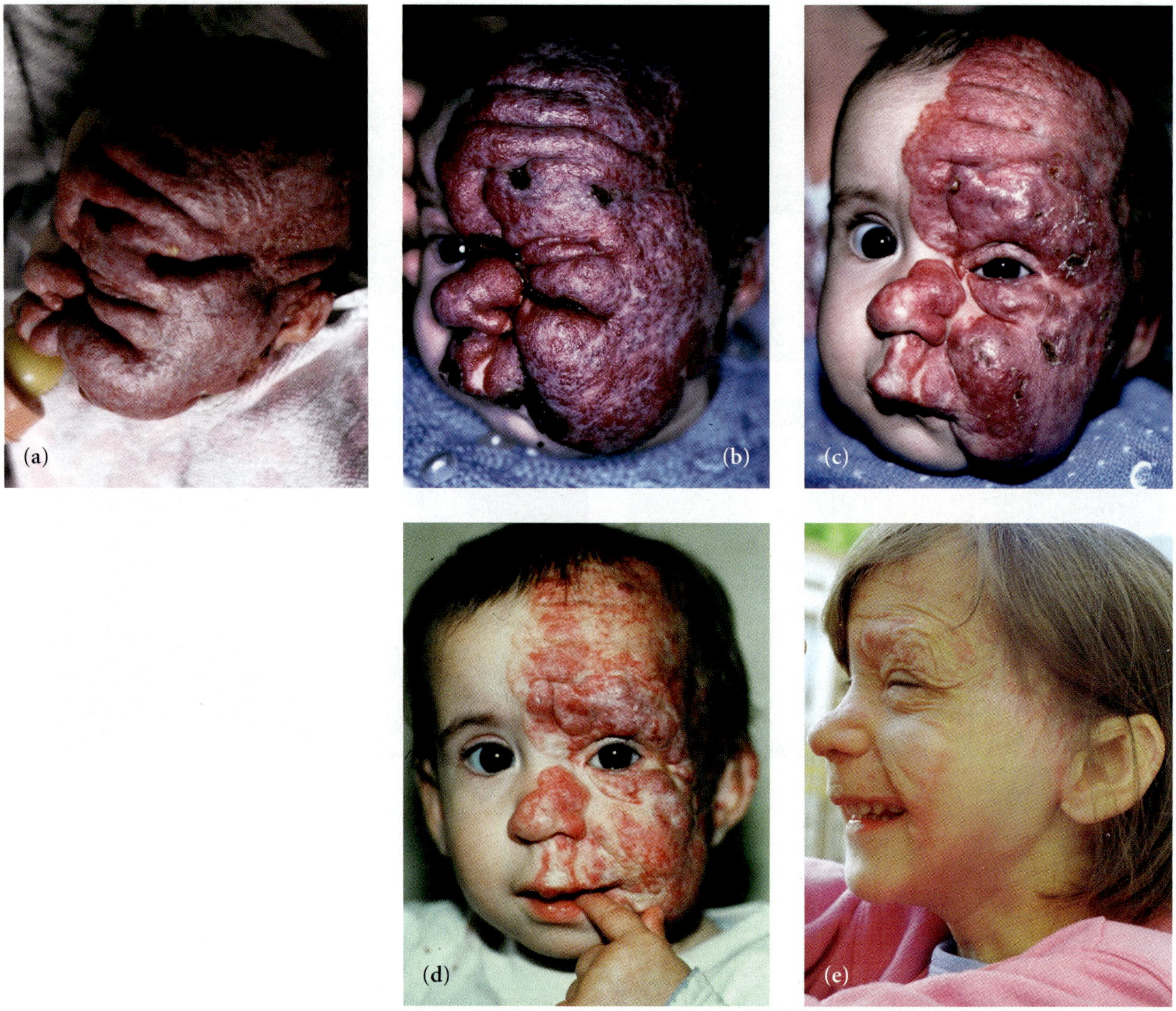

This monozygotic twin girl (the other twin did not develop IH) had a red stain of the left hemiface at birth. She came to us at 3 months of age (a) with this huge, ulcerated, purple facial and scalp IH. The family doctor having said that this "goes spontaneously" the parents were waiting. We initiated oral glucocorticosteroid (GS) treatment but it was poorly effective, giving only slight whitening one month later (b). Pain linked to ulcers was extreme and not soothed by morphine. Interferon alpha 2a (IFN (lyophilized sterile powder)) treatment was then introduced and GS stopped over a period of 1 month. INF was continued for 13 months. The results were excellent, with re-opening of the eye and fading of the tumor ((c) appearance after 4 months of IFN; (d) appearance at the end of IFN treatment at 18 months of age). No neurological side-effects occurred. At 4 years of age the IH had fully vanished but the skin was badly wrinkled and yellowish. A first surgical procedure brought normal skin from the neck to the mandibular area (e) but the repair of the damaged skin of the eyelids will be a tricky task.

Clinical Aspects, Investigations, and Treatment

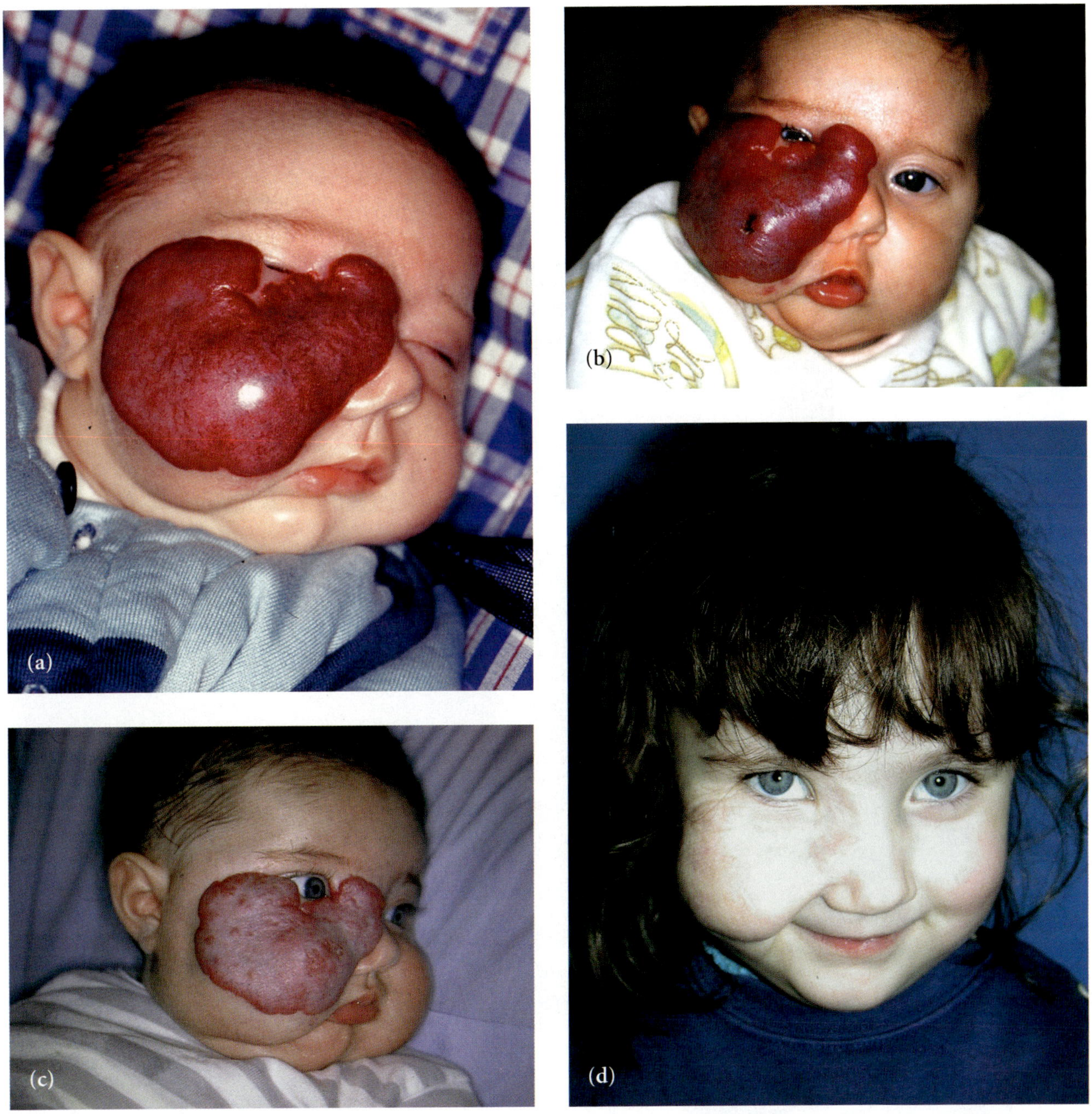

This girl had a sight-threatening IH, still growing under glucocorticosteroid treatment: in (a) she had received prednisone 2 mg/kg/day for 3 weeks; it was changed to betamethasone 0.20 mg/kg/day but growth of the IH continued; (b) is the appearance after a total of 6 weeks of steroids, with the tumor nearly closing the right visual field, and filling the floor of the orbit on MRI. No PHACE syndrome was present. Tapering of steroid was decided on and she received vincristine treatment (a total of 20 weekly IV injections, over 4½ months). A clear improvement with reopening of the eye was visible after the sixth injection (c). The treatment was well tolerated, except for increased esophageal reflux and infection of the central line. Two years later, the IH was in the involuted stage (d). Surgical repair of excess skin could begin at 3 years, while vision was still improving with glasses and patching.

Clinical Aspects, Investigations, and Treatment

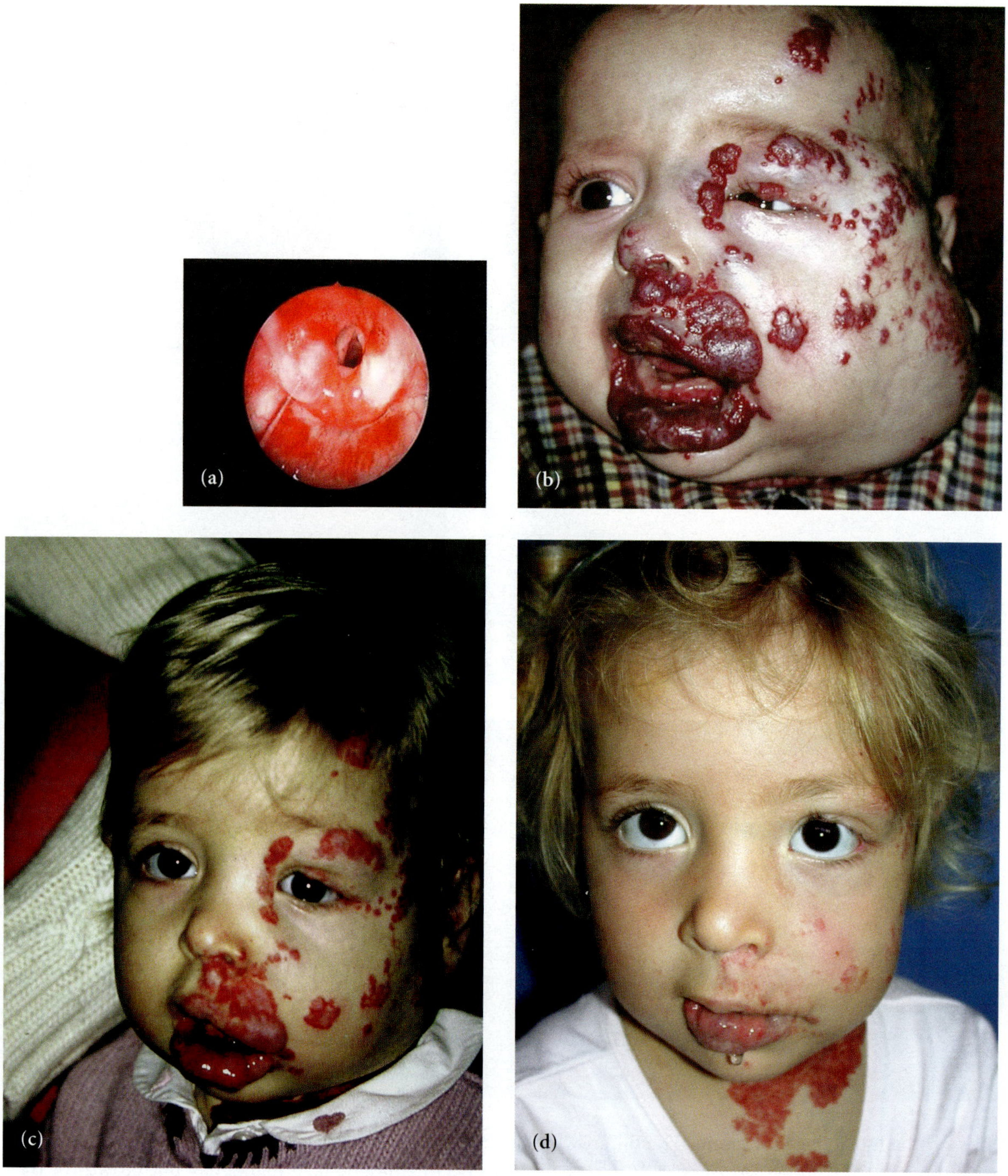

This girl was referred for progressive laryngeal dyspnea, in the context of a diffuse facial and neck IH. Laryngotracheal endoscopy disclosed a diffuse pharyngeal, laryngeal (a) and tracheal IH (courtesy of Dr. Gilles Roger, Hôpital Armand Trousseau, Paris, France). MRI of the brain and cardiac US were normal. No PHACE(S) syndrome was detected. Prednisolone started at 2 then 3 mg/kg/day was unable to control the breathing problem. At 6 weeks of age, open-approach excision of the subglottic IH was performed. A graft of auricular cartilage was preventively used to enlarge the subglottis. Glucocorticosteroid treatment (GS) was

Clinical Aspects, Investigations, and Treatment

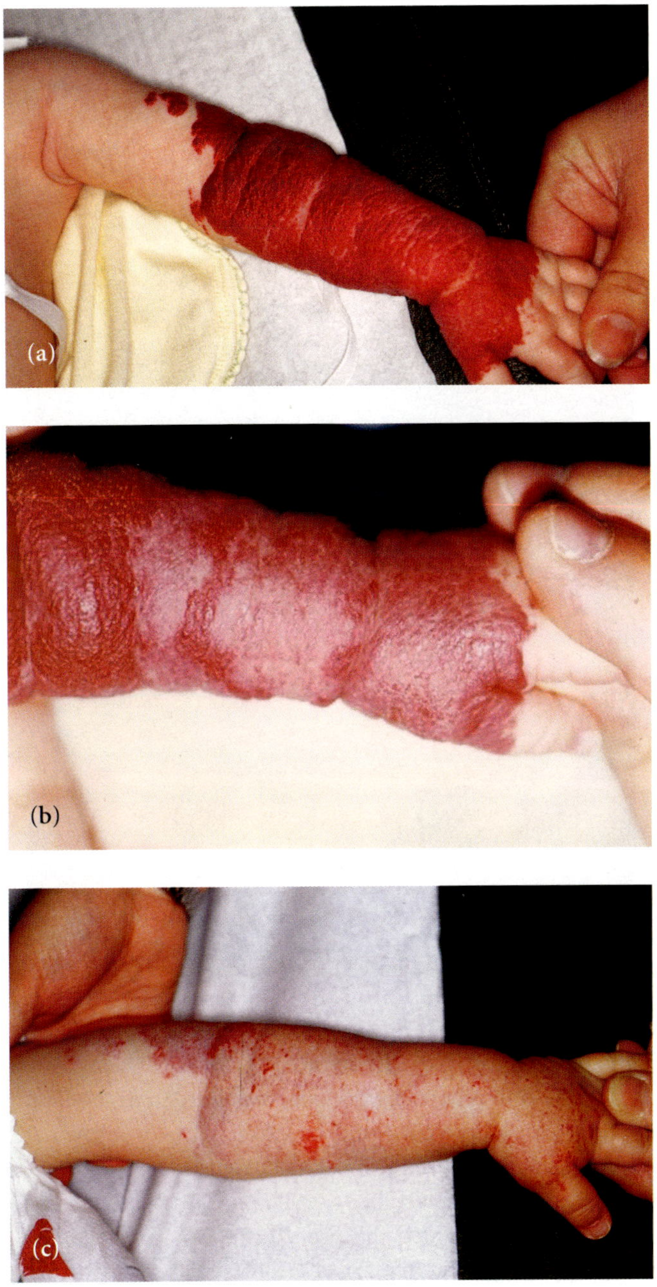

This large hemangioma of the forearm and hand was seen at 1 month of age (a); glucocorticosteroid (GS) and flashlamp pumped-pulsed dye laser (PDL) treatments (operator: Dr. Virginie Fayard, Paris, France) were simultaneously started; 2 months after the first laser treatment, and while beginning tapering of GS, the area treated with laser was clearly fading compared to the rest of the IH (b). She had two additional laser sessions on the whole surface of the IH. Significant regression was obtained before 1 year of age (c) with no further rebound growth. PDL treatment seemed to have boosted the response of IH to GS.

poorly effective: at 3 months a bulky superficial IH had developed with orbital involvement, ulcers, major neck and upper thorax location, as well as extension of the tracheal IH on laryngotracheoscopy. At 4 months of age interferon alpha 2a treatment was initiated (3 million units/m^2/day subcutaneously) while GS treatment was progressively stopped over 4 weeks. Initially, there was clear improvement but secondary rebound growth of the facial IH occurred 4 months later (b) and obstructive dyspnea worsened. Therefore, weekly vincristine treatment was introduced (and interferon stopped) and given over 8 months (24 injections) and stopped (c). Results were clearly good on both the superficial and airway IH. The residual involuting IH slowly improved over the next 3 years of follow-up (d).

Clinical Aspects, Investigations, and Treatment

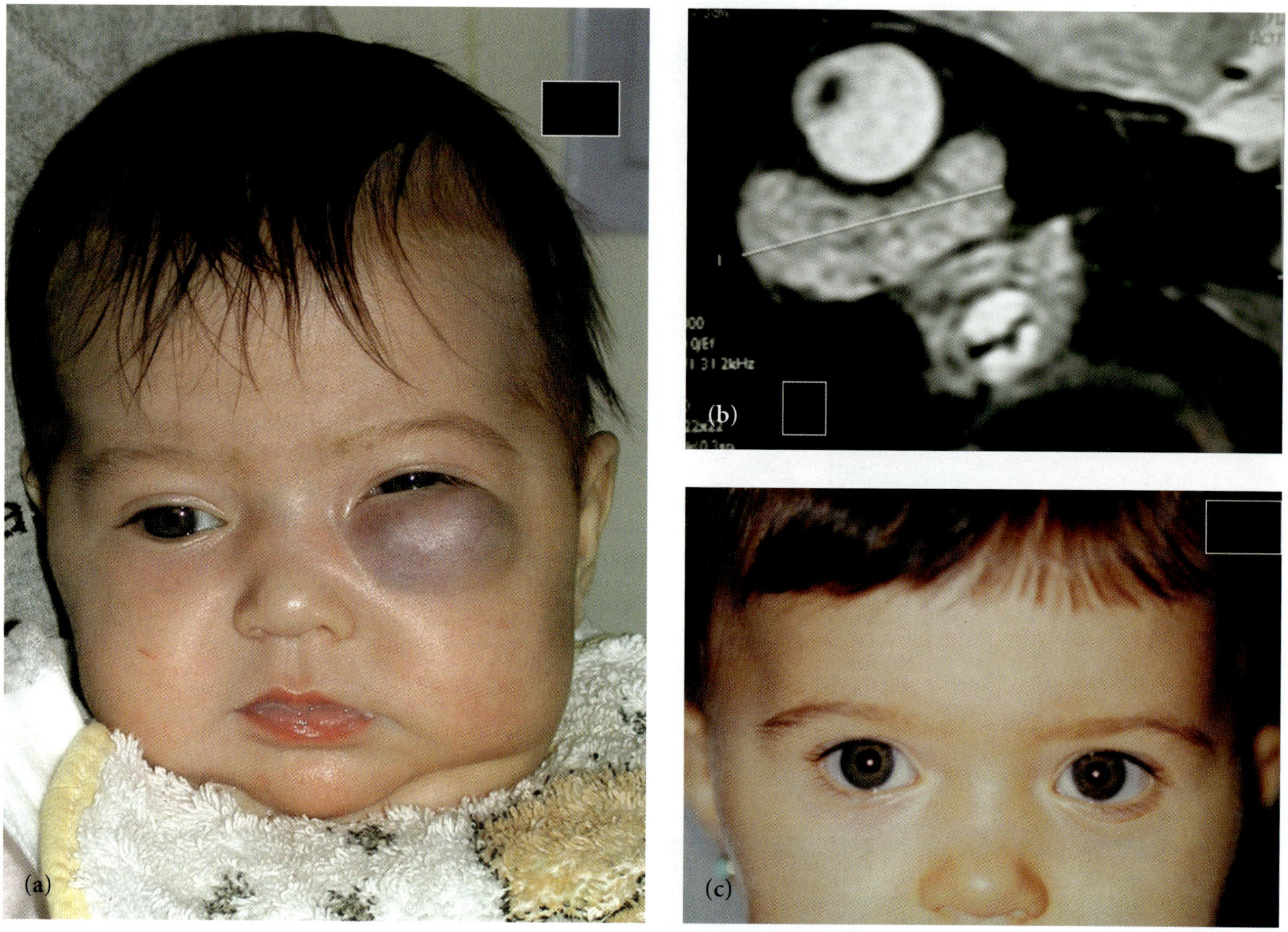

The IH in this girl rapidly proliferated. At 2 months she had upward displacement of the eye and her visual axis was nearly occluded (a). MRI T2-weighted sagittal image showed deep orbital extension along the floor of the orbit (b). No PHACE syndrome was detected. Surgical excision was the preferred therapeutic option to relieve the pressure and burden of the IH on the globe and prevent permanent visual deficit. Both the lid and orbital part of the IH could be extracted with immediate good results (operator: Dr. Patrick Diner, Hôpital Armand Trousseau, Paris, France). Six months later no rebound growth had occurred and the incision scar along the inferior line of eyelashes was barely detectable (c). The use of the electronic dissector CUSA (cavitron ultra sonic aspirator) (Cavitron® and Dissectron®) facilitated the procedure. This technique minimizes intra-operative hemorrhage and postoperative complications (25, 88). Early surgical treatment prevents the development of amblyopia, but post-operative patching, or atropine drops (to blur the normal eye) and/or glasses, are often required to correct the already established refractive error (astigmatism or myopia) (19, 52, 78, 89).

Clinical Aspects, Investigations, and Treatment

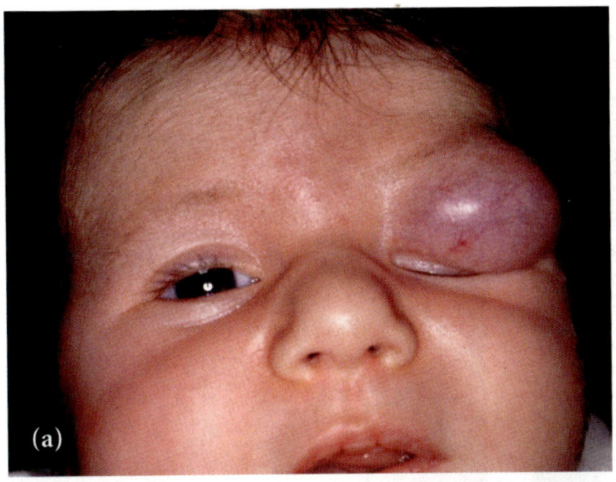

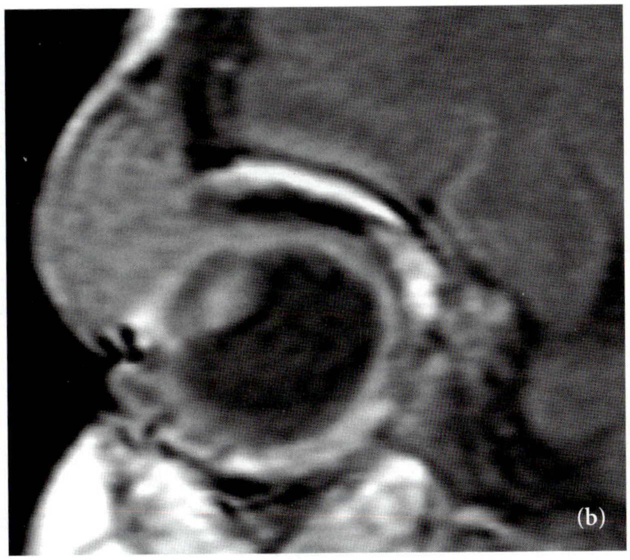

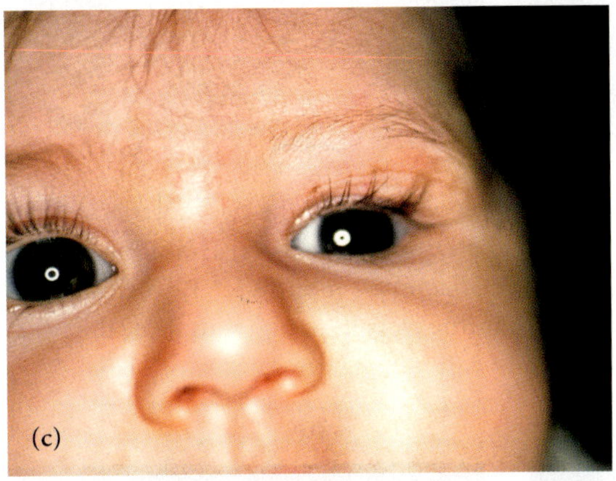

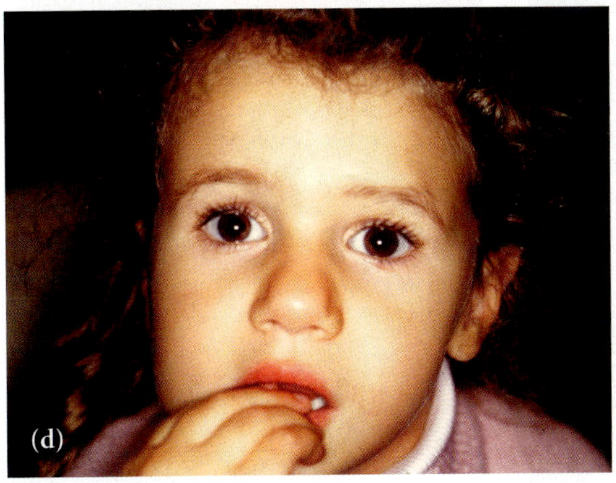

This upper eyelid hemangioma closed the visual field and was growing as a deep IH without superficial red component (a). A bolus of glucocorticosteroid and then daily oral treatment (prednisolone 3 mg/kg/day) did not re-open the eye. MRI indicated that there was no orbital extension (b). Thus surgical excision using an ultrasonic device (Dissectron®) was performed at 2 months of age, to avoid amblyopiogenisis (operator: Dr. Patrick Diner, Hôpital Armand Trousseau, Paris, France). The outcome was excellent 1 month later (c) and perfect 3 years later (d) with a barely visible scar. As soon as the visual axis is re-opened ophthalmologic evaluation is essential, to look for residual palpebral occlusion if any, strabismus secondary to extraocular muscle infiltration, ocular motility, objective refraction, and amblyopia; if necessary, re-education aims at improving vision.

Clinical Aspects, Investigations, and Treatment

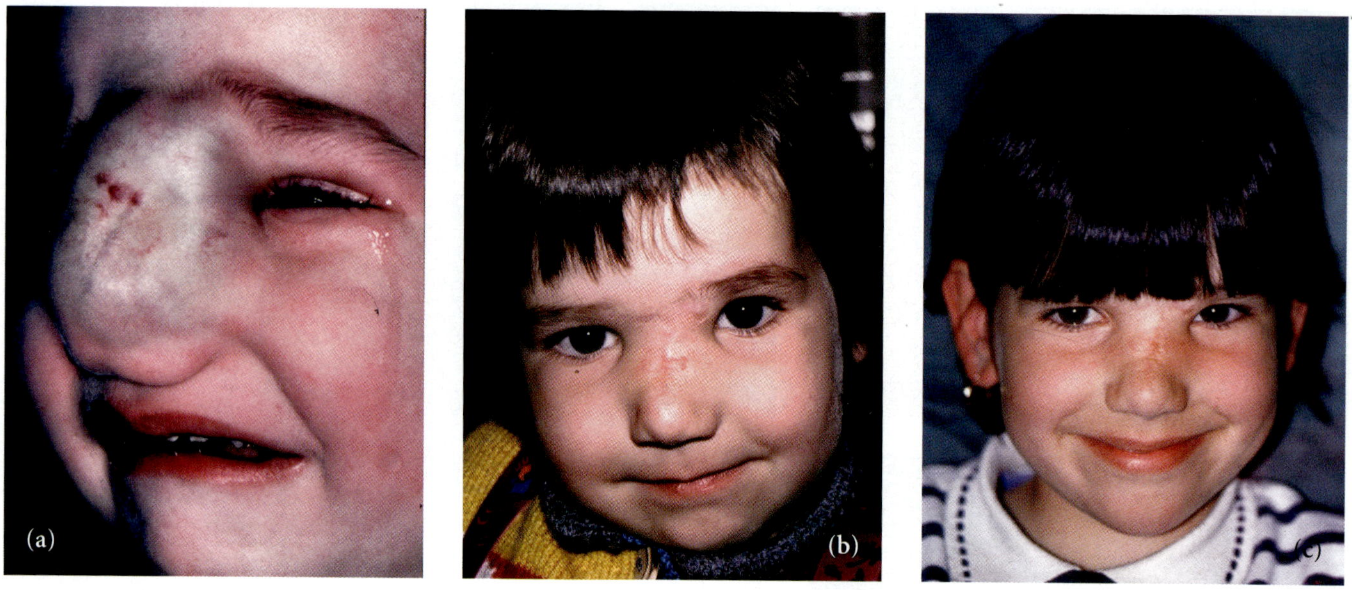

Surgical excision (at 11 months of age) was decided on because this bulky full nose IH was closing the two nostrils (a) and had responded poorly to high-dose and protracted prednisolone treatment (operator: Dr. Patrick Diner, Hôpital Armand Trousseau, Paris, France). Reopening of the nostrils and cosmetic appearance were satisfactory 2 months later, with some IH still involuting in the glabellum (b). Although the scar from incision line was visible in the glabellum and middle of the nose, 8 years later, the overall aspect, the development of the nasal bones and the shape of the nose were satisfactory (c).

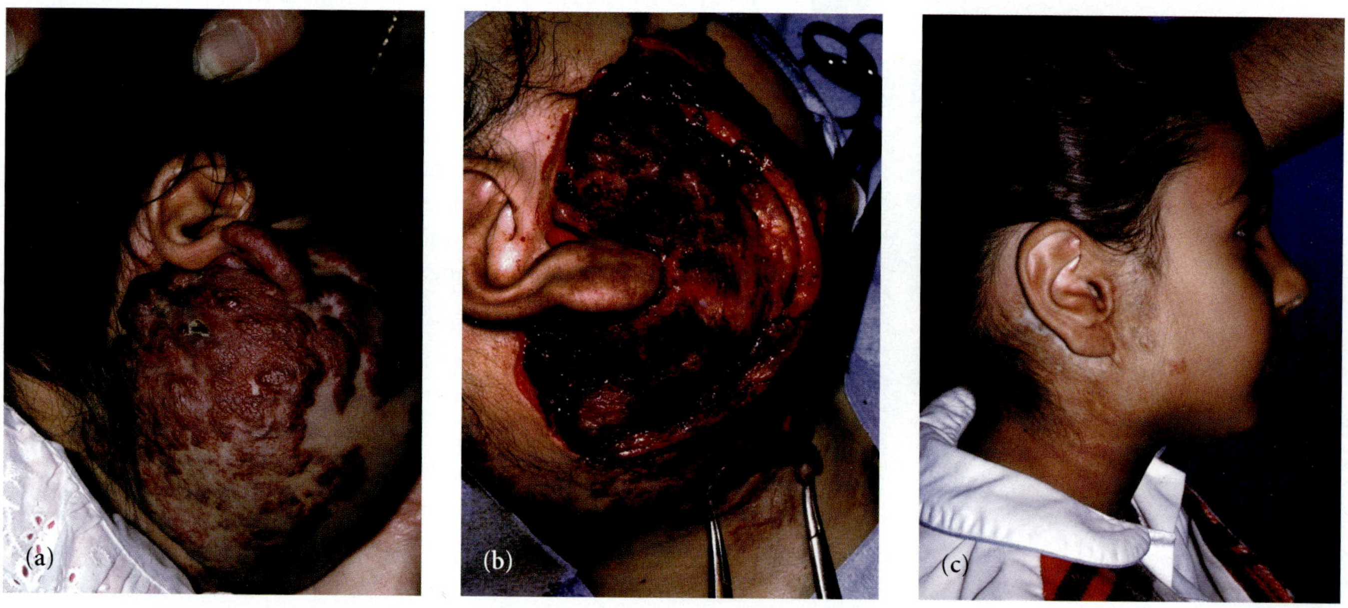

This huge parotid hemangioma obstructed the external auditory canal and had frequent painful ulceration; glucocorticosteroid treatment failed and the mass was still growing and ulcerating (a). Surgical reduction of the bulk of the tumor was performed at 2 years (b) and the ear lobule was replaced. Post-operative healing was complicated by some necrosis of the retroauricular suture. No facial palsy occurred. A minor residual parotid IH was left to involute (operator: Dr. Jacques Buis, Hôpital Armand Trousseau, Paris, France). The final outcome was good ((c) aspect at 4½ years of age). Nevertheless,

Clinical Aspects, Investigations, and Treatment

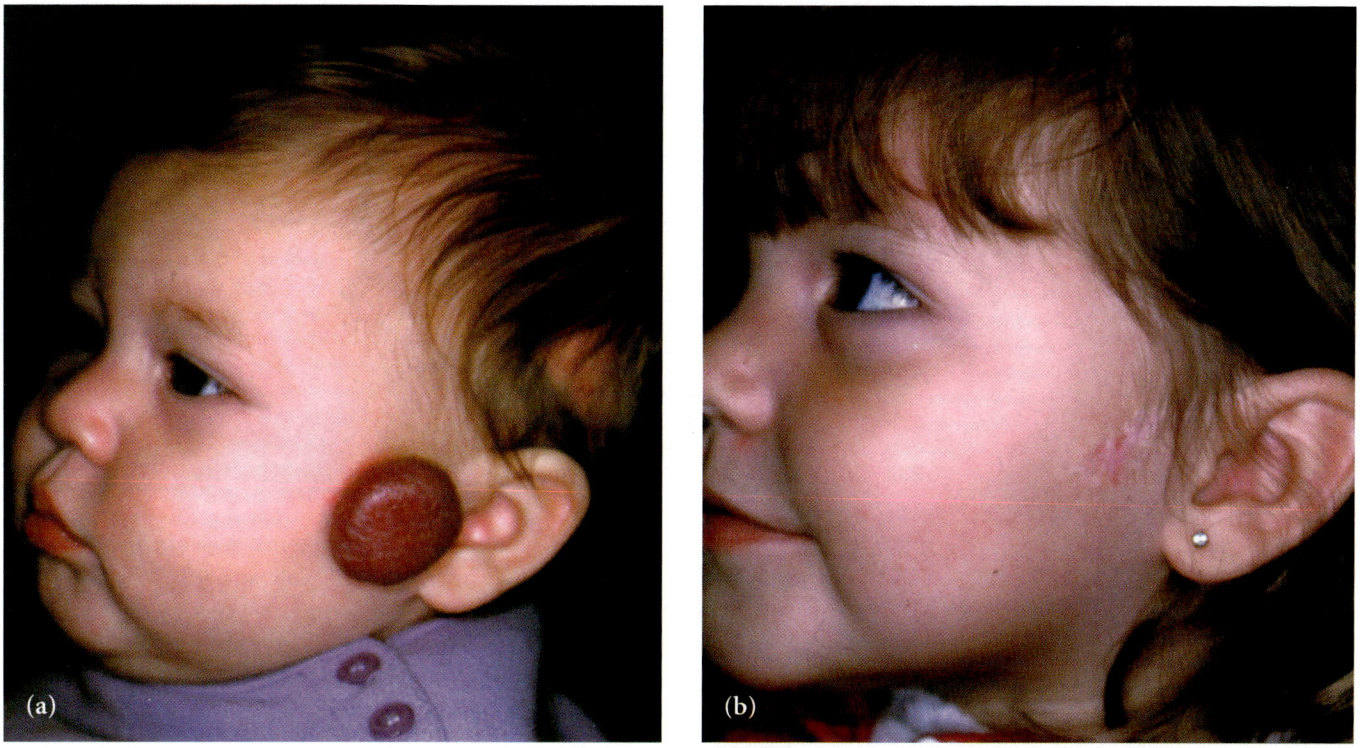

Circular excision and purse string suture (operator: Professor John B. Mulliken, the Children's Hospital, Boston, USA): an 8-month-old girl with proliferating phase hemangioma on the left cheek (a). Skin is irrevocably expanded and sequelae (anetoderma) are expected; the decision was taken to proceed prior to formation of facial image and memory of an operation. Circular excision and purse-string closure were made at 1 year 3 months, and (b) shows the appearance at 2½ years of age.

surgical excision of parotid IH is usually not recommended because of the risk of damage to the facial nerve. Pharmacological treatments are preferred, including corticosteroid, interferon, or vincristine. Reconstructive procedures take place in the involuted stage (excision of excess skin and fibro-fatty residuum, auricular reduction or remodeling). These late surgical procedures were used in two-thirds of patients with parotid hemangioma in a report of 100 cases (48).

Clinical Aspects, Investigations, and Treatment

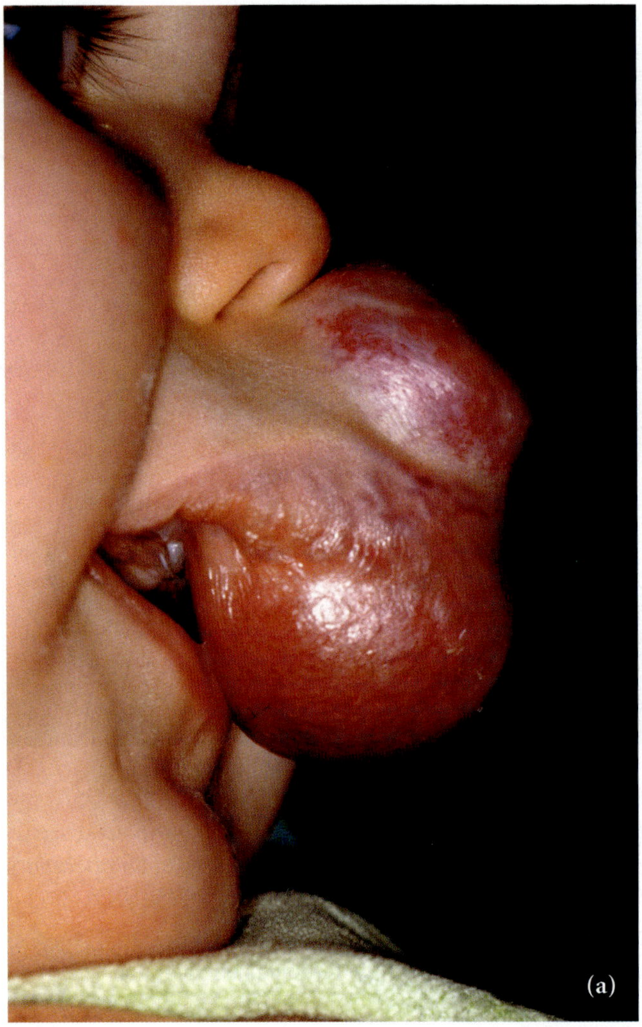

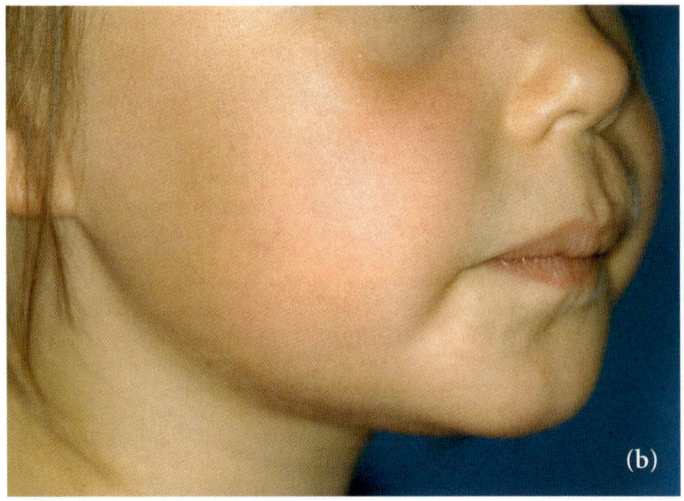

This very large upper lip hemangioma developed in the left part of the upper lip, to the midline, and it involved the full thickness of the lip. After three intralesional injections of a long-lasting corticosteroid (triamcinolone) the tumor was still proliferating; therefore, at 1 year of age (a) a surgical protocol was planned, to prevent mass effect on the underlying bone and dental–alveolar process, and to minimize permanent morphological and functional impact. It included five consecutive procedures. Four years later, at 5 years of age, an excellent cosmetic and functional outcome was attained (b) (operators: Dr. Veronique Soupre and Dr. Patrick Diner, Hôpital Armand Trousseau, Paris, France). Early surgical management helped the parents to cope with the psychological distress created by the facial tumor of their child.

References

1 Adams D. in: Infantile hemangiomas: current knowledge, future directions. Proceedings of a Research Workshop on Infantile Hemangioma. Bethesda Maryland, April 7–9, 2005. *Pediatr Dermatol* 2005; **22**: 383–406.

2 Akyuz C, Yaris N, Kutluk MT, Buyukpamukcu M. Management of cutaneous hemangiomas: a retrospective analysis of 1109 cases and comparison of conventional dose prednisolone with high-dose methylprednisolone therapy. *Pediatr Hematol Oncol* 2001; **18**: 47–55.

3 Allen RM, Sandquist MA, Piatt JH Jr, Selden NR. Ultrasonographic screening in infants with isolated spinal strawberry nevi. *J Neurosurg* 2003; **98**: 247–50.

4 Amir J, Metzker A, Krikler R, Reisner SH. Strawberry hemangioma in preterm infants. *Pediatr Dermatol* 1986; **3**: 331–2.

5 Ashinoff R, Geronemus RG. Failure of the flashlamp-pumped dye laser to prevent progression to deep hemangioma. *Pediatr Dermatol* 1993; **10**: 77–80.

6 Aviles R, Boyce TG, Thompson DM. Pneumocystis carinii pneumonia in a 3-month old infant receiving high-dose corticosteroid therapy for airway hemangiomas. *Mayo Clin Proceed* 2004; **79**: 243–5.

7 Barlow CF, Priebe CJ, Mulliken JB, Barnes PD, MacDonald D, Folkman J. Spastic diplegia as a complication of interferon alfa 2a treatment of hemangiomas of infancy. *J Pediatr* 1998; **132**: 527–30.

8 Batta K, Goodyear HM, Moss C, Williams HC, Hiller L, Waters R. Randomised controlled study of early pulsed dye laser treatment of uncomplicated childhood hemangiomas: results of a 1-year analysis. *Lancet* 2002; **360**: 521–7.

9 Bauland CG, Steijlen PM, Rieu PNMA, Spauwen PHM. The pathogenesis of hemangiomas: a review. *Plast Recontr Surg* 2006; **117**: 29e–35e

10 Bennett ML, Fleischer AB Jr, Chamlin SN, Frieden IJ. Oral corticosteroid use is effective for cutaneous hemangiomas: an evidence-based evaluation. *Arch Dermatol* 2001; **137**: 1208–13.

11 Bhattacharya JJ, Luo CB, Alvarez H, Rodesch G, Pongpech S, Lasjaunias PL. PHACES syndrome: a review of eight previously unreported cases with late arterial occlusions. *Neuroradiology* 2004; **46**: 227–33.

12 Bitar MA, Moukarbel RV, Zalzal GH. Management of congenital subglottic hemangioma: trends and success over the past 17 years. *Otolaryngol Head Neck Surg* 2005; **132**: 226–31.

13 Boon LM, MacDonald DM, Mulliken JB. Complications of systemic corticosteroid therapy for problematic hemangiomas. *Plast Reconstr Surg* 1999; **104**: 1616–23.

14 Bouchard S, Yazbeck S, Lallier M. Perineal hemangioma, anorectal malformation, and genital anomaly, a new association? *J Pediatr Surg* 1999; **34**: 1133–5.

14a Girard C, Bigorre M, Guilot B, Bessis D. PELVIS syndrome. *Arch Dermatol* 2006; **142**: 884–8.

15 Bronzetti G, Giardini A, Patrizi A, Prandstraller D, Donti A, Formigari R, et al. Ipsilateral hemangioma and aortic arch anomalies in posterior fossa malformations, hemangiomas, arterial anomalies, coarctation of the aorta, and cardiac defects, and eye abnormalities (PHACE) anomaly: report and review. *Pediatrics* 2004; **113**: 412–15.

16 Bruckner AL, Frieden IJ. Hemangiomas of infancy. *J Am Acad Dermatol* 2003; **48**: 477–93.

17 Burrows PE, Laor T, Paltiel H, Robertson RL. Diagnostic imaging in the evaluation of vascular birthmarks. *Dermatology Clin* 1998; **16**: 455–88.

18 Burrows PE, Robertson RL, Mulliken JB, Beardsley Ds, Chaloupka JC, Ezekowitz RAB, et al. Cerebral vasculopathy and neurologic sequelae in infants with cervicofacial hemangioma: report of eight patients. *Radiology* 1998; **207**: 601–7.

19 Ceisler EJ, Santos L, Blei F. Periocular hemangiomas: what every physician should know. *Pediatr Dermatol* 2004; **21**: 1–9.

20 Chang E, Boyd A, Nelson CC, Crowley D, Law T, Kenough KM, et al. Successful treatment of infantile hemangiomas with interferon alfa-2b. *J Pediatr Hematol Oncol* 1997; **19**: 237–44.

21 Chen MT, Yeong EK, Horng SY. Intralesional corticosteroid therapy in proliferating head and neck hemangiomas: a review of 155 cases. *J Pediatr Surg* 2000; **35**: 420–3.

22 Chiller KG, Passaro D, Frieden IJ. Hemangiomas of infancy. Clinical characteristics, morphologic subtypes, and their relationship to race, ethnicity and gender. *Arch Dermatol* 2002; **138**: 1567–76.

23 David LR, Malek MM, Argenta LC. Efficacy of pulsed dye laser therapy for the treatment of ulcerated haemangioma: a review of 78 patients. *Br J Plast Surg* 2003; **56**: 317–27.

24 Demiri Ec, Pelissier P, Genin-Etcheberry T, Tsakoniatis N, Martin D, Baudet J. Treatment of facial haemangiomas: the present status of surgery. *Br J Plast Surg* 2001; **54**: 665–74.

25 Diner PA, Petit F, Soupre V, Enjolras O, Lemarchand-Venencie F, Moraillon I, et al. Exérèse précoce des hémangiomes de la face: nouvelle technique par ultrasons. *Ann Dermatol Venereol* 1998; **125**: 605–7.

26 Drolet BA, Dohil M, Golomb MR, Wells R, et al. Early stroke and cerebral vasculopathy in children with facial hemangiomas and PHACE association. *Pediatrics* 2006; **117**: 959–64.

27 Dubois J, Garel L. Imaging and therapeutic approach of hemangiomas and vascular malformations in the pediatric age group. *Pediatr Radiol* 1999; **29**: 879–93.

28 Dubois J, Hershon L, Carmant L, Belanger S, Leclerc JM, David M. Toxicity profile of interferon alfa-2b in children: a prospective evaluation. *J Pediatr* 1999; **135**: 782–5.

29 Egbert JE, Paul S, Engel WK, Summers CG. High injection pressure during intralesional injection of corticosteroids into capillary hemangiomas. *Arch Ophthalmol* 2001; **119**: 677–83.

30 Egbert JE, Enjolras O, Elsas FJ, Stalder JF, Lemarchand-Venencie F, Haik Bg, Hamel-Teillac D, Magalon G, Lacour JP. Question du mois: corticothérapie intralésionnelle et hémangiomes orbito-palpébraux. *Ann Dermatol Venereol* 1998; **125**: 754–8.

31 Enjolras O, Riché MC, Merland JJ, Escande JP. Management of alarming hemangiomas in infancy: a review of 25 cases. *Pediatrics* 1990; **85**: 491–8.

32 Enjolras O, Pouplard F, Beucher A, Ginies JL, Verret JL. Toxicité neurologique de l'interferon alfa 2a au cours du traitement d'un hémangiome céphalique grave. Communication Journées Dermatologiques de Paris 1996. *Ann Dermatol Venereol* 1996; **123**: S1: 144–5.

33 Enjolras O, Gelbert F. Superficial hemangiomas: associations and management. *Pediatr Dermatol* 1997; **14**: 173–9.

34 Enjolras O. Neurotoxicity of interferonalfa in children treated for hemangiomas. *J Am Acad Dermatol* 1998; **39**: 1037–8.

35 Enjolras O, Brevière GM, Roger G, Tovi M, Pellegrino S, Varotti E, Soupre V, Picard A, Leverger G. Traitement par vincristine des hémangiomes graves du nourrisson. *Arch Pediatr* 2004; **11**: 99–107.

36 Esterly NB. Cutaneous Hemangiomas, Vascular stains and malformations, and associated syndromes. *Curr Prob Dermatol* 1995; **VII**: 65–108.

37 Ezekowitz RAB, Mulliken JB, Folkman J. Interferon alfa-2a therapy for life-threatening hemangiomas of infancy. *N Eng J Med* 1992; **326**: 1456–63.

38 Faguer K, Dompmartin A, Labbe D, Barrelier MT, Leroy D, Theron J. Early surgical treatment of Cyrano-nose haemangiomas with Rethi incision. *Br J Plast Surg* 2002; **55**: 498–503.

39 Fishman S. in: Infantile hemangiomas: current knowledge, future directions. Proceedings of a Research Workshop on Infantile Hemangioma. Bethesda Maryland, April 7–9, 2005. *Pediatr Dermatol* 2005; **22**: 383–406.

40 Frieden IJ, Reese V, Cohen D., PHACE syndrome: the association of posterior fossa brain malformations, hemangiomas, arterial anomalies, coarctation of the aorta and cardiac defects, and eye abnormalities. *Arch Dermatol* 1996; **132**: 307–11.

41 Frieden IJ, Haggstrom AJ, Drolet BA, Mancini AJ, Friedlander SF, Boon L, Chamlin S, Baselga E, Garzon M, Nopper AJ, Siegel DH, Mathes EW, Goddard D, Bischoff J, North PE, Esterly NB. Infantile hemangiomas: current knowledge, future directions. Proceedings of a Research Workshop on Infantile Hemangiomas, April 7–9, 2005, Bethesda, Maryland. *Pediatr Dermatol* 2005; **22**: 383–406.

42 Frischer JS, Huang J, Serur A, Kadenhe A, Yamashiro DJ, Kandel JJ. Biomolecular markers and involution of hemangiomas. *J Pediatr Surg* 2004; **39**: 400–4.

43 Garden JM, Bakus AD, Paller AS. Treatment of cutaneous hemangiomas with the flashlamp-pumped pulsed dye laser: prospective analysis. *J Pediatr* 1992; **120**: 555–60.

44 Garmendia G, Miranda N, Borroso S, Longchong M, Martinez E, Ferrero J. Regression of infancy hemangiomas with recombinant IFN alpha-2b. *J Interferon Cytokine Res* 2001; **21**: 31–8.

45 Garzon MC, Lucky AW, Hawrot A, Frieden IJ. Ultrapotent corticosteroid treatment of hemangiomas of infancy. *J Am Acad Dermatol* 2005; **52**: 281–6.

46 George ME, Sharma V, Jacobson J, Simon S, Nopper AJ. Adverse effects of systemic glucocorticosteroid therapy in infants with hemangiomas. *Arch Dermatol* 2004; **140**: 960–9.

47 Gorlin RJ, Kantaputra P, Aughton DJ, Mulliken JB. Marked female predilection in some syndromes associated with facial hemangiomas. *Am J Med Genet* 1994; **52**: 130–5.

48 Greene AK, Rogers GF, Mulliken JB. Management of parotid hemangioma in 100 children. *Plast Reconstr Surg* 2004; **113**: 53–60.

49 Grosso S, De Cosmo L, Bonifazi E, Galluzzi P, Farnetani MA, Loffredo P, et al. Facial hemangioma and malformation of the cortical development: a broadening of PHACE spectrum or a new entity? *Am J Med Genet* 2004; **124A**: 192–5.

50 Guggisberg D, Hadj-Rabia S, Viney C, Bodemer C, Brunelle F, Zerah M, et al. Skin markers of occult spinal dysraphism in children. A review of 54 cases. *Arch Dermatol* 2004; **140**: 1109–15.

51 Haggström A, Lammer E, Schneider R, Marcucio R, Frieden IJ. Patterns of infantile hemangiomas: new clues to hemangioma pathogenesis and embryonic facial development. *Pediatrics* 2006; **117**: 698–703.

52 Hastings MM, Milot J, Barsoum-Homsy M, Hershon L, Dubois J, Leclerc JM. Recombinant interferon alfa-2b in the treatment of vision-threatening capillary hemangioma in childhood. *J AAPOS* 1997; **1**: 226–30.

53 Herman TE, McAlister WH, Dehner LP. Posterior mediastinal capillary hemangioma with extradural extension resembling neuroblastoma. *Pediatr Radiol* 1999; **29**: 517–19.

54 Hersh JH, Waterfill D, Rutleedge J, Harrod MJ, O'Sheal SF, Verdi G, Martinez S, Weisskopf B. Sternal malformation/vascular dysplasia association. *Am J Med Genet* 1985; **21**: 177–86.

55 Hohenleutner S, Badur-Ganter E, Landthaler M, Hohenleutner U. Long-term results in the treatment of childhood hemangioma with the flashlamp-pumped pulsed dye laser: an evaluation of 617 cases. *Lasers Surg Med* 2001; **28**: 273–7.

56 Hohenleutner U, Landthaler M. Laser treatment of childhood hemangioma: progress or not. *Lancet* 2002; **360**: 502–3.

57 Huang SA, Tu HM, Harney JW, Venihaki M, Butte AJ, Kozakewich HPW, Fishman SJ, Larsen PR. Severe hypothyroidism caused by type 3 iodothyronine deiodinase in infantile hemangioma. *N Eng J Med* 2000; **343**: 185–9.

58 Iwata J, Sonobe H, Furihata M, Ido E, Ohtsuki Y. High frequency of apoptosis in infantile capillary hemangioma. *J Pathol* 1996; **179**: 403–8.

59 Jang YC, Isik FF, Bibran NS. Nerve distribution in hemangiomas depends on the proliferative state of the microvasculature. *J Surg Res* 2000; **93**: 144–8.

60 Kassarjian A, Zurakowsky D, Dubois J, Paltiel HJ, Fishman SJ, Burrows PE. Infantile hepatic hemangiomas, clinical and imaging findings and their correlation with therapy. *Am J Roentgenol* 2004; **182**: 785–95.

61 Kniestedt C, Landau K, Brodsky MC, North PE, Waner M. Infantile orofacial hemangioma with ipsilateral peripapillary excavation in girls: a variant of PHACE syndrome. *Arch Ophthalmol* 2004; **122**: 413–15.

62 Konrad D, Ellis G, Perlman K. Spontaneous regression of severe acquired infantile hypothyroidism associated with multiple liver hemangiomas. *Pediatrics* 2003; **112**: 1424–6.
63 Kraling BM, Razon MJ, Boon LM, Zurakowski D, Seachord C, Darveau RP, et al. E-selectin is present in proliferating endothelial cells in human hemangiomas. *Am J Pathol* 1996; **148**: 1181–91.
64 Kronenberg A, Blei F, Ceisler E, Steele M, Furlan L, Kodsi S. Ocular and systemic manifestations of PHACES syndrome. *J AAPOS* 2005; **9**: 169–73.
65 Kushner BJ. The treatment of periorbital infantile hemangioma with intralesional corticosteroid. *Plast Reconstr Surg* 1985; **76**: 517–24.
66 Lasky JB, Sandu M, Balashanmugan A. PHACE syndrome: association with persistent fetal vasculature and coloboma-like iris defect. *J AAPOS* 2004; **8**: 495–8.
67 Leaute-Labreze C, Labbe L, Grenier N, Berge J, Vergnes P, Taieb A. Hémangiomes graves traités par interféron α : 7 cas. *Ann Dermatol Venereol* 1998; **125**: 174–8.
68 Luo CM, Lasjaunias P, Teng MM, Chang FC, Lirng JF, Chang CY. Cervicocerebrovascular anomalies in children with PHACE syndrome. *J Formos Med Assoc* 2003; **102**: 379–86.
69 MacArthur CJ, Senders CW, Katz J. The use of interferon alfa-2a for life-threatening hemangiomas. *Arch Otolaryngol Head Neck Surg* 1995; **121**: 690–3.
70 Mancini AJ, Smoller BR. Proliferation and apoptosis within juvenile capillary hemangiomas. *Am J Dermatopathol* 1996; **18**: 505–14.
71 Metry DW, Dowd CF, Barkovich AJ, Frieden IJ. The many faces of PHACE syndrome. *J Pediatr* 2001; **139**: 117–23.
72 Metry DW, Hawrot A, Altman C, Frieden IJ. Association of solitary segmental hemangiomas of the skin with visceral hemangiomatosis. *Arch Dermatol* 2004; **140**: 591–6.
73 Metry D. Update on hemangiomas of infancy. *Curr Opin Pediatr* 2004; **16**: 373–7.
74 Metry D. Potential complications of segmental hemangiomas of infancy. *Semin Cutan Med Surg* 2004; **23**: 107–15.
75 Metz BJ, Rubinstein MC, Levy ML, Metry DW. Response of ulcerated perineal hemangioma of infancy to beclapermin gel, a recombinant human platelet-derived growth factor. *Arch Dermatol* 2004; **140**: 867–70.
76 Michaud AP, Bauman NM, Burke DK, Manaligod JM, Smith RJ. Spastic diplegia and other motor disturbances in infants receiving interferon alpha. *Laryngoscope* 2004; **114**: 1231–6.
77 Millischer-Bellaiche AE, Enjolras O, André Ch, Bursztyn J, Kalifa G, Adamsbaum C. Les hémangiomes palpébraux du nourrisson. *J Radiol* 2004; **85**: 2019–28.
78 Momtchilova M, Pelosse B, Diner PA, Vazquez MP, Laroche L. Amblyopi et hémangiome capillaire infantile périoculaire. *J Fr Ophtalmol* 2004; **27**: 1135–40.
79 Mulliken JB, Rogers GF, Marler JJ. Circular excision of hemangioma and purse-string closure: the smallest possible scar. *Plast Reconstr Surg* 2002; **109**: 1544–54.
80 Nakayama H. Clinical and histological studies of the classification and the natural course of the strawberry mark. *J Dermatol* 1981; **8**: 277–91.
81 North PE, Waner M, Mizeracki A, Mihm MC Jr. GLUT1: a newly discovered immunohistochemical marker for juvenile hemangiomas. *Hum Pathol* 2000; **31**: 11–22.
82 North PE, Waner M, Mizeracki A, Mrak RE, Nicholas R, Kincannon J, Suen JY, Mihm MC Jr. A unique microvascular phenotype shared by juvenile hemangiomas and human placenta. *Arch Dermatol* 2001; **137**: 559–70.
83 Orlow SJ, Isakoff MS, Blei F. Increased risk of symptomatic hemangiomas of the airway in association with cutaneous hemangiomas in a "beard" distribution. *J Pediatr* 1997; **131**: 643–6.
84 Pascual-Castroviejo I. Vascular and non-vascular intracranial malformations with external capillary hemangiomas. *Neuroradiology* 1978; **16**: 82–4.
85 Pascual-Castroviejo I, Viano J, Moreno F, Palencia R, Fernandez VM, Pascual-Pascual SI, et al. Hemangiomas of the head, neck and chest with associated vascular brain anomalies: a complex neurocutaneous syndrome. *Am J Neuroradiol* 1996; **17**: 461–71.

86 Pascual-Castroviejo I, Pascual-Castroviejo S, Viaño J, Martinez V. Hemangioma cavernoso y mega-arteriosis cerebral: involucion coetanea de ambas malformaciones en un caso. *Patologia Vascular* 1999; **5**: 53–60.

87 Pascual-Castroviejo I, Viaño J, Pascual-Pascual S, Martinez V. Do cutaneous hemangiomas and internal vascular anomalies follow the same evolution? *Neurology* 2003; **61**: 140–1.

88 Picard A, Soupre V, Diner PA, Buis J, Goga D, Vazquez MP. Chirurgie précoce des hémangiomes immatures à l'aide d'un dissecteur à ultrasons. Etude à propos de 81 cas. *Rev Stomatol Chir Maxillofac* 2002; **103**: 10–21.

89 Pienaar C, Graham R, Geldenhuys S, Hudson DA. Intralesional bleomycin for the treatment of hemangiomas. *Plast Reconstr Surg* 2006; **117**: 221–6.

90 Poetke M, Froemmeld T, Berlien HP. PHACE syndrome: new views on diagnostic criteria. *Eur J Pediatr Surg* 2002; **12**: 366–74.

91 Pokorny JJ, Roth F, Balfour I, Rinehart G. An unusual complication of the treatment of a hemangioma. *Ann Plast Surg* 2002; **48**: 83–7.

92 Rahbar R, Nicollas R, Roger G, Triglia JM, Garabedian EN, McGill TJ, Healy GB. The biology and management of subglottic hemangioma: past, present, future. *Laryngoscope* 2004; **114**: 1880–91.

93 Razon MJ, Kräling BM, Mulliken JB, Bischoff J. Increased apoptosis coincides with onset of involution in infantile hemangioma. *Microcirculation* 1998; **5**: 189–95.

94 Reischle S, Schuller-Petrovic S. Treatment of capillary hemangiomas of early childhood with a new method of cryosurgery. *J Am Acad Dermatology* 2000; **42**: 809–13.

95 Ritter MR, Dorrell MI, Edmonds J, Friedlander SF, Friedlander M. Insulin-like growth factor 2 and potential regulators of hemangioma growth and involution identified by large-scale expression analysis. *Proc Natl Acad Sci USA* 2002; **99**: 7455–60.

96 Rothe MJ, Rowse D, Grant-Kels JM. Benign neonatal hemangiomatosis with aggressive growth of cutaneous lesions. *Pediatr Dermatol* 1991; **8**: 140–6.

97 Scheepers JH, Quaba AA. Does the pulsed tunable dye laser have a role in the mangement of infantile hemangioma? Observations based on a 3 years experience. *Plast Reconstr Surg* 1995; **95**: 305–12.

98 Shorr N, Seiff SR. Central retinal artery occlusion associated with periocular corticosteroid injection for juvenile hemangioma. *Ophthalmic Surg* 1986; **17**: 229–231.

99 Takahashi K, Mulliken JB, Kozakewich HPW, Rogers RA, Folkman J, Ezekowitz RA. Cellular markers that distinguish the phases of hemangioma during infancy and childhood. *J Clin Invest* 1994; **93**: 2357–64.

100 The Denat B, Leauté-Labreze C, Boralevi F, Roul S, Labbé L, Marlière V, Taieb A. Surveillance tensionnelle des nourrissons traits par corticothérapie générale pour un hémangiome. *Ann Dermatol Venereol* 2002; **129**: 183–5.

101 Vazquez MP, Diner PA, Picard A, Soupre V, Enjolras O. Les lèvres angiomateuses. *Ann Chir Plast Esthet* 2002; **47**: 561–79.

102 Vazquez-Botet R, Reyes BA, Vazquez-Botet M. Sclerodermiform linear atrophy after the use of intralesional steroids for periorbital hemangiomas: a review of complications. *J Pediatr Ophthalmol Strabismus* 1989; **26**: 124–7.

103 Van Den Abbelee T, Triglia JM, Lescanne E, Roger G, Nocollas R, Ployet MJ, Garabedian EN. Surgical removal of subglottic hemangiomas in children. *Laryngoscope* 1999; **109**: 1281–6.

104 Waner M, North PE, Scherer KA, Frieden IJ, Mihm MC, Suen JY. The non-random distribution of facial hemangiomas. *Arch Dermatol* 2003; **139**: 869–75.

105 Yeh TF, Lin YJ, Huang CC, Chen YJ, Lin CH, Lin HC. Early dexamethasone therapy in preterm infants: a follow-up study. *Pediatrics* 1998; **101**: E7.

106 Yu Y, Fuhr J, Boye E, Gyorffy S, Soker S, Atala A, Mulliken JB, Bischoff J. Mesenchymal stem cells and adipogenesis in hemangioma evolution. *Stem Cells* 2006, Feb epub ahead of print.

CHAPTER II.B

Other Vascular Tumors

Infantile hemangioma (IH) is a common tumor and it is characterized by its distinctive behavior, with growth after birth, on normal skin or on a congenital precursor, proliferation over months during infancy, and slow spontaneous regression over years during childhood. This behavior is less predictable in other, mostly infantile, less-common tumors such as the various congenital hemangiomas, tufted angioma (also known as angioblastoma of Nakagawa) and kaposiform hemangioendothelioma.

II.B.1 Congenital Hemangiomas: RICH, NICH, and Missing Links

The term "congenital hemangioma" (CH) designates a vascular tumor of intrauterine onset, fully grown at birth, which does not exhibit postnatal growth like IH does. In 1996 the vascular anomalies teams in Boston and Paris described CH and presented 31 examples (3). CHs look quite unusual compared to IH, and differ from the various premonitory lesions of IH. In addition, postnatal behaviors of IH and CHs are quite different. We recognize at least two subgroups of CHs, referred to by acronyms:

1. rapidly involuting congenital hemangioma (RICH); and
2. noninvoluting congenital hemangioma (NICH) (2, 5, 9).

There is an equal sex ratio for the two types of CH (3, 5), in contrast to the female preponderance of IH. Distinctive pathological features also differentiate the two types of CH from IH. North and colleagues (10) discovered that the endothelium in IH immunostains for glucose transporter-1 protein (GLUT-1) throughout the tumor's life cycle: neither RICH nor NICH stain with GLUT1 antibody (2, 5, 11).

Table 11 Clinical and histological comparison between infantile hemangioma, RICH, and NICH.

		Common infantile hemangioma	*RICH*	*NICH*
Sex F:M		3–5:1	1:1	1:1
Location		Head and neck in 2/3, 1/4 on trunk	Head and neck = extremities, rare on trunk-(based on biopsied/resected specimens)	Head and neck = extremities, trunk-uncommon
Average size		Variable	6 cm	5 cm
Cutaneous appearance	Proliferative phase	Superficial: bright red, bossed Deep: normal or bluish	Raised and dome-shaped, round or ovoid, telangiectases, often pale rim, central ulcer, scar, or depression	Slightly raised, round or ovoid, purple, well-delineated, telangiectases, central/peripheral pallor
	Involutive phase	Atrophy, telangiectases, dyschromia, anetoderma	Depressed, pale, few residual telangiectases, prominent veins	
General architecture	Proliferative phase	Lobules closely spaced or confluent	Unknown	Lobules separated by dense fibrous tissue, prominent interlobular vasculature, usually no zonation
	Involutive phase	Intralobular and interlobular fibrous tissue	Interlobular fibrous tissue, often zonation with advanced involution in lesional center	
Lobules	Proliferative phase	Usually large	Unknown	Usually large with curved channels and prominent centrilobular draining vessels(s)
	Involutive phase	Small-to-large	Small, medium, or large with prominent centrilobular draining channel(s)	
Endothelium	Proliferative phase	Markedly prominent, GLUT-1 positive	Unknown	Hobnailed, cytoplasmic inclusion, GLUT-1 negative
	Involutive phase	Flat, GLUT-1 positive	Moderately prominent, rarely hobnailed, GLUT-1 usually negative	
Capillary basement membrane	Proliferative phase	Thin	Unknown	Thin, focally thickened
	Involutive phase	Thick	Thin, thickened in late stage	
Extralobular vasculature	Proliferative phase	Minimally or moderately prominent arteries and veins	Unknown	Prominent arteries and abnormal veins, arteriolobular and arteriovenous fistulae
	Involutive phase	Feeding arteries and veins may not regress completely	Large and abnormal draining channels, particularly in lesional center	
Additional features	Proliferative phase		Unknown	Thrombi
	Involutive phase	Fat	Thrombi, infarction, hemosiderin, calcification, cysts, aneurysms, extramedullary hematopoiesis	

RICH=rapidly involuting congential hemangioma; NICH=noninvoluting congential hemangioma; GLUT-1=glucose transporter-1 protein.
Reproduced with permission from: Berenguer B, Mulliken JB, Enjolras O, Boon LM, Wassef M, Josset P, Burrows PE, Perez-Atayde AR, Kozakewich HPW. Rapidly involuting congenital hemangioma: clinical and histopathologic features. *Ped Dev Biol* 2003; **6**: 495–610 (Table 1).

NICH and RICH have distinct clinical and pathological features (Table 11). However, in a number of infants, a RICH may to some extent regress but it results in a lesion similar to NICH: we call these cases "missing links" as they probably indicate some relationship between both tumors, or at least a subset of these congenital hemangiomas.

II.B.1.1 RICH

RICH are fully grown in utero and full-blown at birth, no postnatal proliferation happens, and regression quickly follows over 6 to 14 months. This clinical pattern and course are unique and differ from those of IH. Because of their remarkable postnatal accelerated regression we called these tumors **R**apidly **I**nvoluting **C**ongenital **H**emangioma (RICH) to stress this distinctive behavior, quite different from the protracted regression of a large IH (2, 3, 6). Six analogous tumors were called "congenital nonprogressive hemangioma" by North and colleagues in a study that focused on histological findings; none of the six congenital tumors had vascular immunoreactivity for GLUT1 and Lewis Y antigen; conversely the 25 IH tested in parallel demonstrated strong lesional endothelial immunoreactivity for these two antigens (11).

Due to their fast-flow nature RICH are more and more commonly detected during antenatal ultrasonographic evaluations (6). Most of the lesions discovered during the fetal life were tumors of the scalp or neck, and less frequently of an extremity. In the literature there are various examples of RICH detected during the second or third trimester by antenatal ultrasonography and/or prenatal MRI (2, 3, 8). Tumors discovered during fetal life either exhibited rapid postnatal regression (14) or were excised in infancy (4). In rare instances, the neonate died of complications of the tumor (13).

All tumors initially exhibit fast-flow on ultrasonography and magnetic resonance imaging (3, 12). The ultrasonic characteristics of RICH were reported by Rogers et al. in a group of 10 patients: all lesions were uniformly hypoechoic, confined to the subcutaneous fat and traversed by multiple vascular channels (12). MRI and angiographic characteristics of RICH have both similarities and differences from those of infantile hemangioma. MRI shows a dense tumor with, or without, tortuous large flow voids, usually located near the surface of the tumor, and sometimes areas of inhomogeneity. Angiographic features indicate a fast-flow lesion, which, unlike IH, may include inhomogeneous parenchymal staining, direct AV fistulae, large and irregularly organized feeding arteries, multiple arterial aneurysms, cyst, intralesional bleeding and thrombi; because of significant intratumoral arteriovenous shunting some newborns with RICH may present with high-output cardiac failure (7).

Although RICH have a slightly variable morphology depending on the patients, common features include: a protuberant round lump, pink or purple in color, with coarse often radiating telangiectasia, and habitually a thin surrounding whitish halo. Some have central ulceration or a linear scar or depression. Others exhibit a few central red nodules. Rarely, a nearly normal slightly blanched overlying skin is observed. There is increased local warmth and in some patients dilated veins and pulsations. After regression the involved area is left with either an area of lipoatrophy, or an area of dermal atrophy with persisting blanching-bluish hue. Some lesions leave a rather prominent telangiectatic round macule or plaque. The most typical locations are the extremities, close to a joint (by frequency: mainly the knee, then ankle, shoulder, hip, and wrist) and the head around the ear (forehead, cheek, or scalp). So far, centrofacial lesions of RICH have not been observed.

Management

Most lesions are left to shrink spontaneously. Some are excised early in life, specifically if large arterial vessels are detected close to the surface by ultrasonic and MRI investigation, or if they have a thick central crust with a risk of ulceration: in both cases the aim is to avoid profuse hemorrhage (1). In our experience, none of the excised tumors recurred. Also, as some RICH are now known to result in a pink plaque of telangiectasia with increasing veins over the years, the achievability of excision early in life must be discussed with the pediatric plastic surgeon.

II.B.1.2 NICH

Not all congenital hemangiomas spontaneously shrink in the first year of life. Some do not regress at all. We call these **N**on-**I**nvoluting **C**ongenital **H**emangioma (NICH), as opposed to the RICH behavior (5, 6).

NICH has an almost equal sex distribution. It is solitary, and like RICH it has a predilection for the head or a limb close to a joint. Lesions on the trunk are uncommon. In a group of 53 patients followed from 2 to 30 years of age – mean age at last consultation = 10 years – 43% of the tumors were in the cephalic area, 38% in the limbs and only 19% on the trunk (5). NICH are round or oval, pink-to-purple, plaque-type or slightly raised, and always warm on palpation. There is a rim of peripheral white or bluish pallor, or a bluish hue of the whole surface, punctuated by more or less conspicuous telangiectasia.

NICH persists indefinitely, with a slight tendency to worsening. NICH remains a fast-flow lesion, as documented by duplex Doppler examination often exhibiting arteriovenous fistulas. MRI and angiographic findings in NICH are reminiscent of those of a common IH in the proliferating phase. On MRI a NICH is iso-intense on T1, hyperintense on T2, and it is enhanced with gadolinium injection.

In the past, NICH was misdiagnosed arteriovenous malformation (AVM) or called "arteriolo-capillary malformation" because angiography demonstrates fast-flow and rapid arterial filling, but no early venous return could be documented, as in AVM.

Management

NICH can usually be excised without recurrence, and, unlike AVM, they do not re-expand in cases of partial or serial excision (5, 6). For large lesions we prefer to have pre-operative angiography, and, if arterial feeders are numerous, arterial embolization with particles is performed the day before surgery to limit intra-operative bleeding.

II.B.1.3 MISSING LINKS

RICH, NICH and IH have some overlapping clinical and/or pathological features. This has led us to consider that they may be variations of a single tumoral entity (2, 6, 9). A number of RICH or NICH, present at birth, are later associated with a growing IH. Rare cases show the superposition of an IH growing on top of a RICH. In some of our patients, the postnatal course of some RICH suggests the possibility that NICH could be a late in utero-stage of RICH. The typical story is as follows: an infant is born with a large congenital hemispherical lump typical of a RICH. The lesion involutes over 6 to 12 months, then it ceases to regress. Lastly, a pink telangiectatic plaque, with a white peripheral rim, resembling a NICH will persist indefinitely. In addition, in some NICH excised early in life the histology may be indistinguishable from RICH or there are combined features of NICH and RICH. Based on these postnatal observations we hypothesized that the same phenomenon may arise in utero and that NICH may be the end result of a RICH that has regressed during the end of the intrauterine life. Better prenatal ultrasonic detection and prenatal US follow-up should confirm or refute this hypothesis that RICH can transform to NICH before birth, and that at least some subtypes of RICH are a precursor of NICH.

Figures

CONGENITAL HEMANGIOMAS (RICH AND NICH)
Pathology of RICH

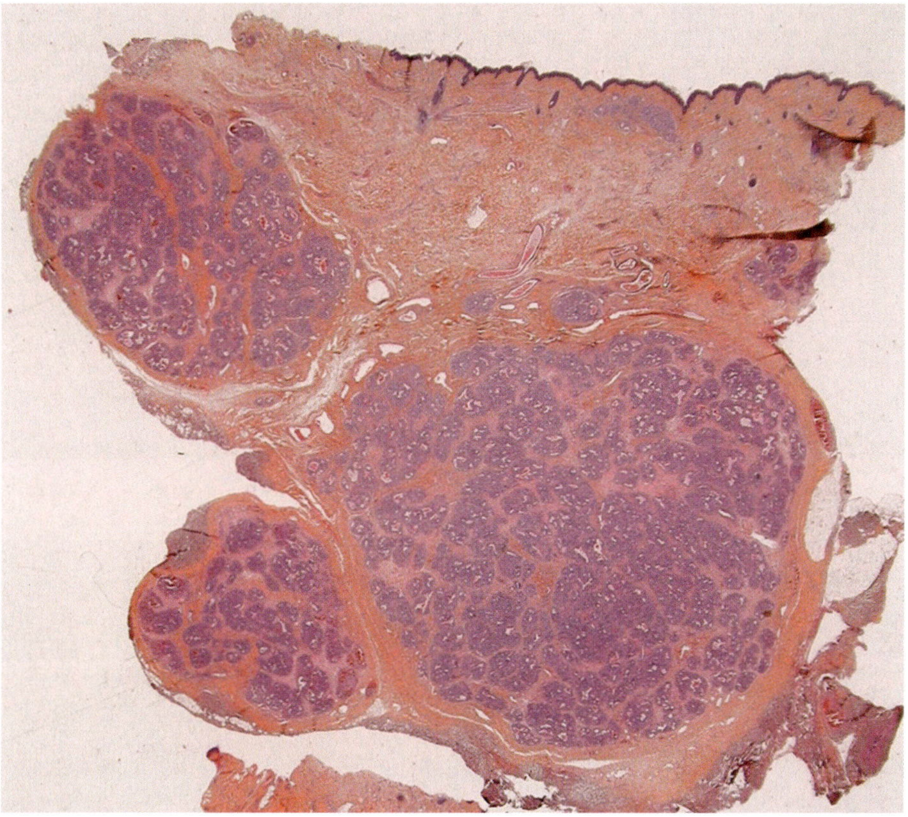

Several large nodules are present in the dermis of a resected RICH, each of them being made of small capillary lobules embedded in fibrosis.

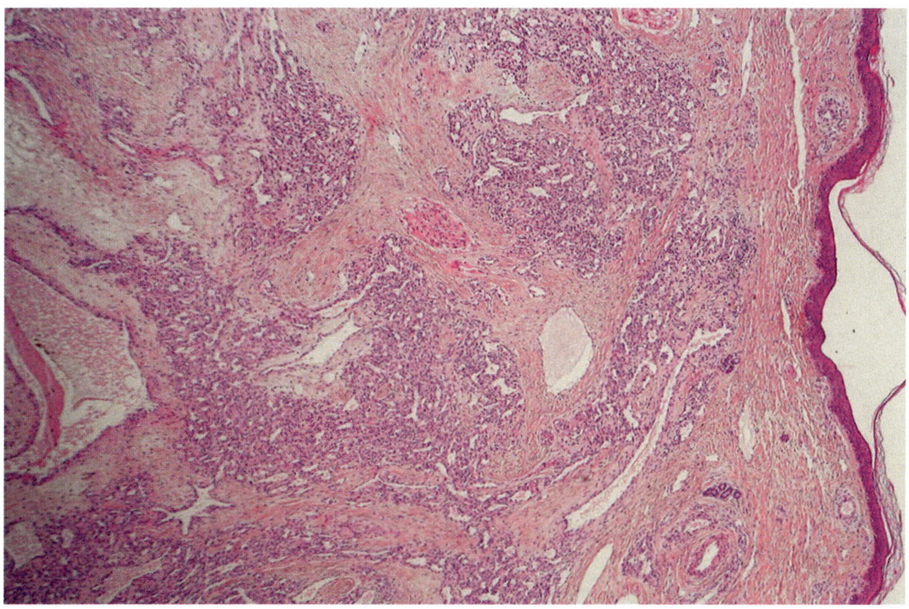

RICH is made up of large-, medium- or small-sized channels grouped in lobules. Extralobular large abnormal vessels are also seen.

Pathology of RICH

RICH contains areas of small lobules with fibrosis. Vessels have a moderately plump endothelium.

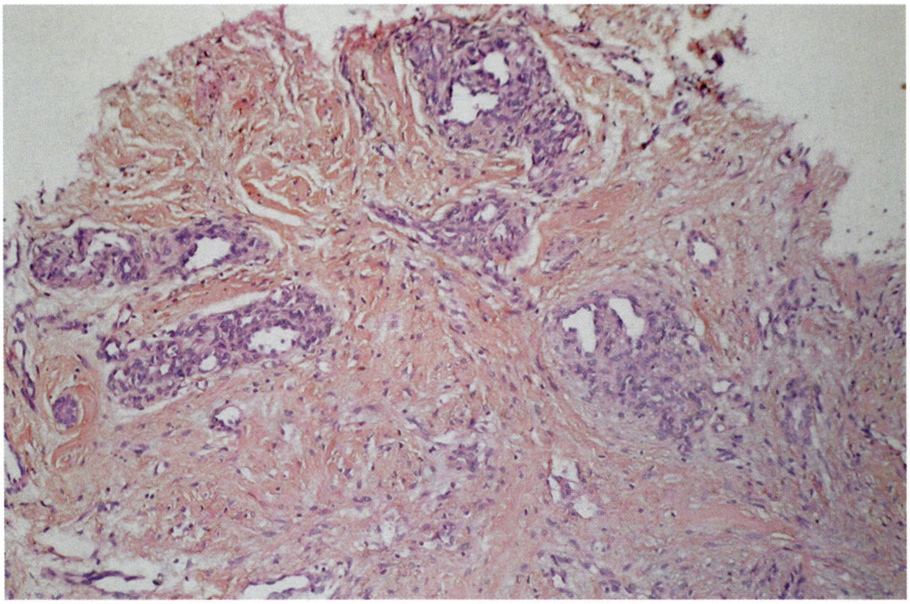

At a higher magnification some endothelial cells appear plump and a mild anisocaryosis is evident.

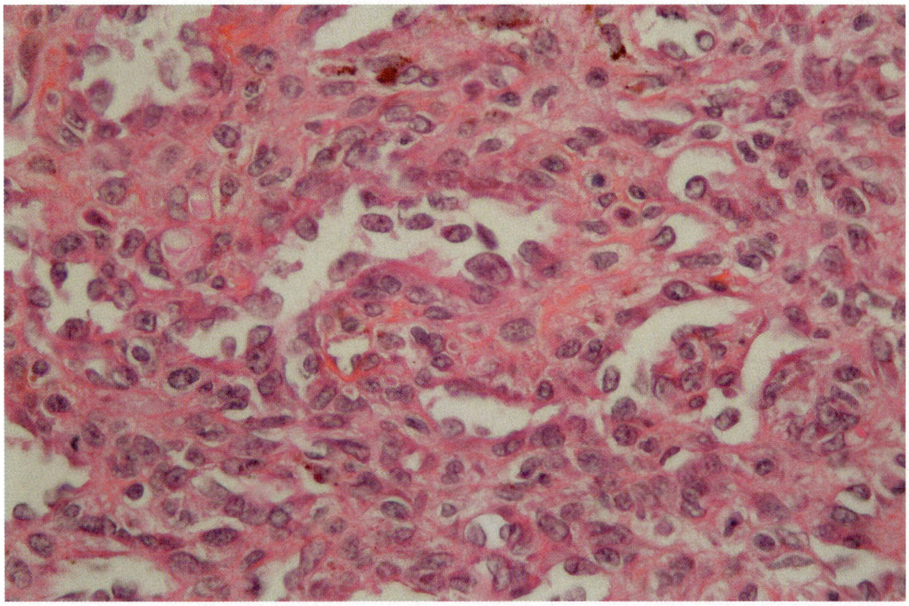

Pathology of NICH

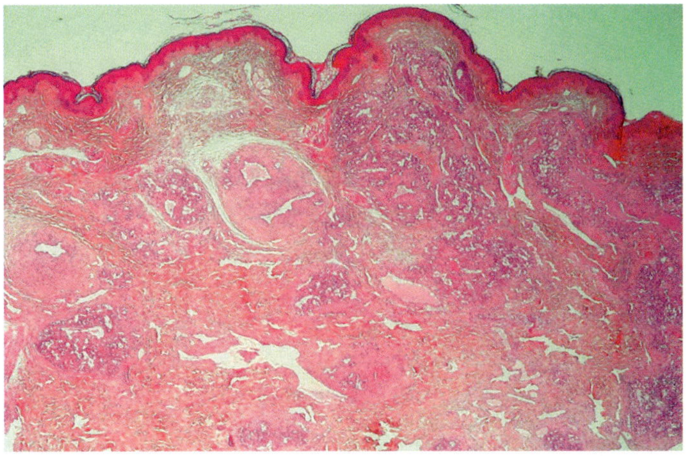

Low-power view of NICH shows cellular capillary lobules and numerous extralobular large vessels (veins, arteries, and lymphatics).

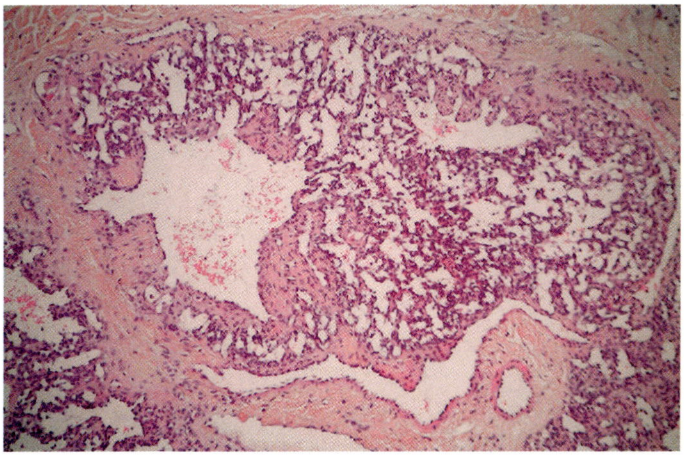

Lobules of NICH are usually made up of large and curved channels, and a centrolobular, irregular, prominent, often stellate vessel is noticed. The wall of the larger vessel lacks well-defined media.

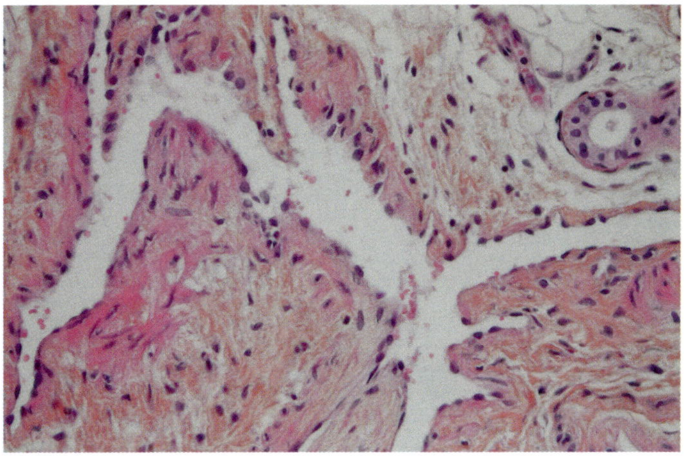

Prominent distorted extralobular vasculature is observed in NICH. This venous-like distorted channel shows an irregular media, composed of areas of normal thickness and thin areas focally lacking smooth muscle cells. This channel morphology is usually evocative of venous malformation.

Pathology of NICH

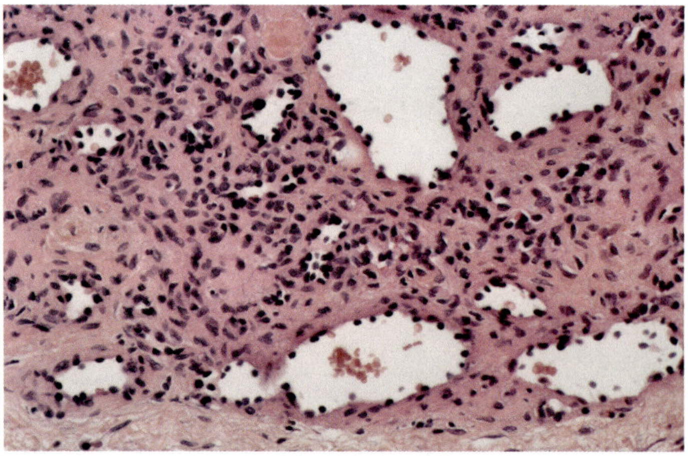

Hobnailed endothelial cells in NICH are observed: the endothelium shows round dark nuclei protruding in the lumen with a hobnail pattern. Some anisocaryosis is present.

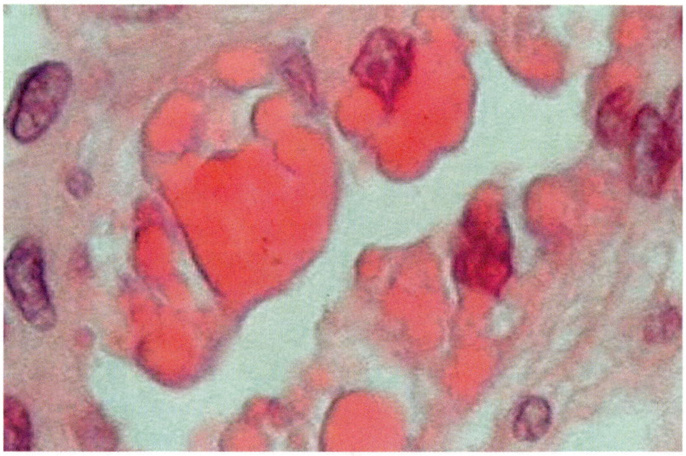

Endothelial cells in NICH may exhibit large eosinophilic cytoplasmic hyaline inclusions. The endothelial cells containing these inclusions are often seen in clusters.

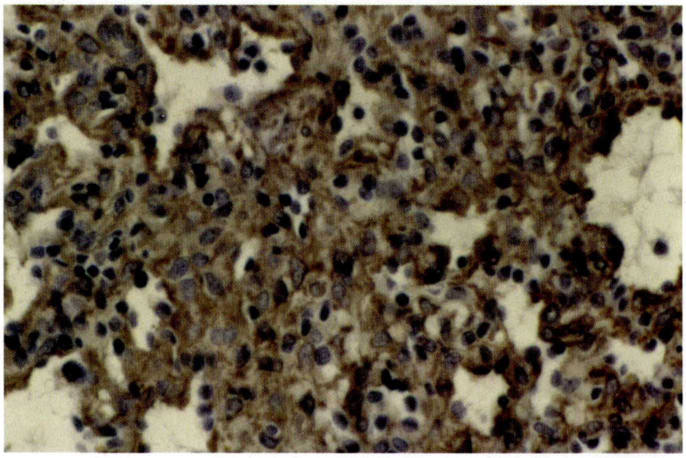

Abundant alpha-actin positive cells are stained in the cellular lobules of NICH. These cells are not well arranged around each capillary, contrasting with their organization in infantile hemangioma.

Clinical Features of Congenital Hemangiomas

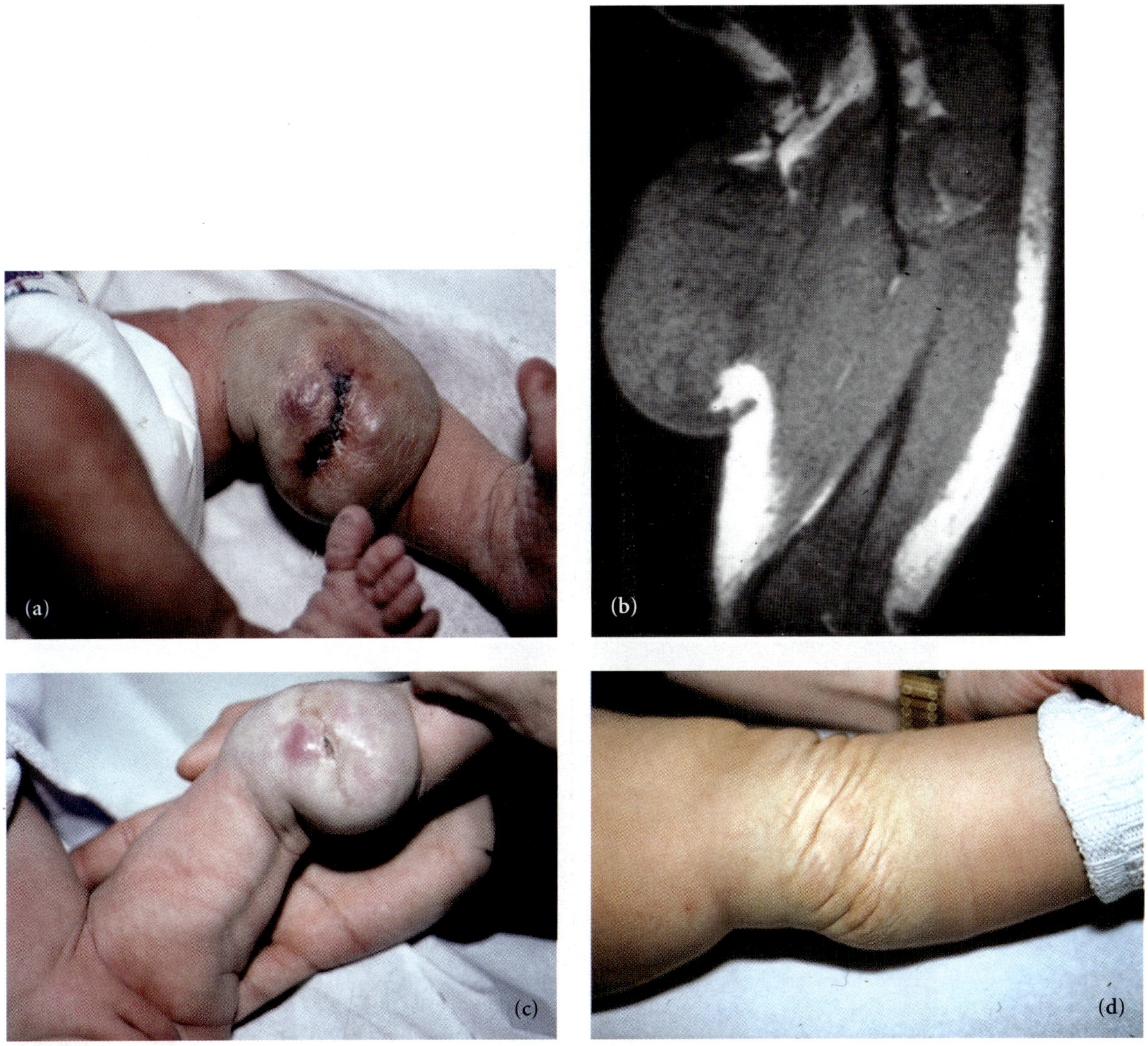

This RICH was detected by prenatal ultrasonographic screening at 23 weeks of pregnancy. At birth the large tumor, located close to the knee joint, had a central thick crust (a). MRI did not indicate numerous fast-flow vessels (b), and we decided to wait. To facilitate healing and protect the lesion we used a thin hydrocolloid adhesive dressing. One month later cure of the wound was obtained. A large draining vein, seen at birth in the thigh, between the tumor and the groin (c) spontaneously disappeared. At 8 months of age the tumor had regressed leaving some excess creased skin in the internal aspect of the knee (d) and the large vein was no longer detectable. At 6 years of age the residuum was occasionally painful and the parents asked for excision. At 10 years of age the girl developed numerous varicose veins under the knee: we hypothesize that these varicose veins are probably the consequence of both the spontaneous closure of the large congenital vein and of the surgical excision which removed venous collectors.

Clinical Features of Congenital Hemangiomas

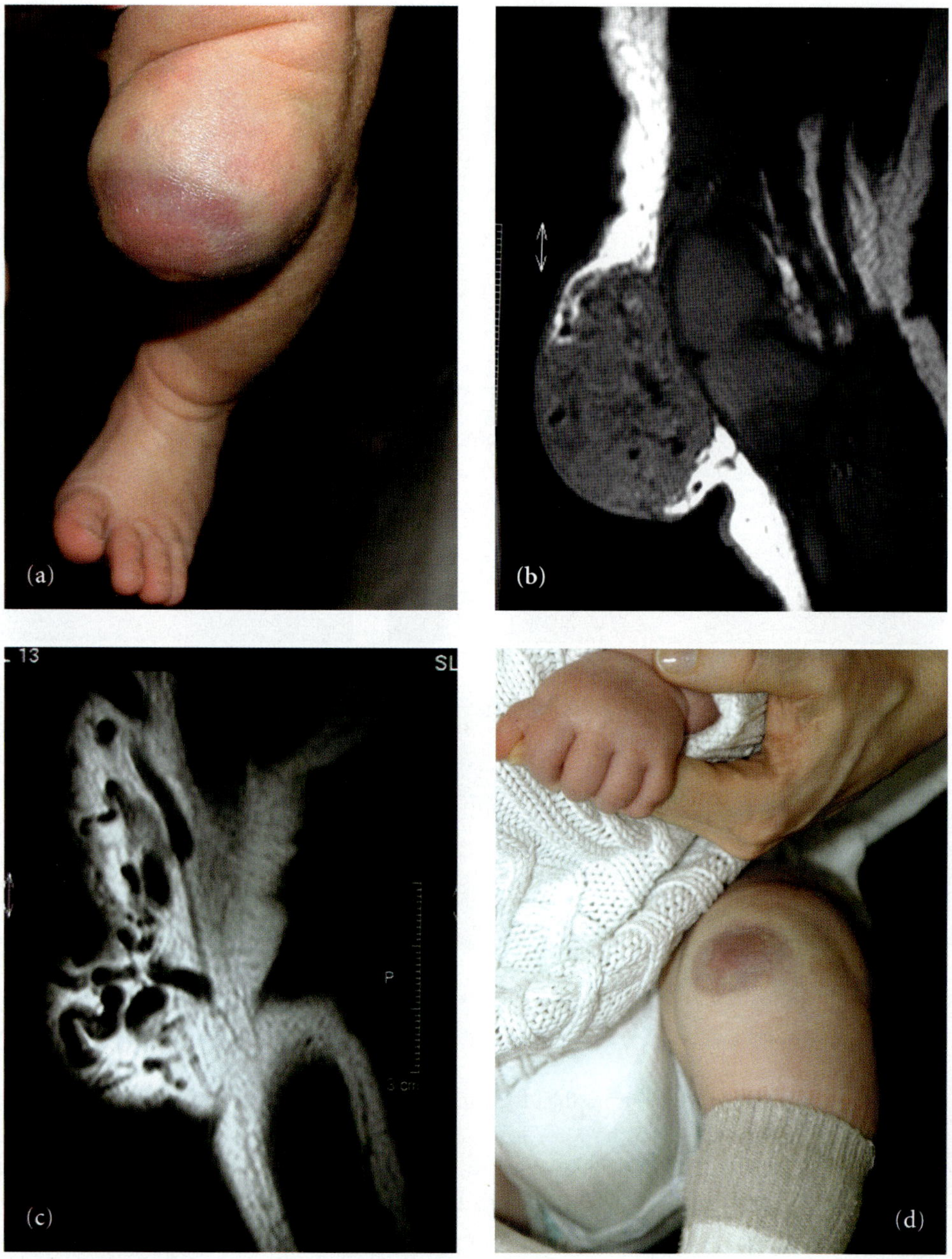

This bulging RICH over the knee joint was red and shiny in the center of the lesion, with two concentric circular halos: purple and pale (a). It was warm on palpation. MRI indicated a parenchymal tumor (b) appearing as a well-circumscribed mass on T1, but also flow voids indicating large fast-flow vessels, more numerous near the surface of the tumor in the surrounding fat (c). This finding was fairly worrisome because of the risk of rupture and life-threatening hemorrhage (1). We protected the skin with thin Opsite Flexigrid® dressings changed once a week, and we were considering surgical resection, but involution began quite quickly. By 6 months of age (d) the lesion was flat, purple and firm in the center with a pink halo and a soft blanching margin. It was clearly less warm on palpation, and vascularization was much reduced on US/Doppler observation.

Clinical Features of Congenital Hemangiomas

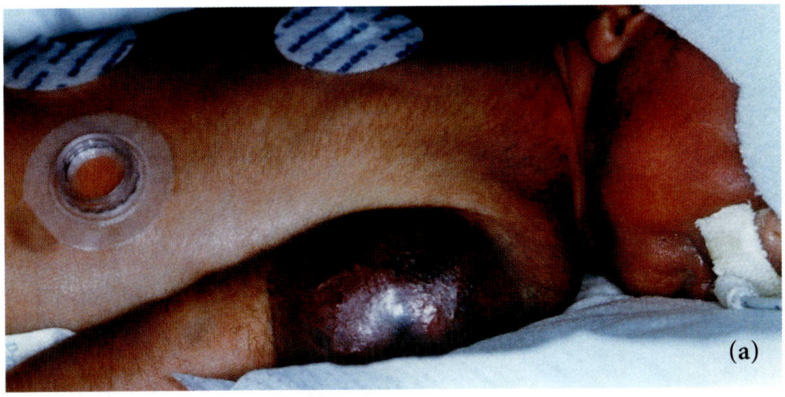

(a)

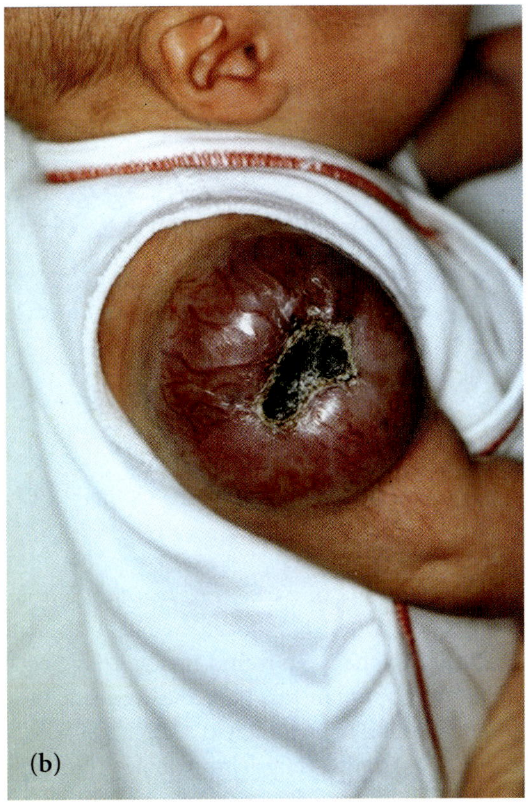

(b)

This premature 3 lb boy had a purple tumor on the arm at birth, with black pre-necrotic areas (a). Fast-flow was clinically evident, as movement of the tumor due to arterial throbbing was visible. Because of the low weight of the newborn excision was postponed. As the infant was cared for in the neonatal premature baby department, he was closely monitored for the risk of bleeding. Excision was decided when he reached a satisfactory weight. The tumor was less purple, more telangiectatic, and had a thick central crust (b) still presenting a risk of hemorrhage. The scar after surgical excision was cosmetically acceptable despite its length and an underlying muscle atrophy (operator: Dr. Frederic Zazurca, Hôpital Armand Trousseau, Paris, France).

Clinical Features of Congenital Hemangiomas

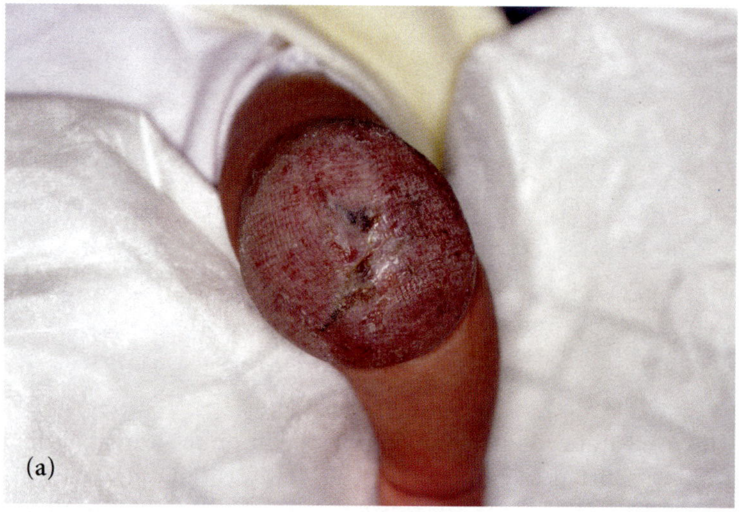
(a)

A typical example of partial regression of a telangiectatic-type RICH located close to the knee joint: at birth the large round mauve telangiectatic bump had a spontaneous thin linear crusted crease in the center and a faint blanched margin (a). The center healed in 1 month using hydrocolloid dressing. Regression progressed over a year. In the meantime radiated telangiectasia and a white margin became prominent, and normal skin appeared at the basis of the lesion (b1, b2). Then involution stopped and the residual lesion, reminiscent of a thick NICH, was excised at 18 months. It presented aspects of both RICH and NICH on pathology.

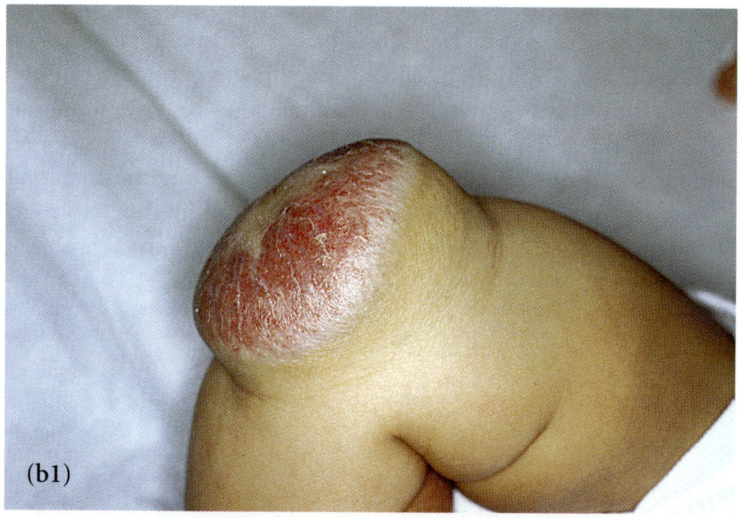
(b1)

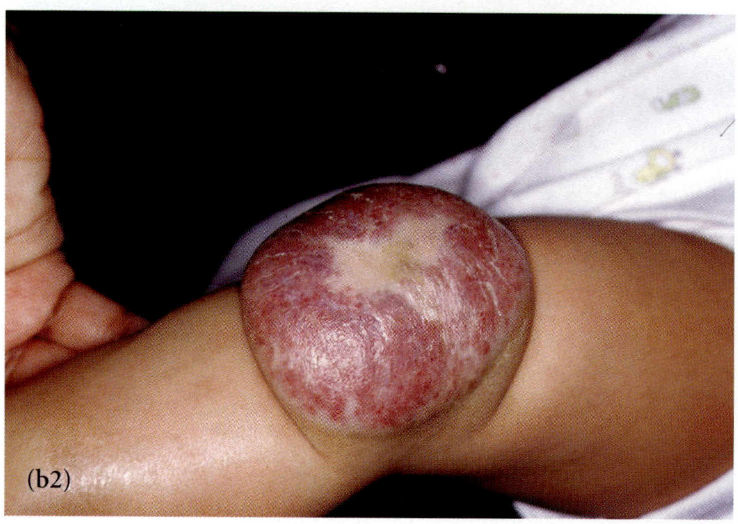
(b2)

Clinical Features of Congenital Hemangiomas

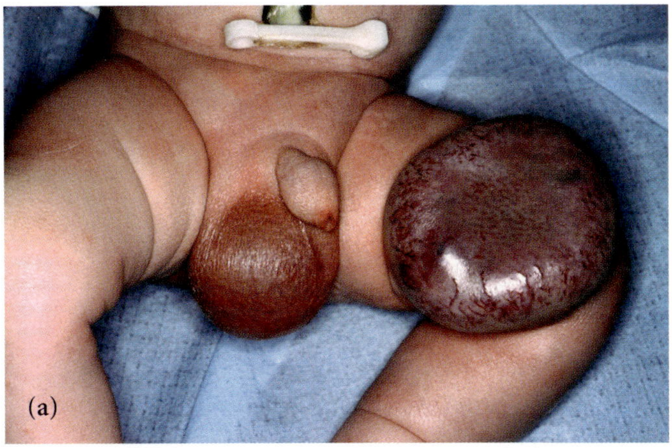
(a)

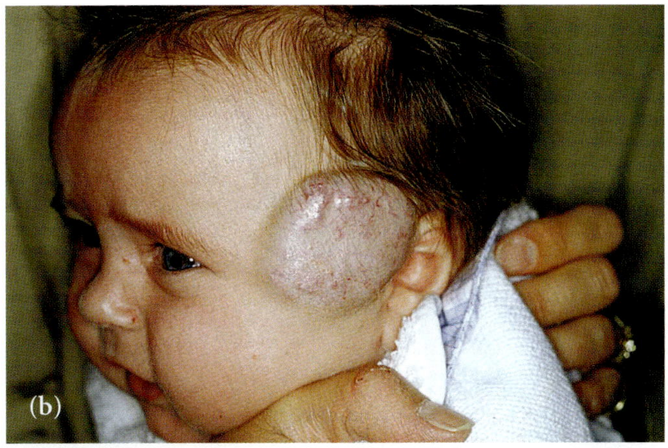
(b)

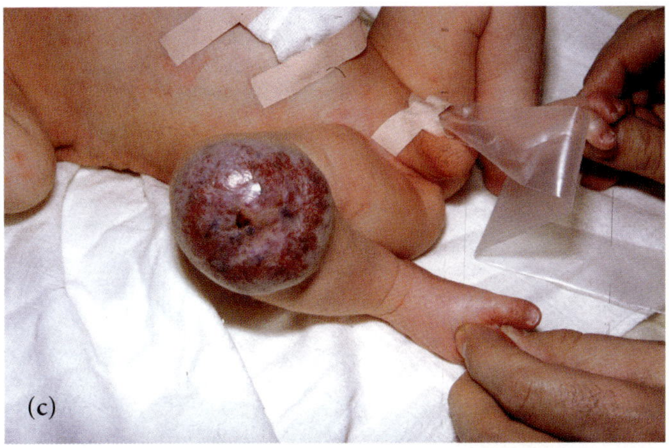
(c)

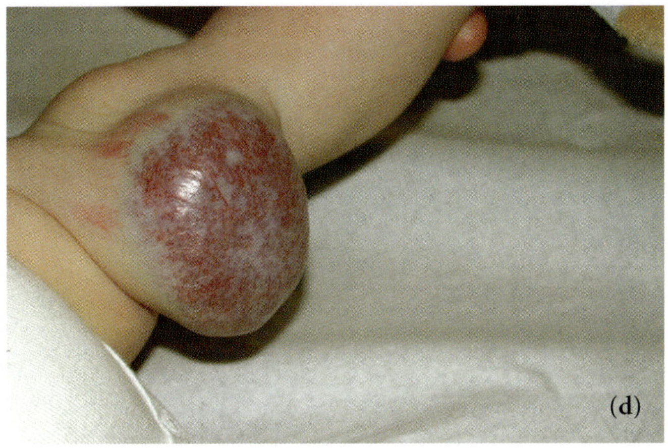
(d)

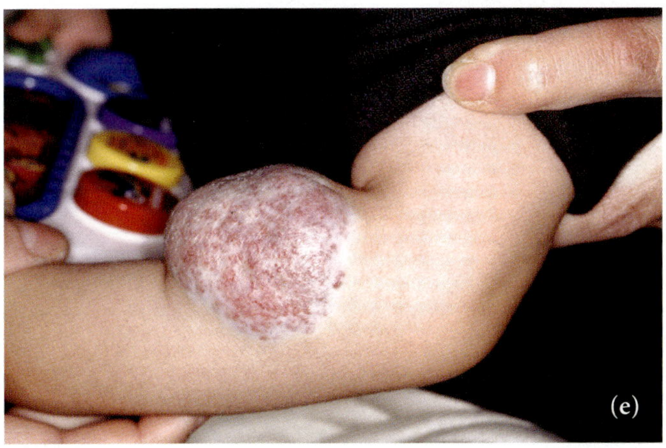
(e)

These RICH presenting as large bulging tumors, purple or bluish, always with coarse radiated telangiectasia, a linear central scar or a flattened center, and often a thin pale peripheral rim, tend to only partially involute and result in a plaque telangiectatic NICH-like residuum. This residuum is often cosmetically problematic. Therefore, if the tumor can be excised in infancy, with an anticipated satisfactory surgical scar, surgical treatment should be considered in infancy or early childhood.

Clinical Features of Congenital Hemangiomas

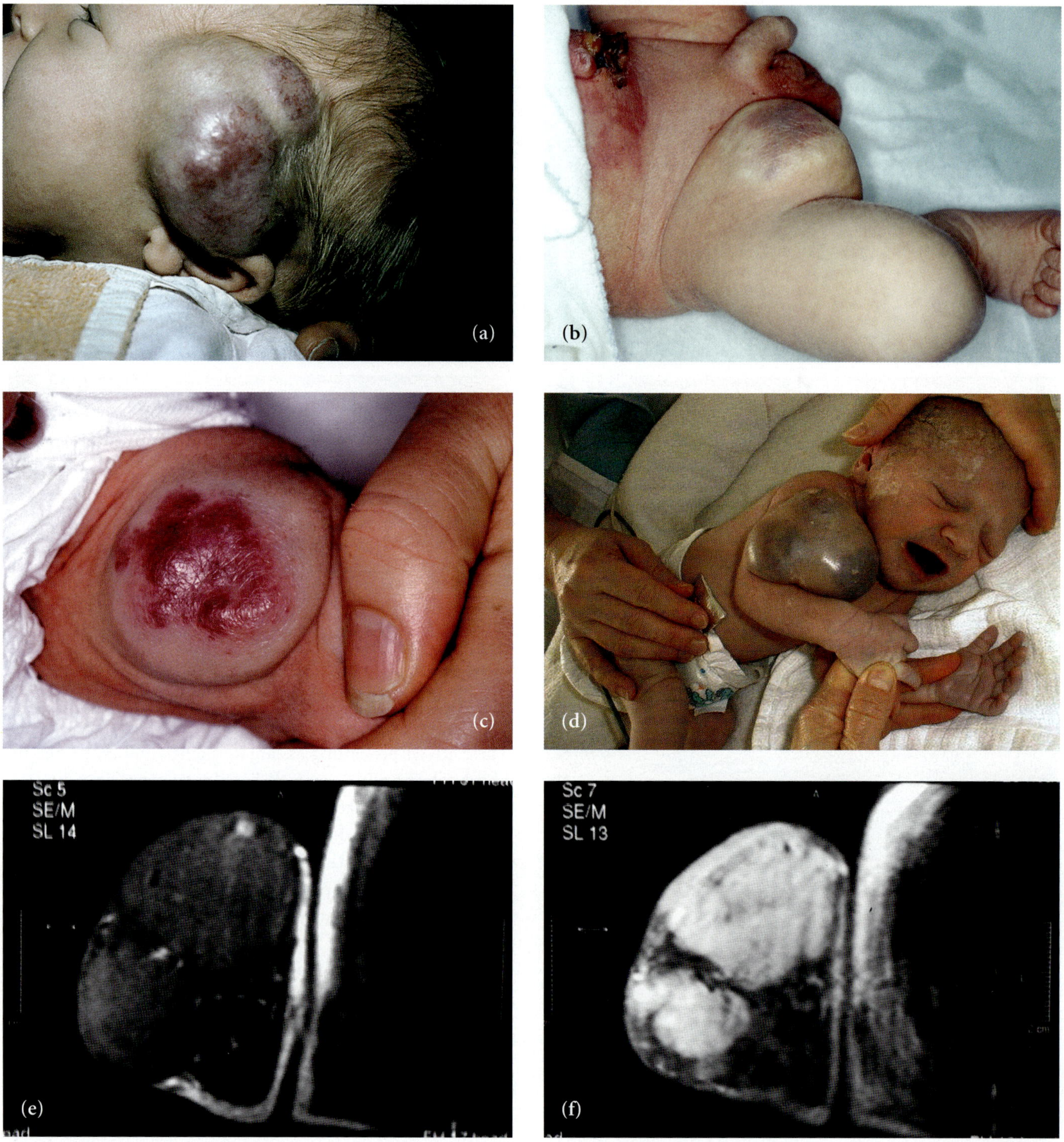

These nodular presentations of RICH are more worrying. All four were diagnosed as RICH based on MRI or Doppler fast-flow findings. However, because they had small (b, c) or large nodules (d) it was considered necessary to have pathology tests to rule out malignancy. The tumors were biopsied (a) or excised early in infancy (b, c, d). In the infant in (d) the bulky tumor in the arm was prenatally diagnosed during the third trimester of pregnancy; it had large nodules on palpation, and three separate vascular masses on MRI, these being T1-isointense (e) and T2-hyperintense (f).

Clinical Features of Congenital Hemangiomas

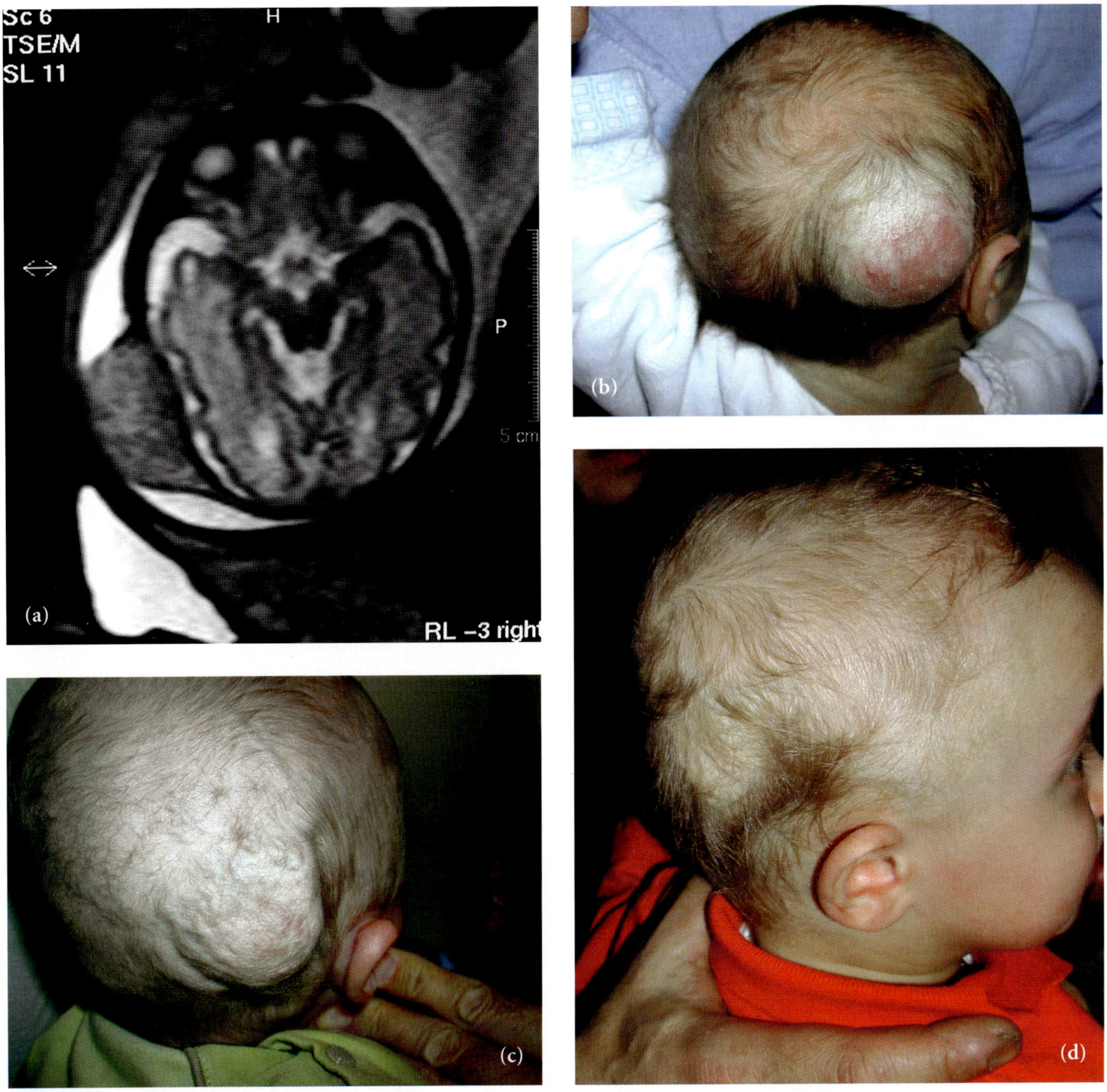

The prenatal ultrasonic detection of this large vascularized occipital tumor was followed by prenatal MRI evaluation. A diagnosis of congenital hemangioma was made (a), and a cesarean delivery was decided on. At birth the appearance was that of a RICH (b). The tumor was left to spontaneously disappear. And, at 6 months of age, its size had reduced by more than 50% but alopecia was still present (c). At 1 year of age complete resolution was obtained and hair was normally growing (d). A highly vascularized mass detected prenatally is usually suggestive of RICH (7), but misdiagnosis is possible: in our experience, an infantile myofibromatosis in the nape, and a large congenital fibrosarcoma of the thigh were misinterpreted as congenital hemangiomas, based on their load of vessels.

Clinical Features of Congenital Hemangiomas

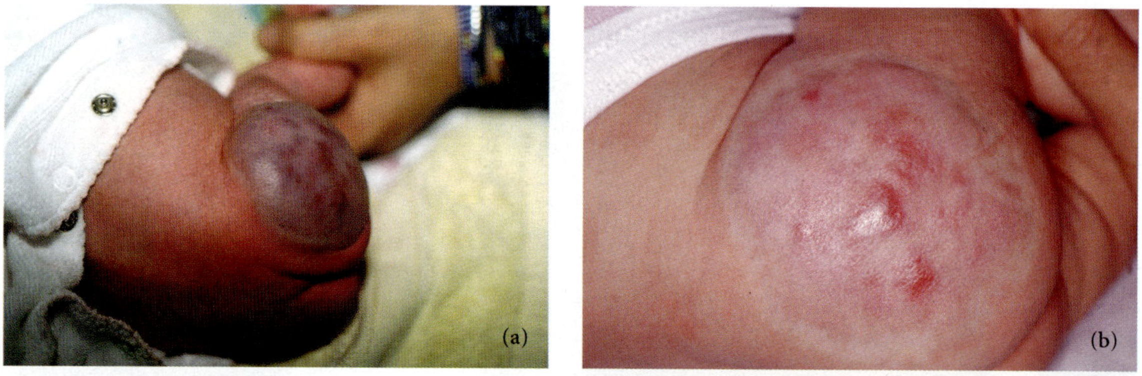

This large round and prominent tumor of the ankle was of a deep purple and blue color (a) at birth; the diagnosis of RICH was made; the appearance rapidly turned into a less impressive red plaque-type tumor, with a thin white margin, and some small nodules in the center (b); at 8 months of age the tumor was fully involuted and a large area of lipoatrophy with focal telangiectasia and a thin white edge persisted in the buttock (c).

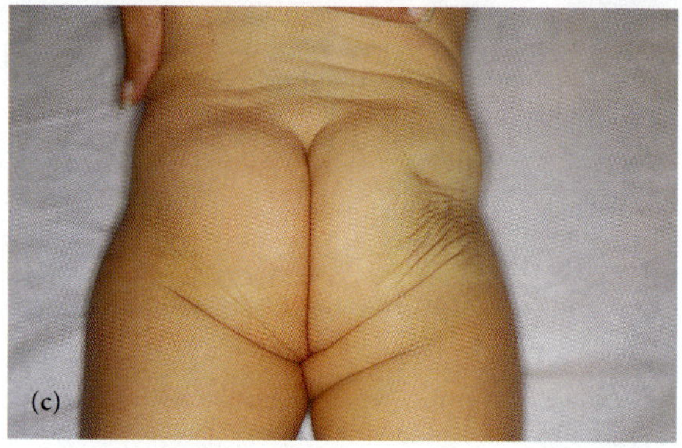

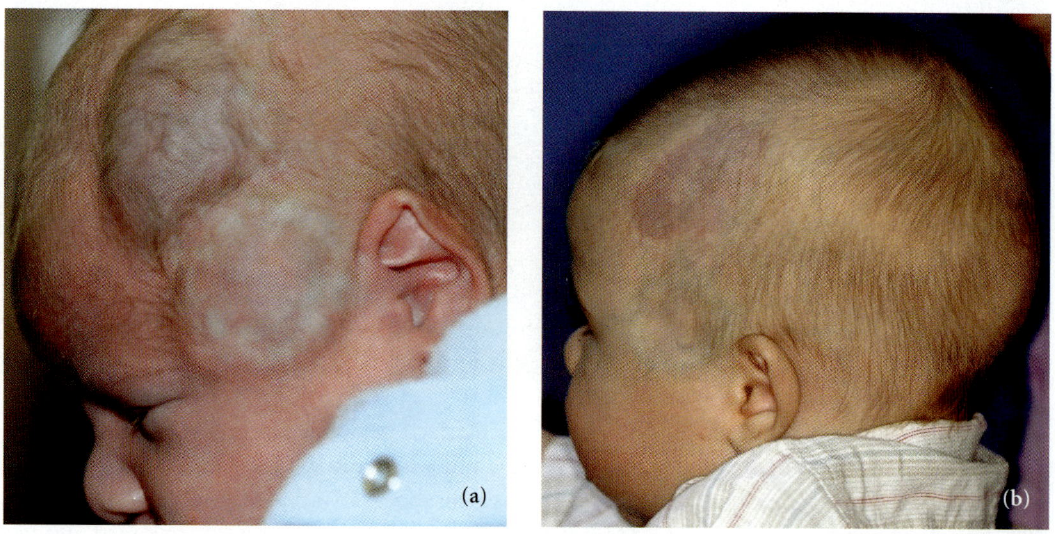

A rare presentation of RICH: twin tumors of the scalp, slightly different clinically (a), detected prenatally because of fast-flow, a finding that led to the decision to have a cesarean delivery. Both tumors promptly involuted in 6 months resulting in two slightly different residual macules (b). RICH are single in the vast majority of cases and this presentation is quite unusual.

Clinical Features of Congenital Hemangiomas

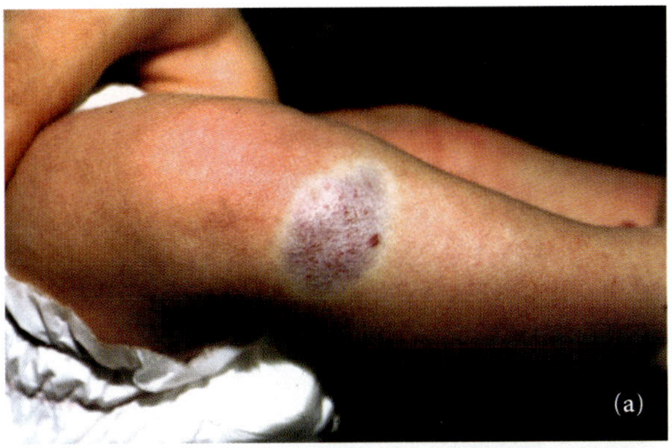

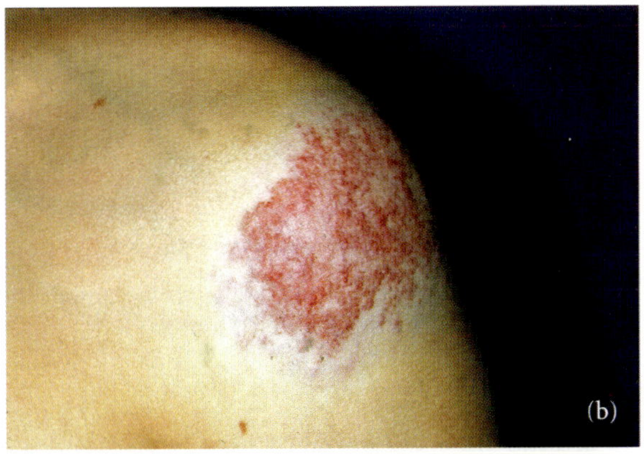

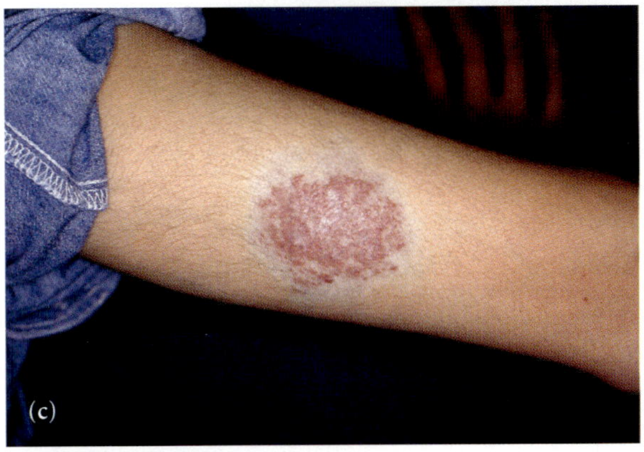

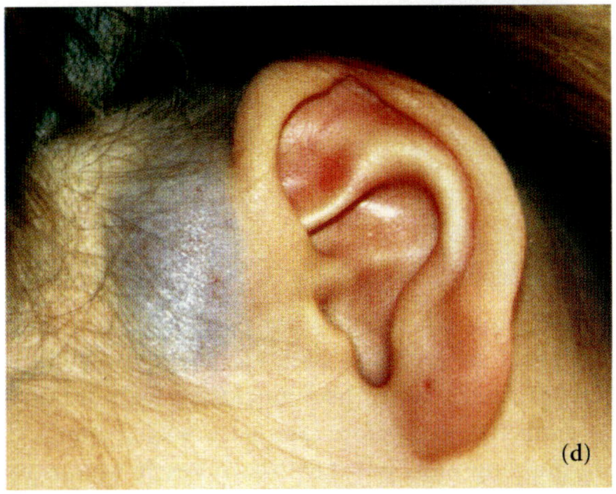

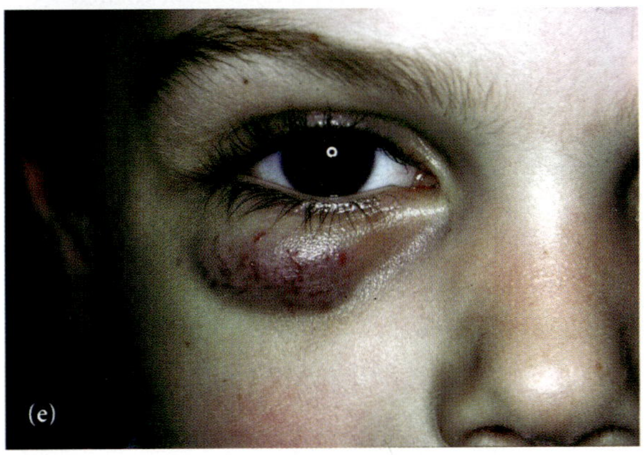

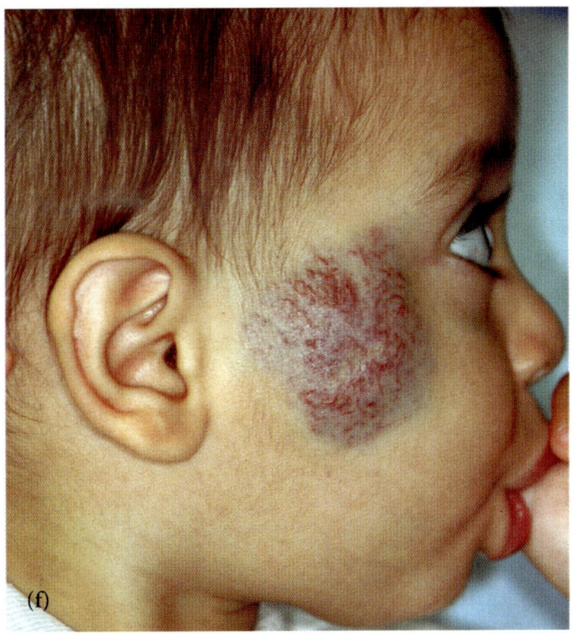

Various presentations of NICH: all these lesions were present at birth, and persisted. Some are round, others are ovoid. Their morphology is slightly variable: some are flat with a white peripheral halo (a, b, c), others are slightly bulging with a bluish unique color (d, e, f). Telangiectasia are constantly significant. Lesions are warm on palpation.

Clinical Features of Congenital Hemangiomas

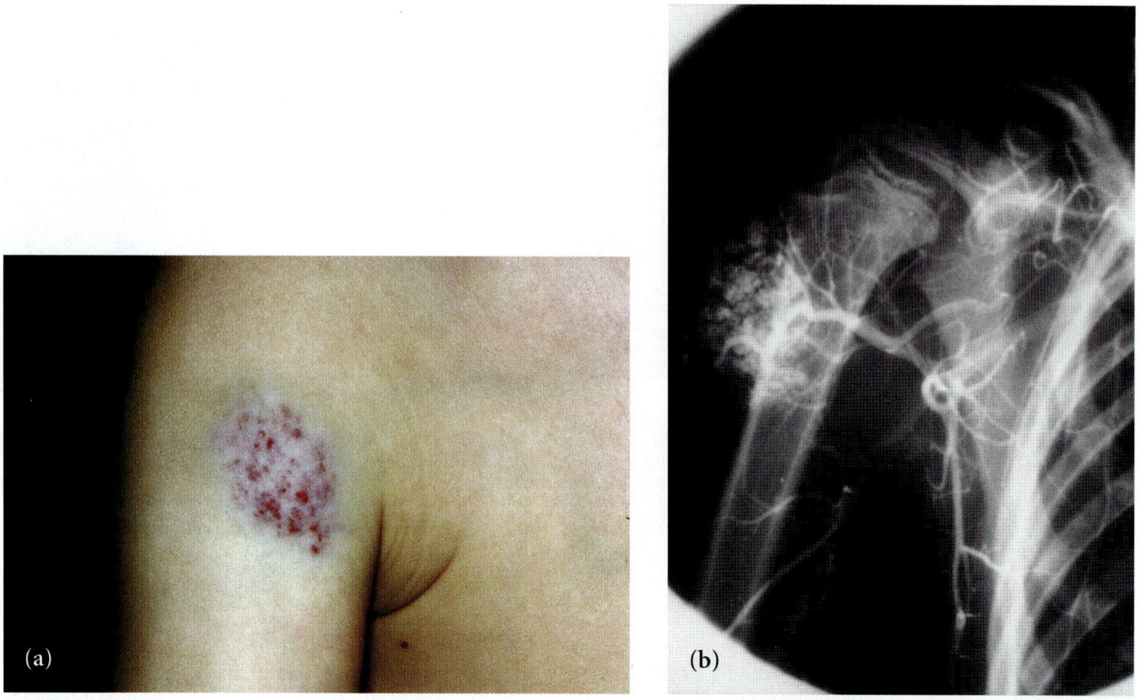

NICH in this boy had been present from birth on the arm. It was reminiscent of an involuting IH. NICH are round or oval, and fairly well delineated. There is often a rim of peripheral pallor or, as in this case, a bluish hue punctuated by more or less coarse telangiectasia. The angiogram performed for embolization, before excision, revealed a large arterial feeder, a tumor-like capillary blush, dilated draining veins but there was no early venous opacification.

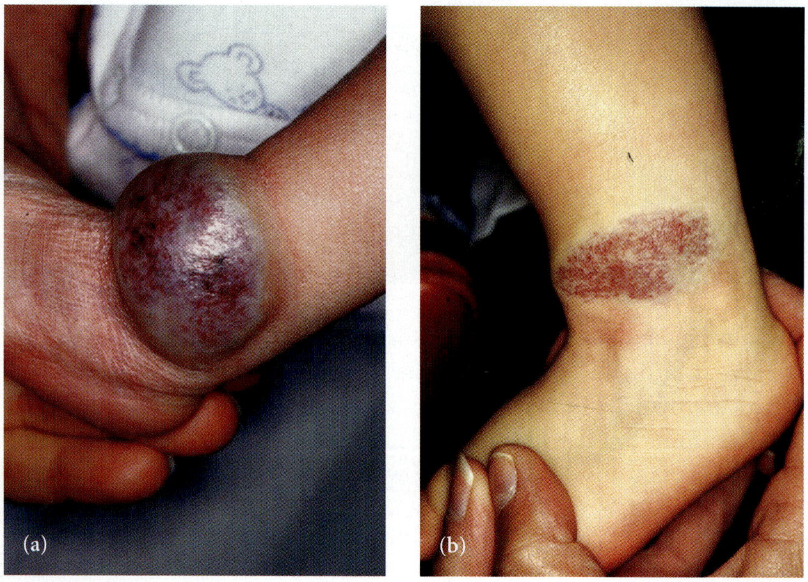

An example of what we call the "missing links" (9), cases showing the possible transformation after birth of a RICH (a) into a NICH (b) suggesting that NICH could be a late, intrauterine stage of a RICH involuted before birth. The large telangiectatic bluish lump present at birth (RICH) involuted over a few months and left a slightly atrophic telangiectatic residuum with a thin peripheral pale halo reminiscent of NICH, which persisted and was excised.

Clinical Features of Congenital Hemangiomas

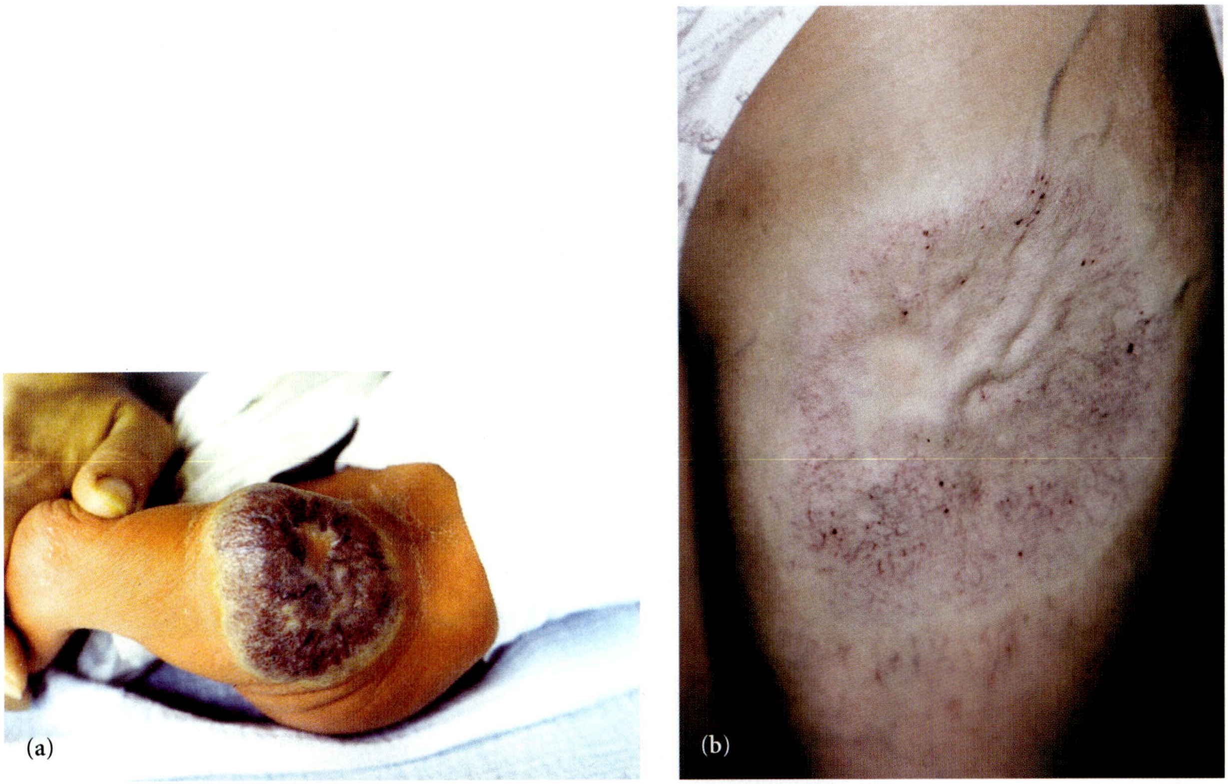

This boy had at birth a large bossed tumor of the thigh with a central scar and large telangiectasia (a). At 8 months of age the tumor had involuted (RICH) and a telangiectatic large macular stain was left. During childhood this residuum not only grew proportionately with the thigh but also developed large veins, an increasing pale halo of vasoconstriction, and pain (b). Excision was performed at 12 years. Preceding cutaneous expansion permitted closure of the large surgical wound. Both RICH and NICH aspects were present in the pathology samples.

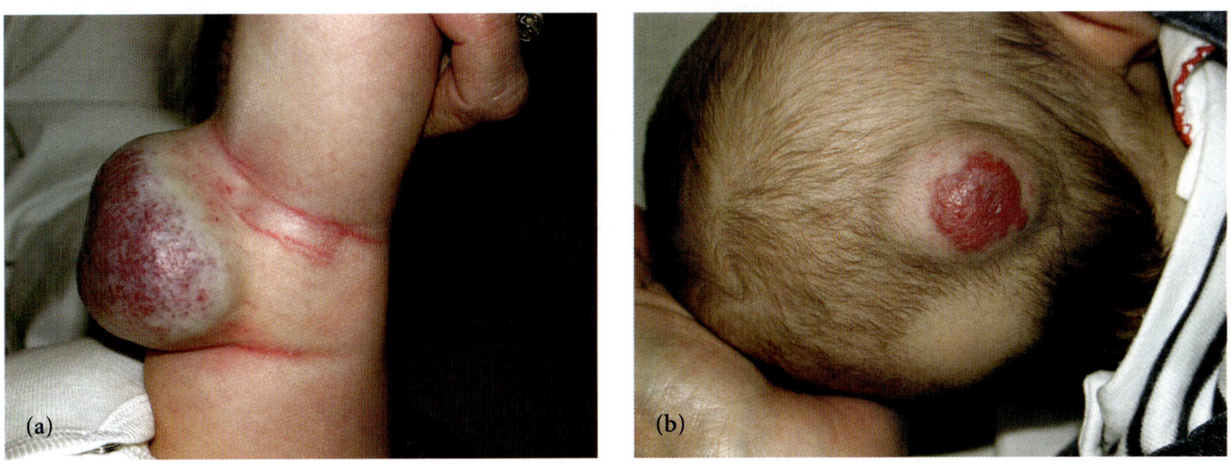

An example of association of RICH and IH: this infant had this large warm telangiectatic RICH (a) of the knee joint at birth and then he developed a common infantile hemangioma on the scalp (b).

Clinical Features of Congenital Hemangiomas

Another striking example indicating possible links between RICH and IH: this girl had at birth a deep blue tumor of the cheek close to the ear (a); then she developed, exactly on top of this RICH, papules typical of an IH; some of these papules had aggressive growth mimicking pyogenic granuloma and were photocoagulated. In the meantime the underlying congenital tumor had involuted at 6 months of age (b), without any pharmacological treatment, while the red strawberry-mark type IH grown on the surface of the RICH took 3 years to fully vanish.

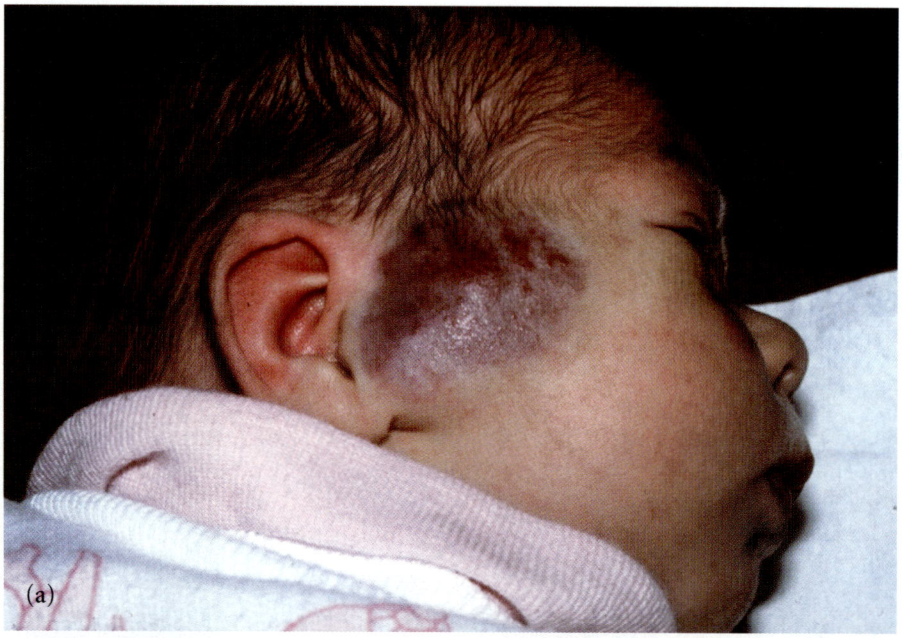
(a)

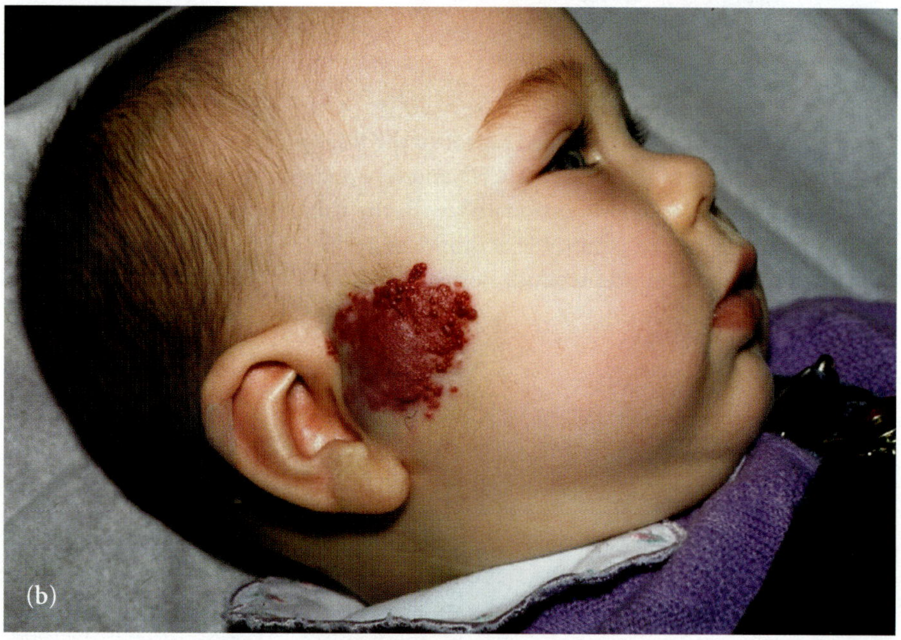
(b)

Clinical Features of Congenital Hemangiomas

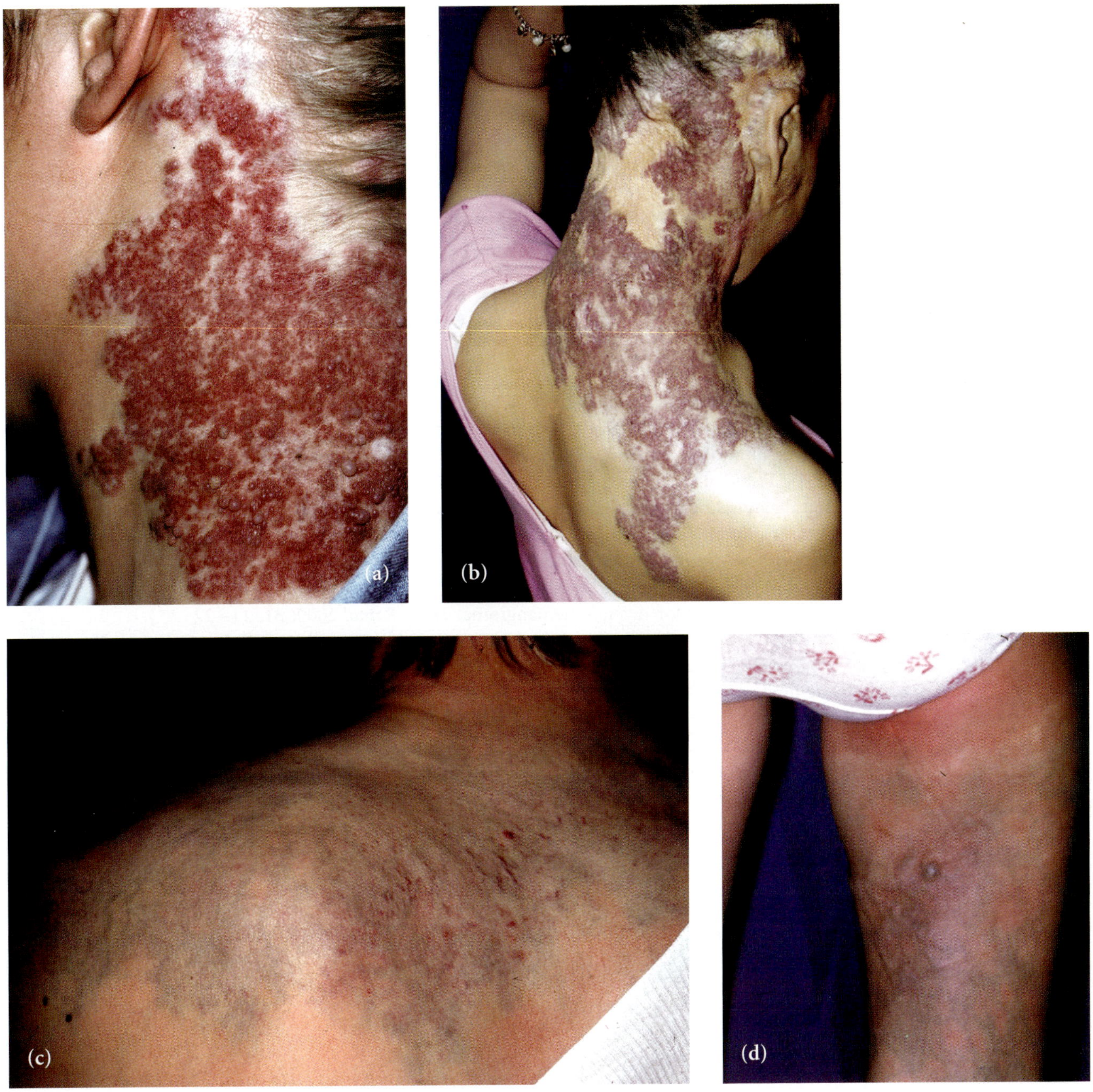

Pathological features of NICH were present in a subset of congenital vascular tumors, creating large, unevenly distributed, and irregularly colored plaques mimicking involuting hemangioma (a, b), often, however, with a number of firm papules on top, spontaneously varying over the years of follow-up (a). Some had a thin white margin and others exhibited a bluish hue of the whole surface (15). They were located mainly on the lateral neck, shoulder and upper back (a, b, c), and rarely in the thigh (d). They had a proportionate growth over the years and persisted from birth into adulthood. Due to their size and site they can only be partially excised. Excision resulted in large scars (b, courtesy of Dr. Aicha Salhi, Hôpital Ain Nadja, Alger, Algeria) but no local recurrence was observed in the treated areas. All these lesions fulfilled the pathological characteristics of NICH and where GLUT1 negative.

References

1 Agesta N, Boralevi F, Sarlangue J, Vergnes P, Grenier N, Léauté-Labreze C. Life-threatening hemorrhage of a congenital haemangioma. *Acta Paediatr* 2003; **92**: 1216–18.

2 Berenguer B, Mulliken JB, Enjolras O, Boon LM, Wassef M, Josset P, Burrows PE, Perez-Atayde AR, Kozakewich HPW. Rapidly involuting congenital hemangioma: clinical and histopathologic features. *Pediatr Dev Biol* 2003; **6**: 495–610.

3 Boon LM, Enjolras O, Mulliken JB. Congenital hemangioma: evidence for accelerated regression. *J Pediatr* 1996; **128**: 329–35.

4 Bulas DI, Johnson D, Allen JF, Kapur S. Fetal hemangioma. Sonographic and color flow Doppler findings. *J Ultrasound Med* 1992; **11**: 499–501.

5 Enjolras O, Mulliken JB, Boon LM, Wassef M, Kozakewich HP, Burrows PE. Noninvoluting congenital hemangioma: a rare cutaneous vascular anomaly; *Plast Reconstr Surg* 2001; **107**: 1647–54.

6 Enjolras O. Hémangiomes congénitaux. *Ann Dermatol Venereol* 2003; **130**: 367–71.

7 Konez O, Burrows PE, Mulliken JB, Fishman SJ, Kozakewich HP. Angiographic features of rapidly involuting congenital hemangioma RICH. *Pediatr Radiol* 2003; **33**: 15–19.

8 Marler JJ, Fishman SJ, Upton J, Burrows PE, Paltiel HJ, Jennings RW, Mulliken JB. Prenatal diagnosis of vascular anomalies. *J Pediatr Surg* 2002; **37**: 318–26.

9 Mulliken JB, Enjolras O. Congenital hemangiomas and infantile hemangioma: missing links. *J Am Acad Dermatol* 2004; **50**: 875–82.

10 North PE, Waner M, Mizeracki A, Mihm MC Jr., GLUT1: a newly discovered immunohistochemical marker for juvenile hemangioma. *Hum Pathol* 2000; **31**: 11–22.

11 North PE, Waner M, James CA, Mizeracki A, Frieden IJ, Mihm MC Jr., Congenital nonprogressive hemangioma. A distinct clinicopathologic entity unlike infantile hemangioma. *Arch Dermatol* 2001; **137**: 1607–20.

12 Rogers M, Lam A, Fischer G. Sonographic findings in a series of Rapidly Involuting Congenital Hemangiomas (RICH). *Pediatric Dermatol* 2002; **19**: 5–11.

13 Shiraishi H, Nakamura M, Ichihashi K. MRI in a fetus with a giant neck hemangioma: a case report. *Prenat Diagn* 2000; **20**: 1004–7.

14 Viora E, Grassi PP, Comoglio F, Bastonero S, Campogrande M. Ultrasonic detection of fetal cranio-facial hemangioma: case report and review of the literature. *Ultrasound Obstet Gynecol* 2000; **15**: 431–4.

15 Wassef M, Salhi A, Kozakewich HPW, Brevière GM, Mulliken JB, Enjolras O. *Atypical cervical NICH: report of 11 cases.* Communication 15th Workshop ISSVA, Wellington (NZ), 22–25 Feb 2005.

Tufted Angioma, Kaposiform Hemangioendothelioma, Kasabach–Merritt Phenomenon (KMP)

TUFTED ANGIOMA

Wilson-Jones and Orkin in 1989 described a distinctive cutaneous lesion as "tufted angioma" (TA), because of the "tufts of hypertrophied endothelial cells" scattered through the whole dermis "in a cannonball distribution" (38). These aggregates of endothelial cells are more prominent in the middle and lower part of the dermis, going down to the fat (28). It is clear today that TA is identical to "angioblastoma of Nakagawa" in the Japanese literature (4, 17, 26).

TA is congenital or acquired usually before 5 years of age. The same pathological features characterize congenital, infantile or "acquired" TA, as well as TA associated with Kasabach–Merritt phenomenon (KMP) (8–10).

TA seems more common in the limbs (16, 39). Herron and colleagues (16) stressed the various clinical patterns and course in infancy. TA is often tender to touch to a variable degree, and it may change its size and shape over time. Pink, reddish or brownish, single or multiple, macules or variably infiltrated plaques, some with hyperhidrosis or hypertrichosis, or tiny red papules on the surface, are observed. In some infants TA appears as a congenital lump with a blanching halo; this uncommon aspect is difficult to differentiate from RICH, thus requiring a biopsy.

Although some of these vascular tumors spontaneously regress in about 6 to 24 months, a majority persists indefinitely, becoming more or less indurated and slightly painful (30). TA may worsen during pregnancy in our experience. The platelet-trapping syndrome, KMP, sometimes engrafts on TA, exactly like on kaposiform hemangioendothelioma (see below).

Treatment

No treatment is really satisfactory. Topical corticosteroid, systemic corticosteroid, intralesional interferon alpha 2 or systemic interferon alpha and laser treatments gave both encouraging results and failure (6, 22, 27, 31, 37).

KAPOSIFORM HEMANGIOENDOTHELIOMA

Zukerberg and coworkers (40) used the term "kaposiform hemangioendothelioma of infancy and childhood" for a tumor that could be mistaken for Kaposi sarcoma. This lesion was also called "hemangioma with Kaposi sarcoma features" (24) and "Kaposi-like infantile hemangioendothelioma" of the retroperitoneum (32). The lymphatic nature was long discussed based on pathological features (the presence of lymphatic channels). In 2005, Debelenko et al. demonstrated that the lymphatic vessels present in kaposiform hemangioendothelioma (KHE) and the spindled neoplastic cells exhibit distinct staining for the lymphatic marker D2 40, suggesting lymphothelial differentiation of the proliferation (5).

KHE is aggressive: it permeates soft tissues, muscles, and even bones. There is no report of distant metastatic disease but perinodal infiltration or involvement of the subcapsular sinus in a regional lymph node was observed (18).

Skin location of KHE is uncommon: it develops in skin as a reddish tender plaque or a conglomerate of nodules and macules, with a chronic course (19). Involution rarely occurs. Visceral KHE affects the neck, mediastinum and thymus, or retroperitoneum. These visceral forms are massively infiltrative and usually platelet trapping, and thrombocytopenia engraft on these KHE: the KMP, the identical hematological disorder occurring with TA (see above and below). TA without KMP is not rare, and conversely cutaneous KHE without KMP is exceptional. Based on pathology overlap is commonly observed in superficial cases of KMP, with tumors exhibiting gradation between TA and KHE. These two tumors are now considered to be of the same pathological spectrum and closely related if not identical (8, 18, 29, 36). Considering the visceral KMP, including the retroperitoneal location, all reported cases were linked to KHE, except one case demonstrating overlapping pathological features (KHE + TA) in the retroperitoneal tumor (2).

Treatment

There are no clear guidelines for the treatment of KHE without KMP. Glucocorticosteroids, vincristine, interferon alpha 2 a or 2b or excision may be indicated.

KASABACH–MERRITT PHENOMENON

Since its description by Kasabach and Merritt in 1940, the association of a large vascular tumor and thrombocytopenia has been called "Kasabach–Merritt syndrome" (KMS) or "Kasabach–Merritt phenomenon" (KMP). It was long believed to be a complication of infantile hemangioma. However, the original microscopic report specified that there were: "spindle-shaped cells supported by a delicate fibrillar stroma." It is now established that KMP occurs with distinct vascular tumors, KHE, and TA (8–10, 14, 29, 34, 40).

KHE and TA can be congenital or appear after birth, and KMP develops at birth or in infancy mainly before 5 months of age. Thrombocytopenia is profound (platelets rapidly fall to less than 10000/mm^3). There is anemia, low fibrinogen, and elevated D-dimers.

KMP with KHE and TA has identical clinical appearance. KMP developed on a previously biopsy-proven TA is not less severe in our experience: the tender tumor becomes larger, purple or purplish-blue, often with a shiny smooth fragile surface, and purpura comes out. The sudden development of KMP or the sudden worsening of a minor pre-existing skin lesion is striking. After cure of the hematologic anomalies, three types of residual lesions have been documented (10). Type 1 is a "pseudo port-wine stain." Type II is "red telangiectatic streaks and swelling." Type III is a "firm irregular subcutaneous lesion" or a firm "sclerodermiform infiltration" appraised by palpation, or "a deep infiltration" as demonstrated by CT or MRI. All these lesions are not fixed: they slightly modify their presentation over the years and they occasionally ache, requiring low doses of aspirin to soothe the pain.

Nosology

There is a tendency in the literature to use the term Kasabach–Merritt syndrome (KMS) or KMP for various diseases with associated hematological and coagulation disorder, e.g. coagulation disorder associated with malignancies (infantile fibrosarcoma, angiosarcoma), and the chronic coagulopathy associated with an extensive venous or lymphatic–venous malformation (see page 170 and Table 15 p. 171). This is confusing: the pathological background and prognosis are very different, and there is a more problematic issue: their treatments are also completely different. Such an extension of the use of the label KMS or KMP is inappropriate and dangerous for the management of these patients.

Treatment

Excision, when possible, is curative (7, 33). Heparin is contraindicated. Platelet infusions may boost both the hematologic phenomenon and growth of the tumor (21). Platelet infusions must not be prescribed because of a very low platelet count; they are only indicated in case of life-threatening hemorrhage, or immediately before the resection of the tumor, when surgical treatment is feasible. Platelets are rapidly entrapped within the tumor and they are destroyed. Pharmacological therapy should be given promptly. However, large variations in the platelet counts often occur during the first weeks or months of treatment: this is not an indication for more aggressive treatment with combinations of drugs (1) if no life-threatening symptom emerges. KMP remains a life-threatening disease, although the prognosis has improved. From a review of cases it appeared to us that more deaths resulted from serious side-effects of multimodal pharmacological treatments than from the disease itself and its hemorrhagic risk. The main drugs prescribed for KMP have been glucocorticosteroids (11, 35); interferon alpha 2a or 2b (10, 12, 13, 23, 29); and vincristine (15). Surprisingly, in some patients, pharmacological agents that interfere with hemostasis have been as beneficial as glucocorticosteroids, interferon alpha, or vincristine; the combination of ticlopidine and aspirin has mainly been used, but also dipyridamole, pentoxiphyllin, tranexamic acid, and amicar were occasionally helpful. No medical treatment gives constant results and the pathological features do not provide us with therapeutic indications. Arterial embolization or radiotherapy are infrequently considered.

Figures

TUFTED ANGIOMA, KAPOSIFORM HEMANGIOENDOTHELIOMA, AND THE KASABACH–MERRITT PHENOMENON

Pathology of Tufted Angioma

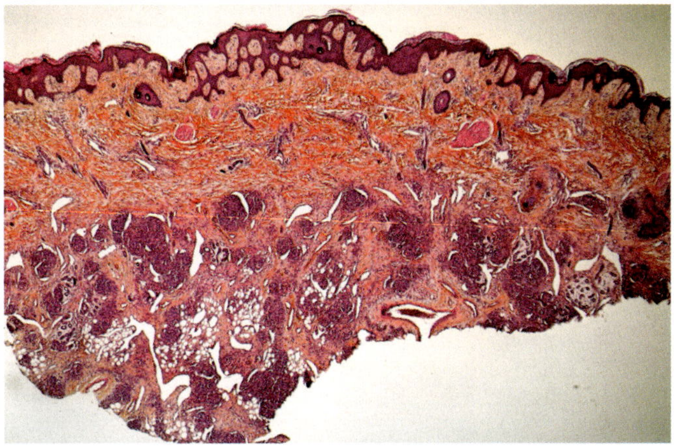

TA is characterized by round small lobules scattered in the mid and deep dermis in a cannonball distribution.

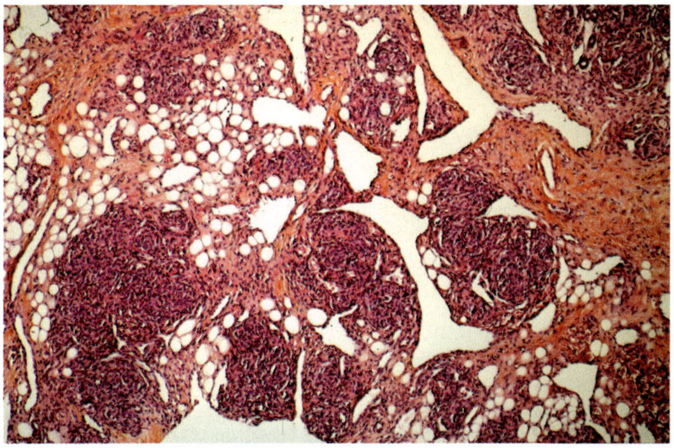

The tufts of capillaries in TA also deeply infiltrate the hypodermis and subcutis.

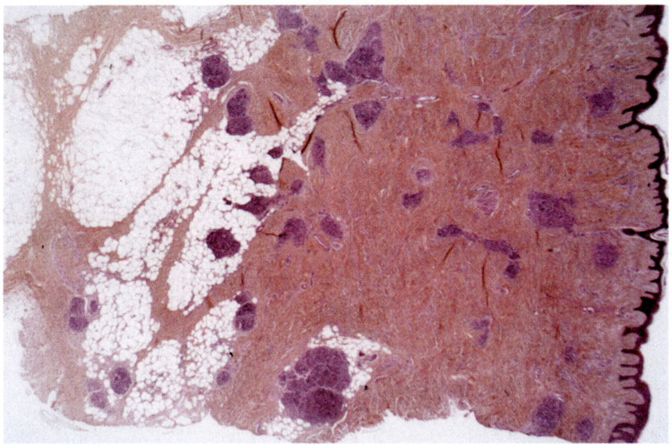

In this TA sample of a biopsy corresponding to a residual plaque-type lesion of the gluteal area, after cure of Kasabach–Merritt phenomenon, fibrosis is noticeable in the dermis and the small capillary tufts are seen in the dermis but also deeply located in the fat.

Pathology of Tufted Angioma

This is the typical appearance of a tuft in TA, with a dense capillary lobule and an empty crescent-like vessel encircling the lobule. Fibrosis is obvious in the surrounding dermis.

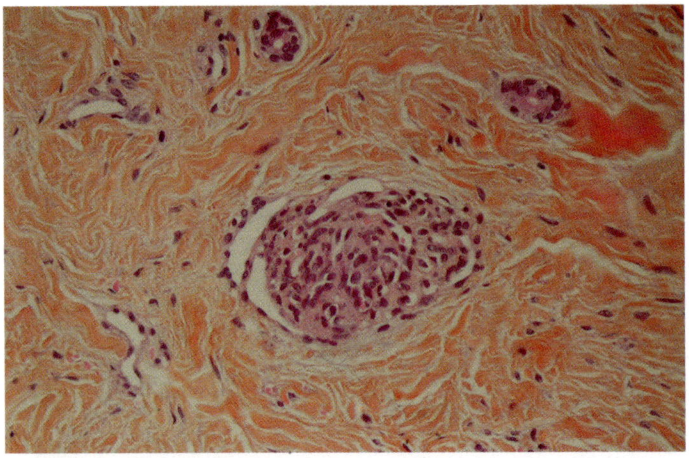

Besides the characteristic capillary tufts, many lesions of TA contain areas with only clusters of vessels with empty lumen. These vessels dissect the tissues. They correspond to lymphatic vessels as confirmed by staining with markers such as D2-40.

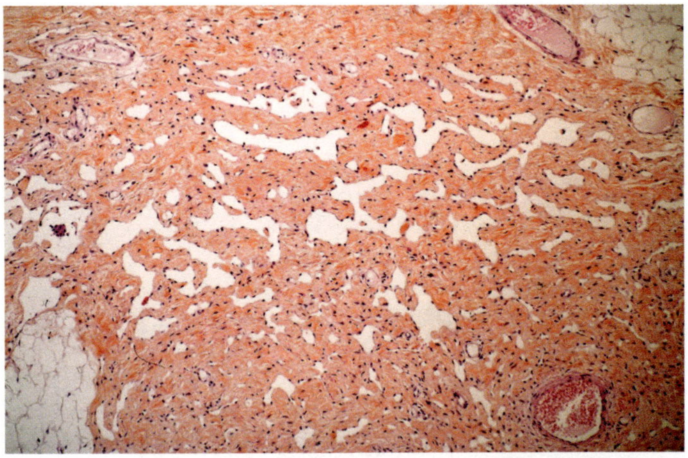

In some areas in a TA biopsy sample, the tufts tend to be larger, ill-defined, and to coalesce, and they contain spindled cells, all findings suggestive of a diagnosis of KHE. In this sample, the large vessels with empty lumen, visible between the lobules, correspond to lymphatics.

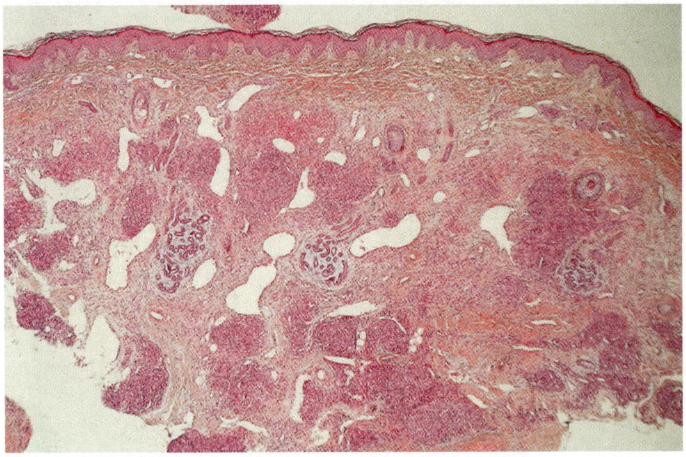

Pathology of Kaposiform Hemangioendothelioma

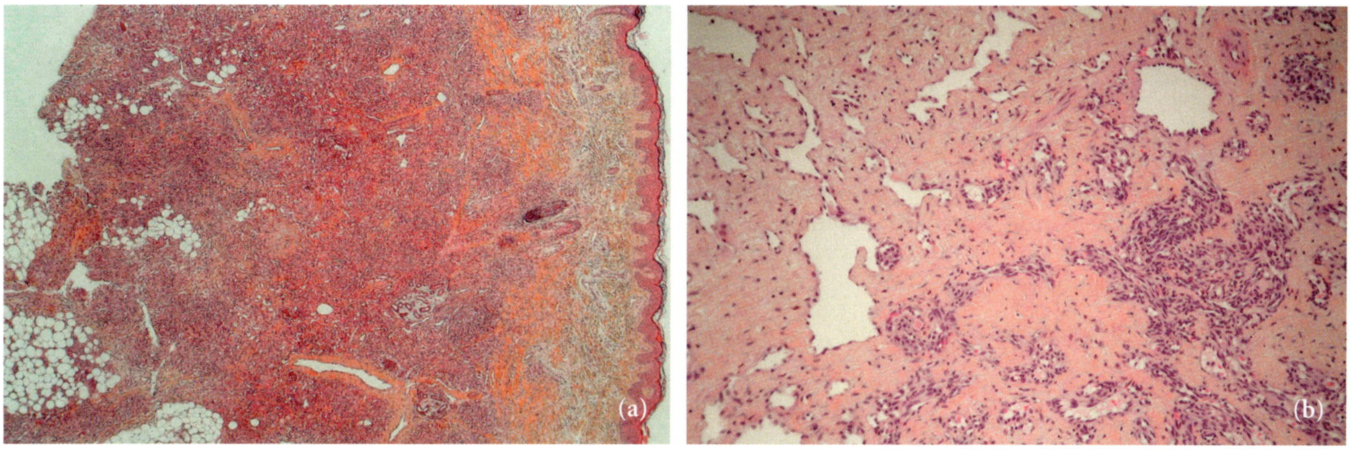

KHE creates massive and often ill-defined lobules made of spindled cells (a). Less-cellular areas with lymphatic vessels and fibrosis are also present (b).

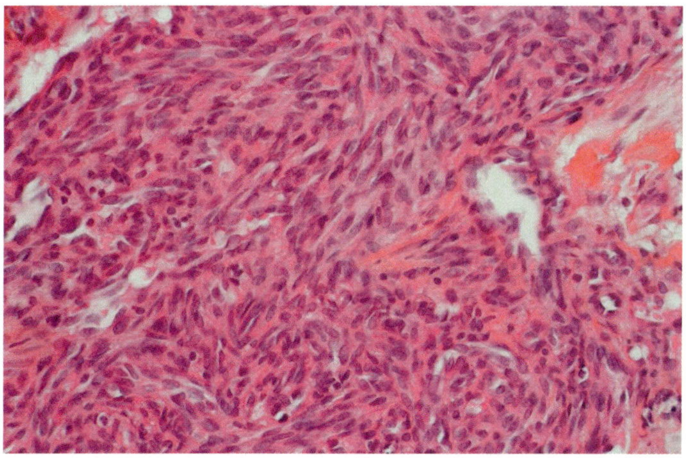

The spindling of the cells is evident at this higher magnification in a KHE biopsy, resembling a Kaposi sarcoma. Spindle cells are separated by slit-like lumina containing few red blood cells. Epithelioid endothelial cells intermingle with the spindle cells.

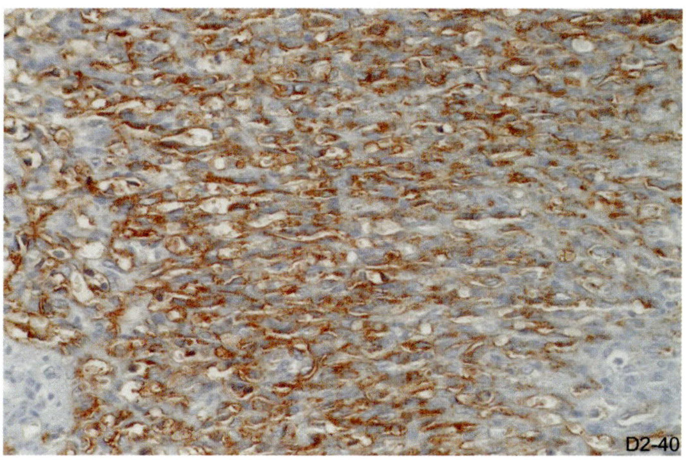

The majority of the spindled cells in KHE are stained with D2-40, a lymphatic marker.

Pathology of Kaposiform Hemangioendothelioma

One can observe better-defined lobules of spindled cells in KHE, with surrounding fibrosis, a pattern reminiscent of 2TA.

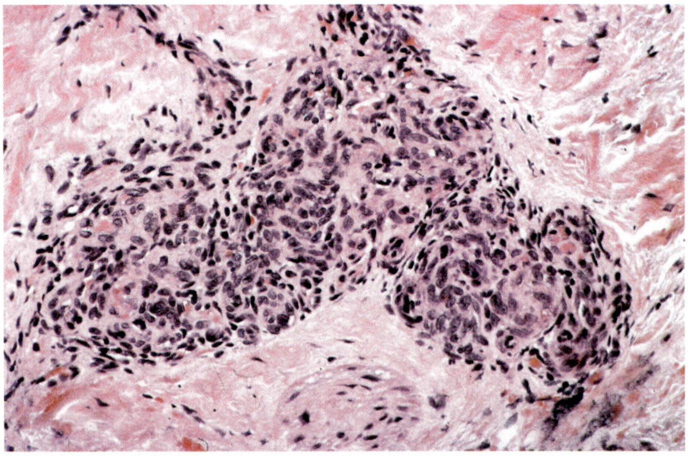

Microthrombi are detected in cellular areas.

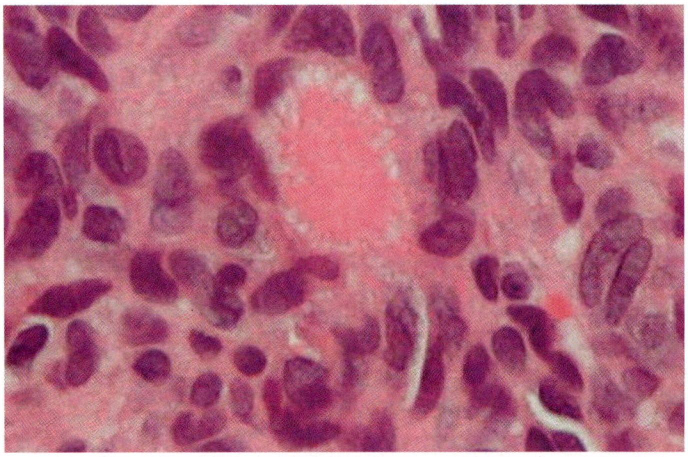

The infiltrating cells may permeate and invade a large lymphatic channel.

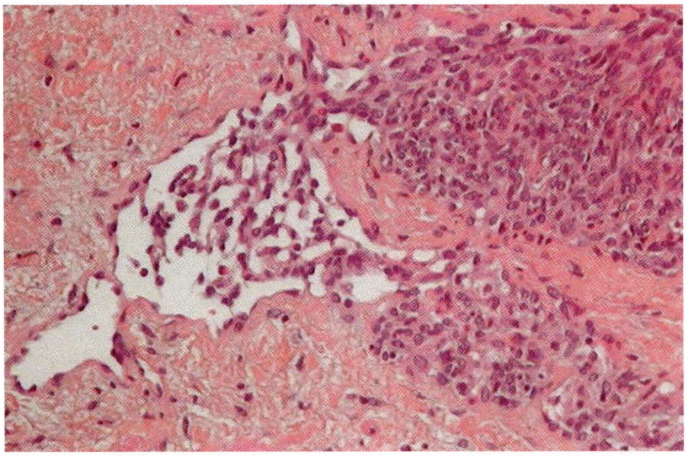

Clinical Aspects of Tufted Angioma, Kaposiform Hemangioendothelioma, and the Kasabach–Merritt Phenomenon

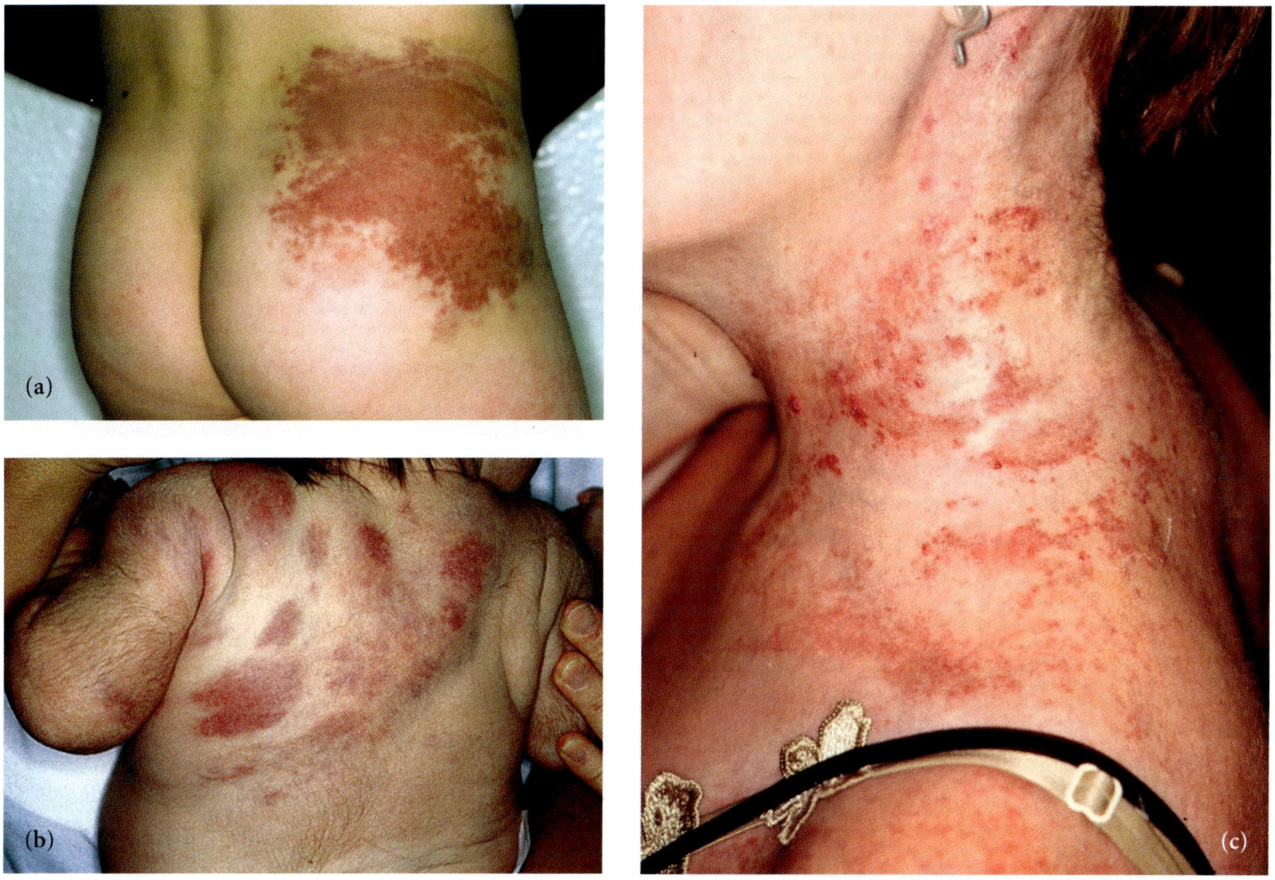

Pink, reddish or brownish, usually single (a), sometimes multiple (b), slightly infiltrated plaques, with a more- or less-well-defined border, are the most common presentations of TA in infancy. You cannot predict from the appearance whether KMP will develop or not.

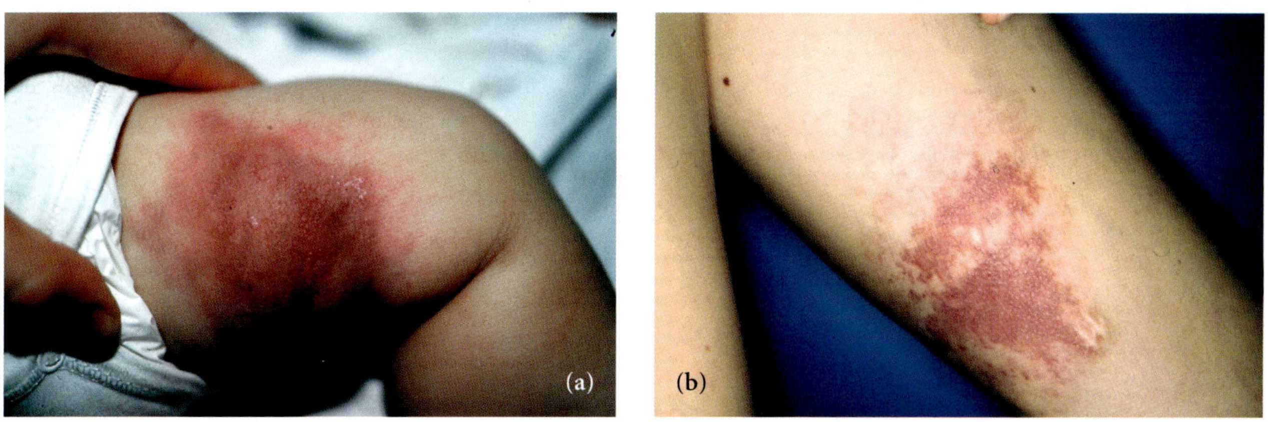

A girl with plaque-like TA of the thigh complained of pain and cosmetic problems. The pictures illustrate the frequent changes in shape, size, and infiltration from 8 months (a) to 10 years of age (b). According to a review by Okada et al. (26), 56% of TA are evident during the first year of life.

Clinical Aspects of Tufted Angioma, Kaposiform Hemangioendothelioma, and the Kasabach–Merritt Phenomenon

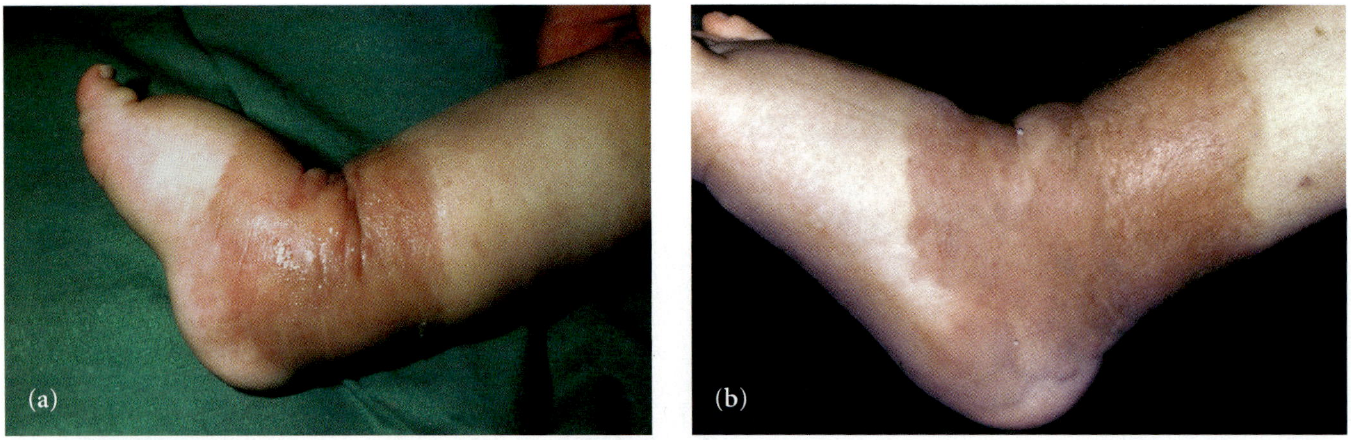

TA infrequently regresses. This congenital lesion had no propensity to recede: on the contrary a sclerosing pattern (3) developed around the ankle. The girl was first seen at 4 months of age (a) with a thick congenital TA of the ankle and foot; TA was still progressing at 7 years of age (b); without treatment, over the years the sclerosing TA generated severe joint and bone complication in the foot and gait impairment when seen again at 24 years of age.

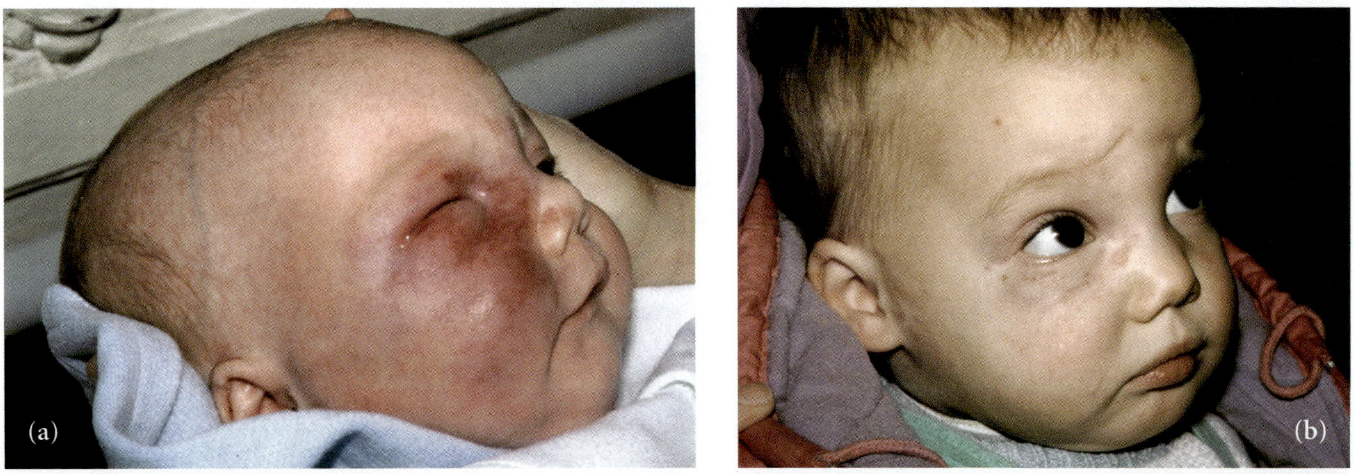

TA usually persists indefinitely, although some congenital lesions regress. This infant had this large purple tumor closing her eye at birth (a); there was no thrombocytopenia. The biopsy indicated TA. She received oral glucocorticosteroid treatment. The visual field was rapidly opened; one year later (b) a bluish minor infiltration persisted.

Clinical Aspects of Tufted Angioma, Kaposiform Hemangioendothelioma, and the Kasabach–Merritt Phenomenon

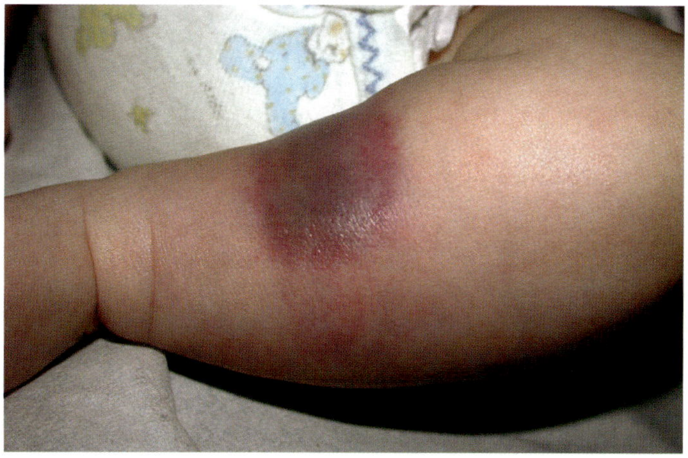

This congenital, biopsy-proven KHE of the leg was slowly enlarging and obviously painful on palpation in this infant. KHE usually presents as a reddish or purplish-blue tender plaque with an ill-defined border, and is clinically difficult to differentiate from TA (20).

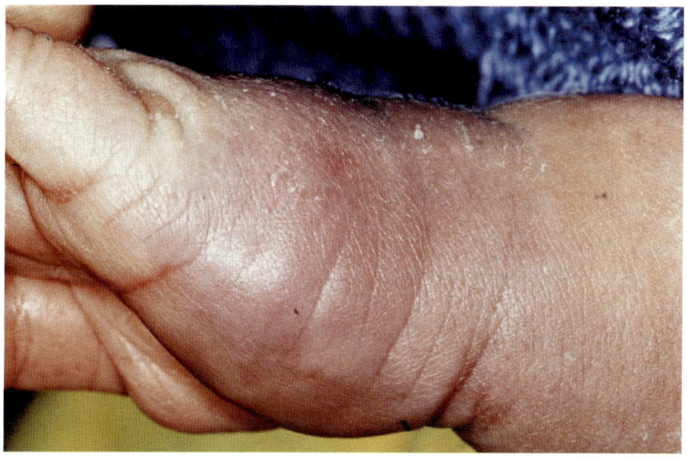

A large congenital plaque-type, biopsy-proven KHE infiltrates the dorsum and lateral aspect of the hand. It first slightly progressed to a more important infiltration in the center. Then spontaneous involution occurred, leaving a minor pink residuum.

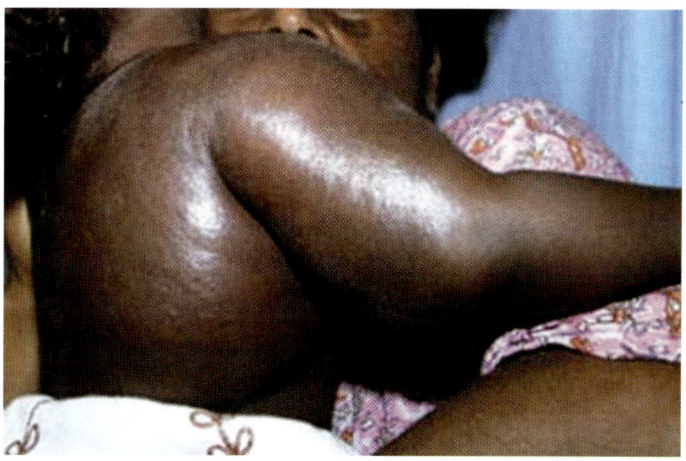

KHE has long been known possibly to grow on a large lymphatic malformation, as in this infant who never developed KMP (40).

Clinical Aspects of Tufted Angioma, Kaposiform Hemangioendothelioma, and the Kasabach–Merritt Phenomenon

This large infiltrating plaque and lump, covering the full right buttock, was of a light purple color with a single blue nodule, and some purpura in the periphery; it had enlarged from birth; at this stage the biopsy evidenced KHE and the platelet count was subnormal; but a few days later a sudden drop of the platelet count confirmed the diagnosis of KMP on KHE.

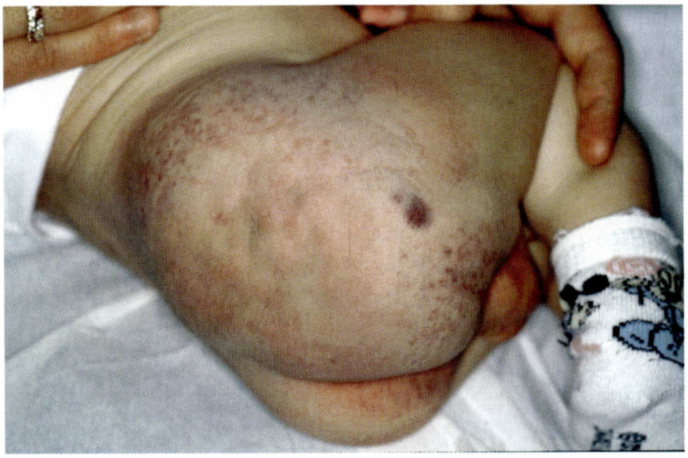

This massive congenital tumor with KMP (courtesy of Dr. Paul Rieu, St. Radboud Hospital, Nijmegen, The Netherlands) had pathological features of TA on the first biopsy and then aspects of both TA and KHE depending on the biopsy sections. Various pharmacological treatments were tried over 4 years, with poor response and local severe deterioration, and finally the boy had amputation at the hip level.

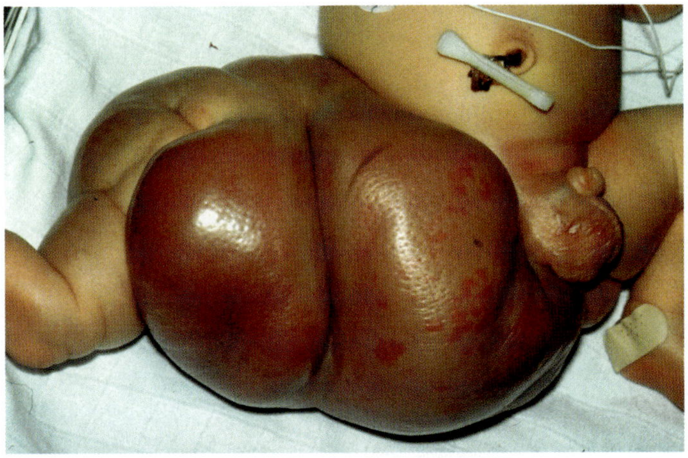

KMP, the severe platelet trapping phenomenon within the pre-existing tumor, suddenly modified the clinical aspects of a lesion described as a minor red infiltrated plaque, present at birth, in a twin boy hospitalized in the neonatal unit because of severe congenital cardiac ventricular septal malformation. Purpura appeared on the arm, distant to the tumor. The KMP was cured with vincristine treatment in association with pentoxyfillin, and the infant could have the cardiac surgery.

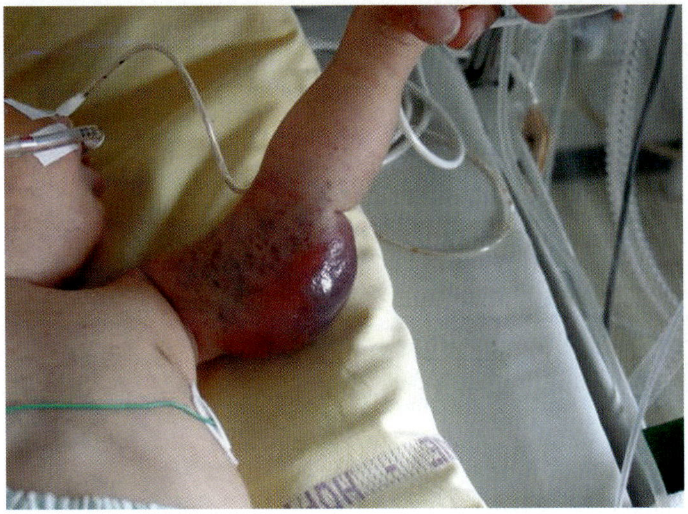

Clinical Aspects of Tufted Angioma, Kaposiform Hemangioendothelioma, and the Kasabach–Merritt Phenomenon

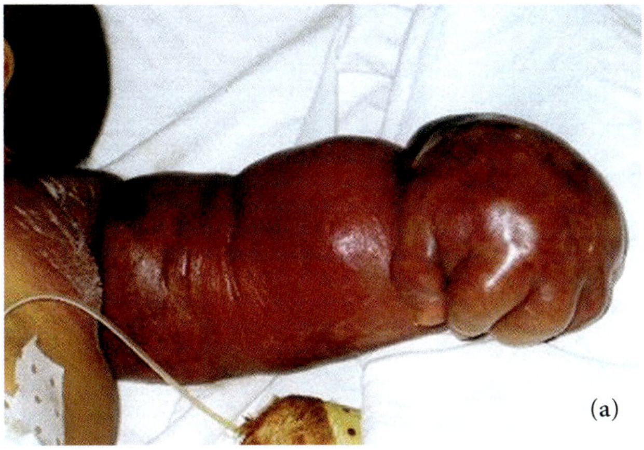
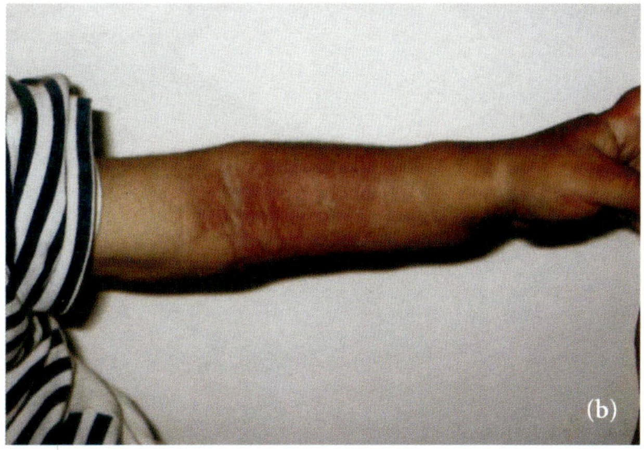

Impressive presentation of KMP in a 6-day-old neonate (a) and the excellent functional and cosmetic results after 9 months of treatment combining ticlopidine and aspirin, and an additional follow-up period of 6 months without treatment and no rebound of the hematologic phenomenon (b) (courtesy of Dr. Aicha Salhi, Hôpital Ain Nadja, Alger, Algeria).

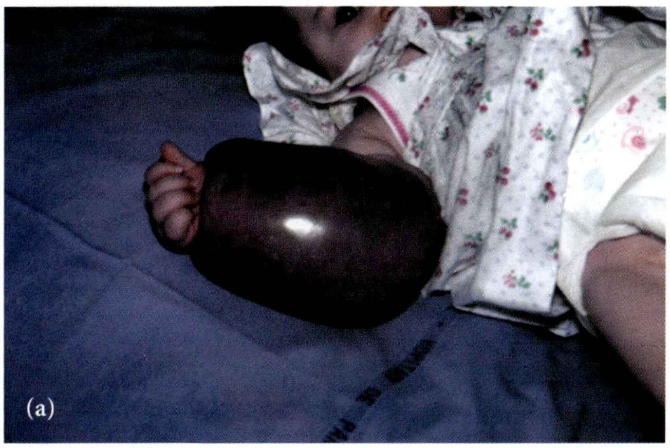
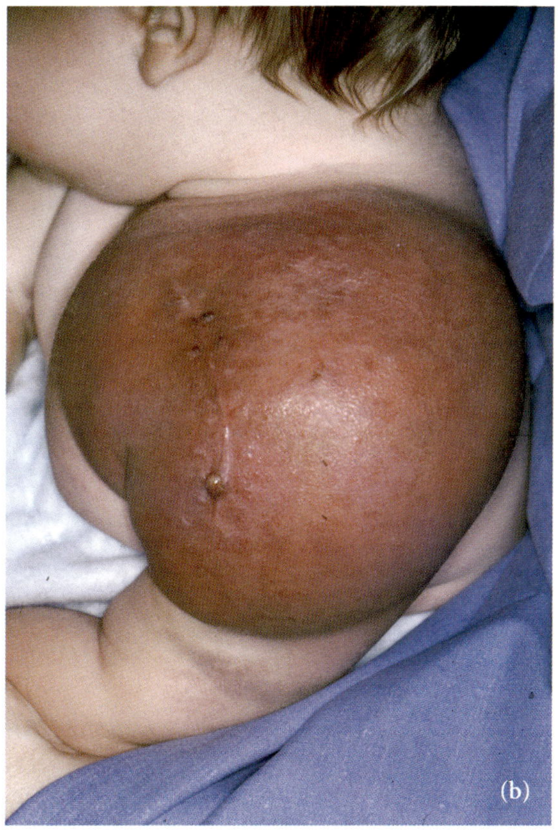

The appearance of the tumor during KMP may be quite different depending on the patient. Here are two major presentations: major bruise (a) in a tumor which was a biopsy-proven TA before the platelet entrapping phenomenon occurred, and a more inflammatory appearance (b) in a large swelling lump of the shoulder, also a TA on a biopsy performed during the KMP.

Clinical Aspects of Tufted Angioma, Kaposiform Hemangioendothelioma, and the Kasabach–Merritt Phenomenon

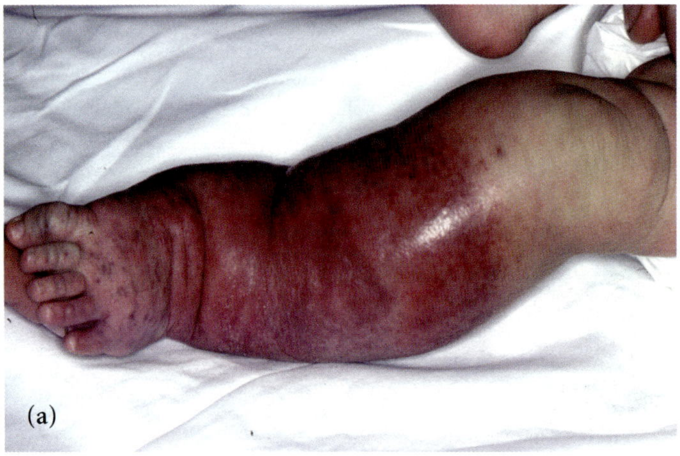

The thrombocytopenia and bulk of the tumor in this boy (a) affected with KMP was controlled after multiple therapeutic approaches including glucocorticosteroids and ticlopidine plus aspirin, and he also received radiotherapy. Years later, a slight "fibrosis" persisted and made the ankle thicker (b): this was considered to be a sequela of radiation therapy until the biopsy indicated residual TA (type III residuum of the KMP tumor).

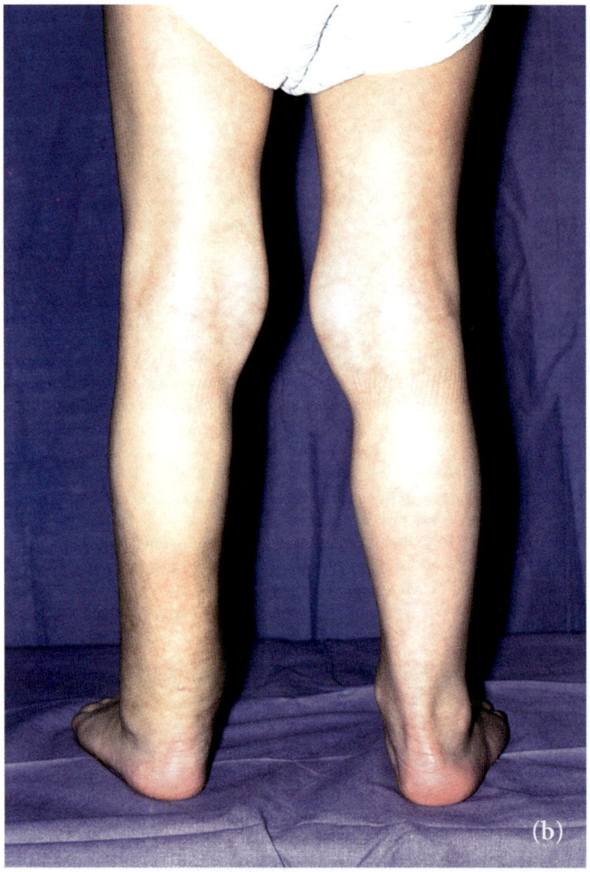

Clinical Aspects of Tufted Angioma, Kaposiform Hemangioendothelioma, and the Kasabach–Merritt Phenomenon

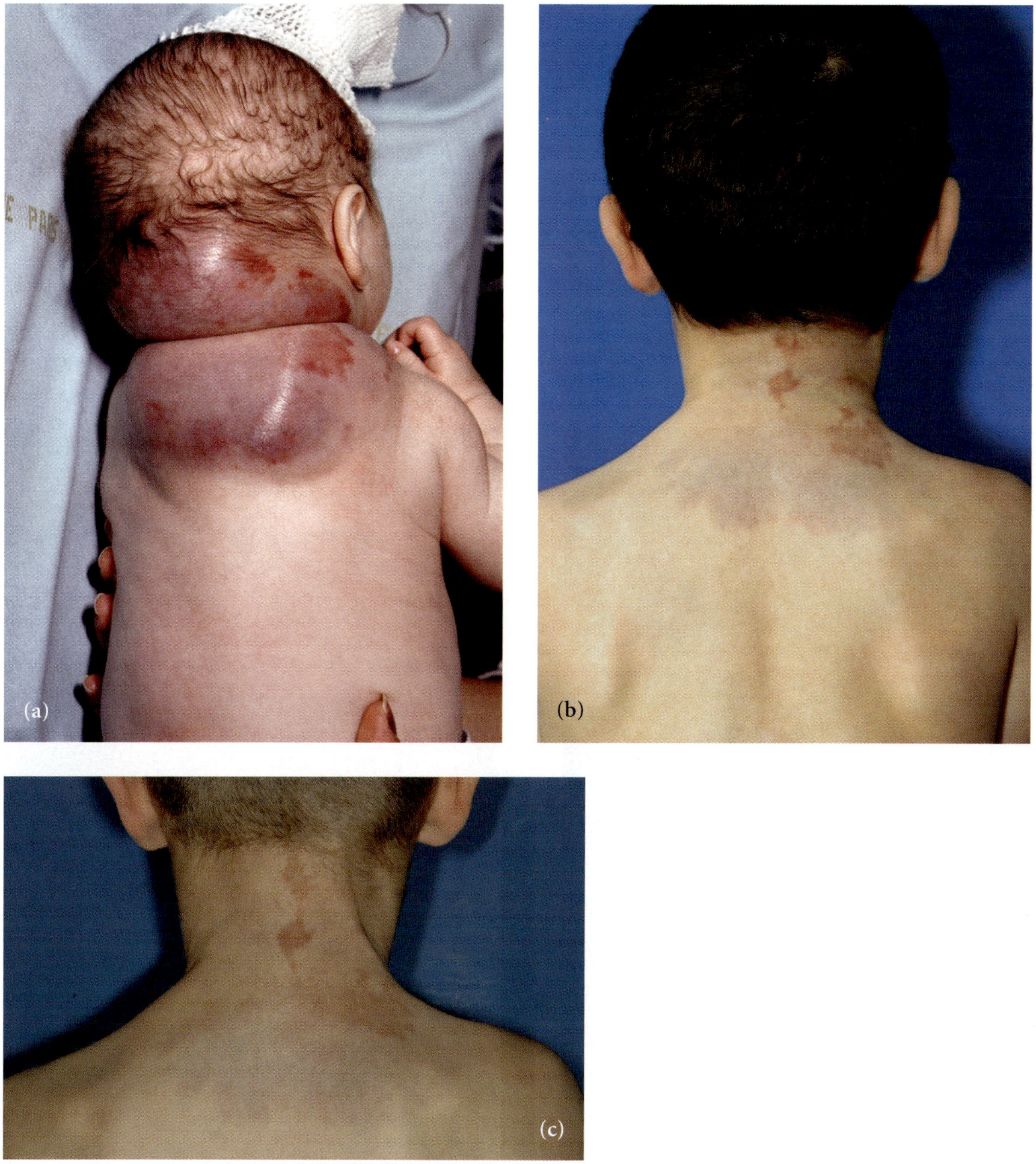

This massive congenital tumor of the nape and upper back with thrombocytopenia was present at birth (a); on MRI it permeated the muscles. Prednisone (5 mg/kg/day) did not improve the platelet count. The KMP was controlled using vincristine treatment. At 7 years of age, the residual lesion was a pseudocapillary malformation (type I residuum of KMP) and MRI showed only minor signal modification of the muscles of the nape. However, comparing the appearance of the nape at 5 years (b) and 7 years (c) it appeared that a fibrotic muscular band had developed. Although the child complained of intermittent pain and weakness of the neck, neurological examination remained normal during the 7 years of follow-up.

Clinical Aspects of Tufted Angioma, Kaposiform Hemangioendothelioma, and the Kasabach–Merritt Phenomenon

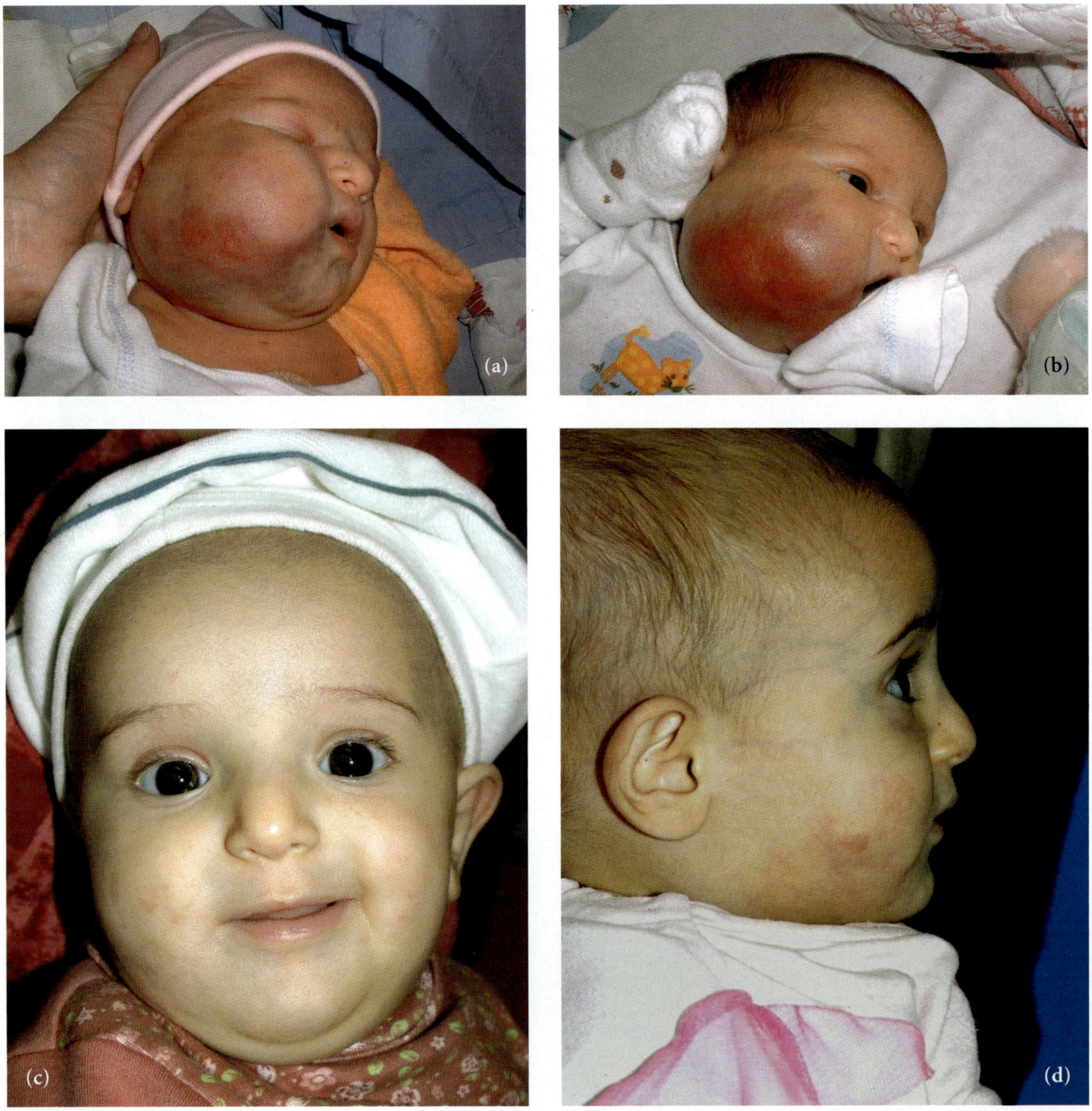

The congenital tumor in the cheek (a) and severe thrombocytopenia were not influenced by glucocorticosteroid treatment; 2 weeks after birth the girl received a platelet infusion and within 24 h the tumor became more tense and shiny (b), and platelet infusions were therefore no longer prescribed. Then the infant received vincristine treatment with an excellent outcome, normalization of the very low platelet counts in a few months, and excellent cosmetic results at 6 months of age at the end of the treatment (c), and better again at 10 months of age (d) with a minor pink stain (type I residuum of the KMP tumor) in the cheek. Platelet infusions are known to accentuate the platelet entrapping within the tumor, clotting and hemorrhage and growth of the tumor; they have a very short half-life in KMP patients and they have no role in management of KMP, except when the patient has visceral bleeding or when biopsy or excision of the lesion is considered (8, 21).

Clinical Aspects of Tufted Angioma, Kaposiform Hemangioendothelioma, and the Kasabach–Merritt Phenomenon

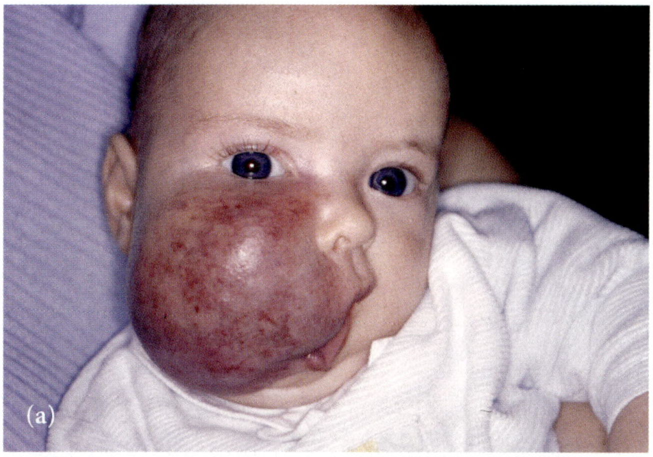

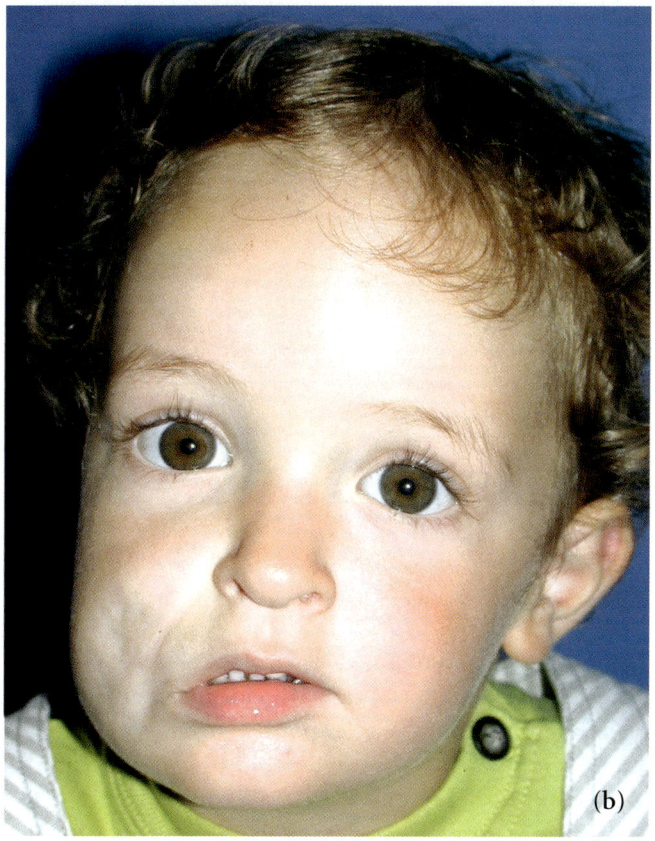

A congenital purple tumor with a double contour was located along the nose in the right cheek at birth. It then slowly enlarged to create a large mauve mass displacing the lips commissure, which was present when the infant was brought to us for diagnostic advice; at that stage (a) the platelet count was very low and KMP was diagnosed. Vincristine treatment was very effective. Three years after the end of treatment, a residual pink infiltration persisted in the lower part of the cheek and nasolabial fold (type III residuum of KMP), but it was still slowly improving (b).

Clinical Aspects of Tufted Angioma, Kaposiform Hemangioendothelioma, and the Kasabach–Merritt Phenomenon

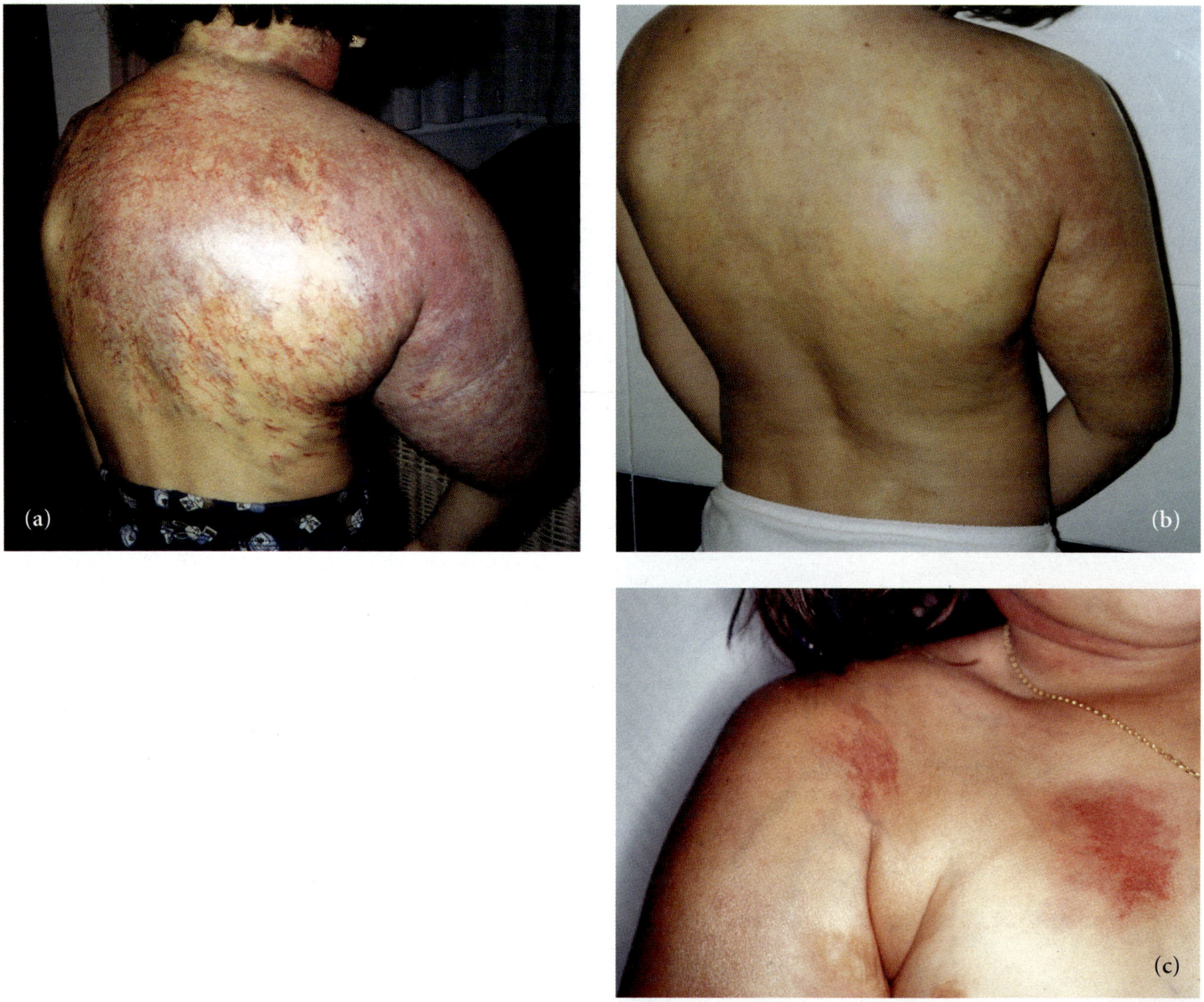

This massive telangiectatic tumor of the right arm and back (a) had not responded to the pharmacological treatments used in infancy. When the girl was seen she had been without treatment for years; she was in a poor general condition, had a severe thrombocytopenia, was bleeding easily, also had lymphatic fluid oozing from vesicles on the lateral aspect of the chest. Among complications, she endured pain, cardiac failure, and scoliosis, and was unable to go to school. Combined ticlopidine and aspirin treatment was initiated (she had never received this before) and she had a dramatic clinical and hematological improvement within a few months (b). The good results were maintained with the same treatment sustained over the next 3 years. Residual lesions in the lateral neck and chest were slightly infiltrated red stains (type I residuum (10)) clinically reminiscent of TA (c); on the trunk telangiectasia were observed as type II residuum of KMP.

Clinical Aspects of Tufted Angioma, Kaposiform Hemangioendothelioma, and the Kasabach–Merritt Phenomenon

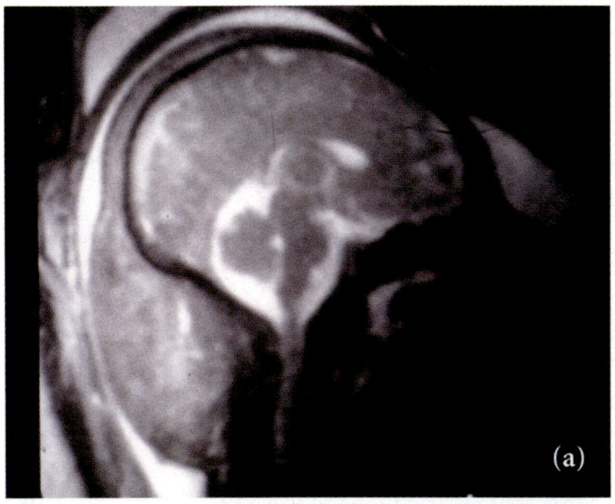

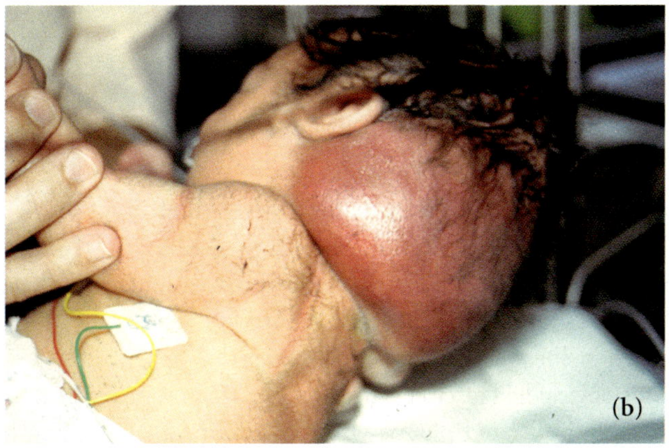

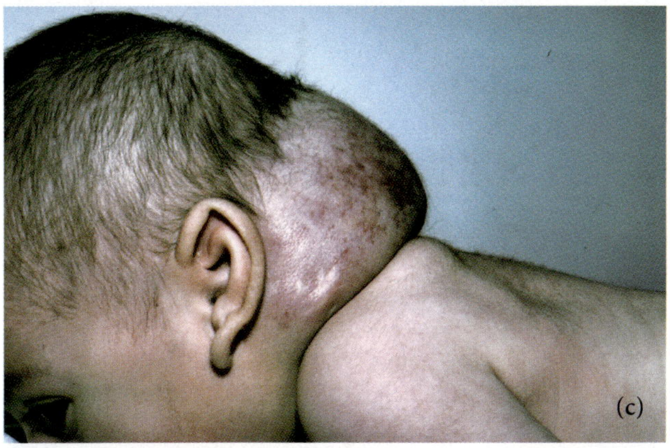

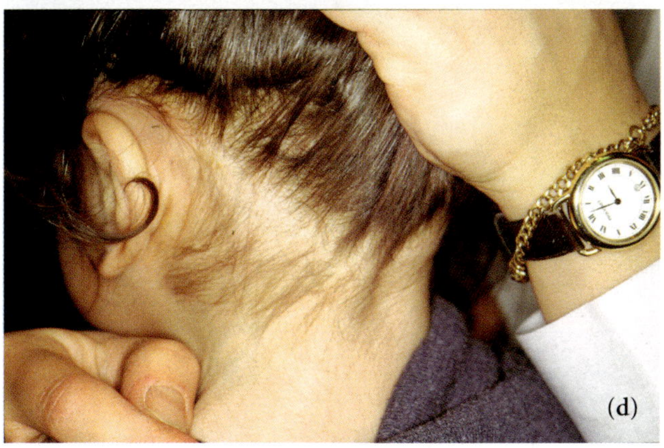

Prenatal diagnosis of the tumor associated with KMP was made in the third trimester: prenatal MRI performed at 7 months of pregnancy shows the bulky tumor in the nape of the neck (a). The tumor at birth (b) was shiny and fragile. No response was observed with steroids, and ticlopidine and aspirin. Effective treatment with vincristine first improved the biological parameters (platelets increased and D-dimers slowly decreased). At the end of treatment the mass was still large with alopecia (c) and was painful on palpation. It progressively reduced its size over 2 years and hair grew normally (d). No unwanted side-effects were observed in 8 years of follow-up. A slight type III residuum of the tumor was evidenced by Doppler and MRI in the skin and muscles of the nape.

Clinical Aspects of Tufted Angioma, Kaposiform Hemangioendothelioma, and the Kasabach–Merritt Phenomenon

This adolescent was treated soon after birth for a congenital KMP with a large bumped thoracic tumor. She received glucocorticosteroids, ticlopidine and aspirin, radiotherapy, and finally remained under ticlopidine and aspirin treatment for years. We saw her when she was 13 years old because of recurrence of thrombocytopenia after cessation of her treatment. Her lesion was a deeply infiltrated plaque with well-defined margins on the lateral thorax. Long telangiectasia were running over her torso. There was also a newly developed bump under normal skin in her back and bony lytic lesions were discovered in her ribs. A biopsy was performed to rule out radiation-induced angiosarcoma, and it indicated KHE. Platelet counts were between 5000 and 15000. She was treated consecutively with vincristine, interferon alpha 2b, thalidomide, and again ticlopidine and aspirin, and topical imiquimod, without any further clinical and hematological improvement over the next 3 years. Relapse of KMP after a long interval is rare (25).

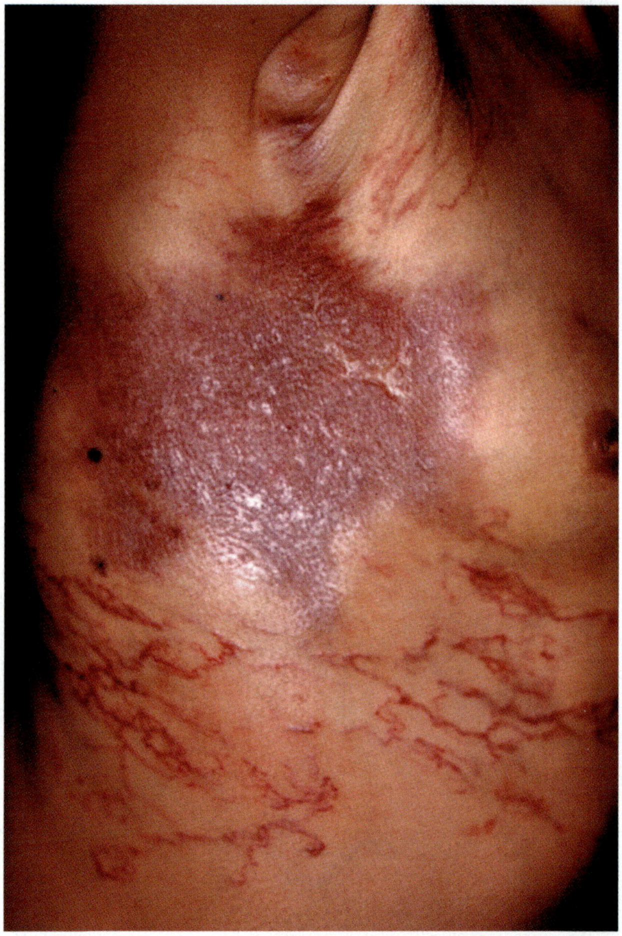

References

1 Blei F, Karp N, Rofsky N, Rosen R, Greco MA. Successful multimodal therapy for kaposiform hemangioendothelioma complicated by Kasabach–Merritt phenomenon, case report and review of the literature. *Pediatr Hematol Oncol* 1998; **15**: 295–305.

2 Brasansac D, Janic D, Boricic I, Jovanovic N, Dokamanovic L. Retroperitoneal kaposiform hemangioendothelioma with tufted angioma like features in an infant with Kasabach–Merritt syndrome. *Pathol Int* 2003; **53**: 627–31.

3 Catteau B, Enjolras O, Delaporte E, Friedel J, Breviere G, Wassef M, Lecomte-Houcke M, Piette F, Bergoend H. Angiome en touffes sclérosant. *Ann Dermatol Venereol* 1998; **125**: 682–7.

4 Cho KH, Kim SH, Park KC, Lee AY, Song KY, Chi JG, Lee YS, Kim KJ. Angioblastoma (Nakagawa) – is it the same as tufted angioma? *Clin Exp Dermatol* 1991; **16**: 110–13.

5 Debelenko, Perz-Atayde AR, Mulliken JB, Liang MG, Archibald TH, Kozakewich HP. D2-40 immunohistochemical analysis of pediatric vascular tumors reveals positivity in kaposiform hemangioendothelioma. *Mod Pathol* 2005; **18**: 1454–60.

6 Dewerdt S, Callens A, Machet L, Grangeponte MC, Vaillant L, Lorette G. Acquired tufted angioma in an adult: failure of pulsed dye laser therapy. *Ann Dermatol Venereol* 1998; **125**: 47–9.

7 Drolet BA, Scott LA, Esterly NB, Gosain AK. Early surgical intervention in a patient with Kasabach–Merritt phenomenon. *J Pediatr* 2001; **138**: 756–8.

8 Enjolras O, Wassef M, Mazoyer E, Frieden IJ, Rieu PN, Drouet L, Taieb A, Stalder JF, Escande JP. Infants with Kasabach–Merritt syndrome do not have 'true' hemangioma. *J Pediatr* 1997; **130**: 631–40.

9 Enjolras O, Wassef M, Dosquet Ch, Drouet L, Fortier G, Josset P, Merland JJ, Escande JP. Syndrome de Kasabach–Merritt sur angiome en touffes congénital. *Ann Dermatol Venereol* 1998; **125**: 257–60.

10 Enjolras O, Mulliken JB, Wassef M, Frieden IJ, Rieu PN, Burrows PE, Salhi A, Leaute-Labreze C, Kozakewich HP. Residual lesions after Kasabach–Merritt phenomenon in 41 patients. *J Am Acad Dermatol* 2000; **42**: 275–9.

11 Esterly N. Kasabach–Merritt syndrome in infants. *J Am Acad Dermatol* 1983; **8**: 504–13.

12 Ettlinger JJ, Fleming PJ, Joffe HS, Kennedy CTC. Cavernous haemangioma with Kasabach–Merritt syndrome: treatment with alpha interferon. *J R Soc Med* 1996; **89**: 55P–56P.

13 Ezekowitz RA, Mulliken JB, Folkman J. Interferon alfa-2a therapy for life-threatening hemangiomas of infancy. *N Engl J Med* 1992; **326**: 1456–63.

14 Fukunaga M, Ushigome S, Ishikawa E. Kaposiform hemangioendothelioma associated with Kasabach–Merritt syndrome. *Histopathology* 1996; **28**: 281–4.

15 Haisley-Royster C, Enjolras O, Frieden IJ, Garzon MD, Oranje A, Gonzalez F, Frangoul H, LeMoine P, Prose NS, Adams D. Kasabach–Merritt phenomenon: a retrospective study of treatment with vincristine. *J Pediatr Hematol Oncol* 2002; **24**: 459–62.

16 Herron MD, Coffin CM, Vanderhooft SL. Tufted angioma: variability in clinical morphology. *Pediatr Dermatol* 2002; **19**: 394–401.

17 Igarashi M, Oh-I T, Koga M. The relationship between angioblastoma (Nakagawa) and tufted angioma: report of four cases with angioblastoma and a literature-based comparison of the two conditions. *J Dermatol* 2000; **27**: 537–42.

18 Lyons LL, North PE, Mac-Moune Lai F, Stoler MH, Folpe AL, Weiss SW. Kaposiform hemangioendothelioma. A study of 33 cases emphasizing its pathologic, immunophenotypic, and biologic uniqueness from juvenile hemangioma. *Am J Surg Pathol* 2004; **28**: 559–68.

19 Mac-Moune Lai F, To KF, Choi PC, Leung PC, Kumta SM, Yuen PP, Lam WY, Cheung AN, Allen PW. Kaposiform hemangioendothelioma: five patients with cutaneous lesions and long follow-up. *Mod Pathol* 2001; **14**: 1087–92.

20 Mentzel T, Mazzoleni G, Dei Tos A, Fletcher CDM. Kaposiform hemangioendothelioma in adults. Clinicopathologic and immunohistochemical study of three cases. *Am J Clin Pathol* 1997; **108**: 450–5.

21 Mulliken JB, Anupindi S, Ezekowitz RAB, Mihm MC Jr. Case 13-2004: a newborn girl with a large cutaneous lesion, thrombocytopenia, and anemia. *N Engl J Med* 2004; **350**: 1764–75.

22 Munn SE, Jackson JE, Russel Jones R. Tufted angioma responding to high dose systemic steroids. *Clin Exp Dermatol* 1994; **19**: 511–14.

23 Nako Y, Fukushima N, Igarashi T, Hoshino M, Sugiyama M, Tomomasa T, Morikawa A. Successful interferon therapy in a neonate with life-threatening Kasabach–Merritt syndrome. *J Perinatol* 1997; **17**: 244–7.

24 Niedt GW, Greco MA, Wieczorek R, Blanc WA, Knowles DM. Hemangioma with Kaposi's sarcoma-like features: report of two cases. *Pediatr Pathol* 1989; **9**: 567–75.

25 Ohtsuka T, Saegusa M, Yamakage A, Yamazaki S. Angioblastoma (Nakagawa) with hyperhidrosis, and relapse after a 10-year interval. *Br J Dermatol* 2000; **143**: 223–4.

26 Okada E, Tamura A, Ishikawa O, Miyachi Y. Tufted angioma (angioblastoma) case report and review of 41 cases in the Japanese literature. *Clin Exp Dermatol* 2000; **25**: 627–30.

27 Park KC, Ahn PS, Lee YS, Kim KH, Cho KH. Treatment of angioblastoma with recombinant interferon-α2. *Pediatr Dermatol* 1995; **12**: 184–6.

28 Requena L, Sangueza OP. Cutaneous vascular proliferation. Part II. *J Am Acad Dermatol* 1997; **37**: 887–919.

29 Sarkar M, Mulliken JB, Kozakewich HPW, Robertson RL, Burrows PE. Thrombocytopenic coagulopathy (Kasabach–Merritt phenomenon) is associated with kaposiform hemangioendothelioma and not with common infantile hemangioma. *Plast Reconstr Surg* 1997; **100**: 1377–86.

30 Satter EK, Graham BS, Gibbs NF. Congenital tufted angioma. *Pediatr Dermatol* 2002; **19**: 445–7.

31 Suarez SM, Pensler JM, Paller AS. Response of deep tufted angioma to interferon alfa. *J Am Acad Dermatol* 1995; **33**: 124–6.

32 Tsang WYW, Chan JKC. Kaposi-like hemangioendothelioma. A distinctive vascular neoplasm of the retroperineum. *Am J Surg Pathol* 1991; **15**: 982–9.

33 Velin P, Dupont D, Golkar A, Valla JS. Syndrome de Kasabach–Merritt neonatal guéri par exérèse chirurgicale complète de l'angiome. *Arch Pediatr* 1998; **5**: 295–7.

34 Vin-Christian K, McCalmont TH, Frieden IJ. Kaposiform hemangioendothelioma, an aggressive locally invasive vascular tumor that can minic hemangioma of infancy. *Arch Dermatol* 1997; **133**: 1573–8.

35 Wananukul S, Nuchprayoon I, Seksarun P. Treatment of Kasabach–Merritt syndrome: a stepwise regimen of prednisolone, dipyridamole and interferon. *Int J Dermatol* 2003; **42**: 741–8.

36 Weiss SW, Goldblum JR (eds). *Enzinger and Weiss's Soft Tissue Tumors.* 4th Edn, St Louis: Mosby; ch. 23: pp. 837–890; ch. 24: pp. 891–915, 2001.

37 Wilmer A, Katz M, Bocker T, Wollina U. Tufted angioma. *Eur J Dermatol* 1999; **9**: 51–3.

38 Wilson-Jones E, Orkin M. Tufted angioma (angioblastoma): a benign progressive angioma not to be confused with Kaposi's sarcoma or low-grade angiosarcoma. *J Am Acad Dermatol* 1989; **20**: 214–25.

39 Wong SN, Tay YK. Tufted angioma: a report of five cases. *Pediatr Dermatol* 2002; **19**: 388–93.

40 Zukerberg LR, Nickoloff BJ, Weiss SW. Kaposiform hemangioendothelioma of infancy and childhood. An aggressive neoplasm associated with Kasabach–Merritt syndrome and lymphangiomatosis. *Am J Surg Pathol* 1993; **17**: 321–8.

PART III

Vascular Malformations

CHAPTER III.A

Capillary Malformations (CM)

Introduction

Capillary malformations (CM) are hemodynamically inactive, slow-flow vascular malformations affecting the capillary network of skin and mucosa, sometimes invading deeper underlying structures specifically in the facial area. They include common CMs also known as "port-wine stains" and "telangiectasia." Both can occur as a single isolated anomaly or in association with other abnormalities. Some are included in complex syndromes, the majority being sporadic and some being familial. We can also include the various "angiokeratomas", localized, systematized or diffuse (angiokeratoma corporis diffusum), familial or not.

III.A.1 Common Capillary Malformations: Port-wine Stains (PWS)

Clinical Aspects

This is the most common type of vascular malformation. Typically a port wine stain (PWS) is present at birth and persists lifelong growing proportionately. However, rare acquired PWSs develop and progress in adolescents or adults; the possible role of trauma has been stressed (1), and reported as Fegeler syndrome (51).

A PWS is a more- or less-extensive well-demarcated red macular stain. Localized segmental PWSs are common on the face. On the face, CMs are commonly sub-classified as lateral CM (PWS) and medial CM (also known as salmon patch). Lateral PWSs of the face always persist whereas medial lesions usually become lighter and some disappear, particularly those of the mid-face. Metameric distribution occurs on the trunk and limbs; on the other hand it seems that PWSs never spread along Blaschko lines. A stain with geographical contour on the lateral aspect of the thigh and knee at birth usually predicts the further development of a complex syndrome (Klippel–Trenaunay syndrome) including capillary, venous, and lymphatic abnormalities (19, 44). Diffusely scattered PWSs all over the body are less common, except in Proteus syndrome.

A PWS often has a bright red, scarlet color at birth, because of the high neonatal hemoglobin content of skin capillaries. Then it fades over 1 or 2 months to reach a pink or red hue. The color is the result of ectatic capillaries in the dermis carrying more blood than small normal channels. Deficiency in perivascular innervation has been reported (61, 62). Some PWSs in adults take on a darker color, tissular hyperplasia gives them a cobblestone appearance: this is obvious in some facial CMs undergoing progressive dilatation of the capillaries, an increasing number of ectatic capillaries, and often sebaceous hyperplasia and fibrosis. A striking nodular hyperplasia may develop in some patients, creating disfigurement (36). According to Sanchez-Carpintero et al. (58), thickening and nodularity can, at least in some cases, be explained by hamartomatous changes in the connective tissue surrounding the dilated engorged capillaries: in addition to the prominent vascular ectasia they found pilo-sebaceous abnormalities, arrector pili-type smooth-muscle bundles, and neural and mesenchymal hamartomatous changes. PWSs of the face, particularly those involving the cheek and lips, are sometimes associated with hyperplasia of underlying soft tissues and bones resulting in macrocheilia, gum hypertrophy, epulis, and bony maxilla hypertrophy in the three planes with dental malocclusion.

Diagnosis

Diagnosis of CM/PWS is made clinically without the need for complementary investigation. However, two vascular lesions may generate confusion: the red, sometimes telangiectatic, congenital stain precursor of hemangioma (see the section on Hemangioma page 53) and an AVM in a quiescent stage (stage 1 AVM) (see the section on AVM, page 261) which requires US/Doppler duplex scan confirmation.

Treatment

Since the 1980s the flashlamp pumped-pulsed dye laser (PDL) has been considered the best laser system for the treatment of PWS. Modified devices enabling longer pulse widths, longer wavelengths, and bigger spot sizes have improved PDL efficacy (43). The use of dynamic surface cooling, reducing the risk of epidermal damage and minimizing the pain of treatment, has permitted the application of more-effective, higher energy fluence. Nonetheless, only one-fifth of PWSs clear completely, although the color of the majority of treated CMs improves significantly (28, 68). Various methods have been tested to try to predict and improve the response to laser treatment, depending on the color of the stain, depth of vessels and size of ectatic capillaries. Spectrophotometry first gave a better correlation between color, clinical appearance, and hemoglobin content. Videomicroscopy permits localization of the ectatic capillary network and allowed

Eubanks and McBurney (21) to correlate areas of poorer response to laser treatment (for example the V2 facial PWS) with the type of ectasia: type 2 pattern (rings) corresponded to ectasia of deeper horizontal plexus. High-frequency ultrasound evaluation confirmed that thicker areas of skin with PWS respond worse to PDL (48). Under confocal microscopy of biopsies of PWSs, decreased nerve density, increased capillary density, and increased mean blood vessel diameter correlated with poor response to PDL (61).

III.A.2 Capillary Malformations and Associations

We will illustrate quite common associations occurring with CM/PWS, such as CM and nevus anemicus, CM and pigmentary disorders with the various types of phakomatosis pigmentovascularis, the problem of CM as a marker of spinal dysraphism, CM with hyperhidrosis due to increased eccrine glands in eccrine angiomatous hamartoma or sudoriparous angioma.

III.A.2.1 PHAKOMATOSIS PIGMENTOVASCULARIS

This association of cutaneous vascular anomalies (CM and nevus anemicus) and epidermal or pigmentary changes (29, 30, 57) is considered to be the result of the "twin-spotting" phenomenon (30). Five types are currently described: type I is CM and epidermal nevus; type II is CM with dermal melanocytosis (aberrant Mongolian spots) a very common finding in skin of color; type III is the association of CM and nevus spilus (54); type IV may combine CM and aberrant Mongolian spots and nevus spilus; type V is the association of cutis marmorata telangiectatica congenita and Mongolian spots (65). Nevus anemicus can be also present in types II, III and IV. Each group is classified as A (without another anomaly) or B (with additional abnormalities, including nevus of Ota, KTS, and SWS (27)). Extracutaneous anomalies have also been reported.

III.A.2.2 ECCRINE ANGIOMATOUS HAMARTOMA (EAH)

This clinically heterogeneous lesion, often congenital or appearing in children (46) is more common on the distal extremities, notably a toe or ankle. Some patients have only a purple or bluish nodule, others have a plaque-type lesion and some have a very large infiltrated blue-purple plaque with increased sweating, occasionally dampening the clothes of the trunk. The lesion is usually solitary and often not well-defined at its edges; it hurts on palpation or contact, and in our experience sweating is obvious if the patient feels anxious during examination. Infiltration is variable. Color varies from yellowish to brownish or pink to bluish-purple. Hypertrichosis can be present. The lesion grows slowly and recurs after incomplete excision. Pain increases in adulthood and it is often because of the pain that patients seek treatment. If surgical excision is reasonably possible, we advise doing it during childhood, when the lesion has a reasonable size. Histopathologic features include closely associated thin-walled irregular capillaries and abundant eccrine glands and ducts; larger channels may be present (veins) as well as fatty tissue, hair follicles, and a hyperplastic overlying epidermis (55).

III.A.3 Syndromic Capillary Malformations

III.A.3.1 STURGE–WEBER SYNDROME (SWS)

This systematized vascular syndrome is likely caused by a somatic mutation in the anterior neural primordium. The "whole" disease includes a facial PWS always staining the so-called V1 area (forehead and upper eyelid) and sometimes extending further, ipsilateral vascular anomalies of the leptomeninges, and ipsilateral ocular abnormalities. The dermis of the face is made of cells originating from the cephalic neural crests (except endothelial cells, of mesodermal origin). SWS is hypothesized to be the result of a very early mutational event arising in the prosencephalic neural crest, a region providing cells to the dermis of the supra-ocular area and nasal bud. This may arise at a time when precursors of the V1 dermis, ocular choroid and piamater are still in the anterior neural primordium, before they start their migration to their final destination. The dermis of the V2 (maxillary) and V3 (mandibular) areas is made of cells from the mesencephalic neural crests, cells not forming leptomeninges: this is why SWS is not linked to a PWS occupying the V2 and V3 skin, without V1 location. However, the limits are not strict at the boundaries of these three regions (20). At these boundaries, cells of various origin may mix together: this explains slight variation in the limits of the so-called V1, V2, and V3 PWSs. It is noteworthy that, although we still retain this terminology of V1, V2, and V3 distribution of facial PWS, the sensitive trigeminal nerve (Vth nerve) has nothing to do with the pathogenesis of facial PWS and SWS, as was thought in the past.

Epilepsy in SWS may be devastating and it usually starts very early in life between birth and one year. About 10% of infants with V1 PWS actually have leptomeningeal vascular anomalies. Cognitive deficit and mental retardation, loss of developmental milestones, and motor deficit contralateral to the

Table 12 Neurological risks associated with vascular anomalies involving the cephalic region.

Diagnosis	*Neurological associations*	*Neurological consequences*
Infantile hemangioma	PHACE(S) syndrome: posterior fossa malformations, arterial intracranial anomalies	Symptom-free or seizures, ischemic attacks, stroke
Sturge–Weber syndrome	Leptomeningeal vascular malformation, cerebral atrophy and calcifications	Epilepsy, hemiplegia, developmental delay, mental retardation, headaches
Proteus syndrome	Hemimegalencephaly, hydrocephalus, abnormal cerebral cortex, tumors	Seizures, developmental delay, and mental retardation
Cutis marmorata–macrocephaly syndrome	Hemimegalencephaly, hydrocephalus	Mental retardation
Ataxia telangiectasia		Ataxia
HHT (Rendu–Osler–Weber disease)	Cerebral AVM, risk of cerebral abscess if pulmonary AVF	Headaches, bacterial emboli, and stroke
Cephalic VM	Developmental venous anomalies (DVA)	Symptom-free or headaches
Bonnet–Dechaume–Blanc or Wyburn-Mason syndrome	Brain AVM	Headaches, seizures, cerebral hemorrhage
Orbital LM	Dural AVF, DVA	Exophthalmos, conjunctival chemosis, intracranial hypertension

HHT=hereditary hemorrhagic telangiectasia; AVM=arteriovenous malformation; AVF=arteriovenous fistula; VM=venous malformation; LM=lymphatic malformation.

meningeal lesions follow the onset of epilepsy, with a correlation between prolonged seizure and further severe developments, and motor and intellectual deficits (Table 12).

Prevention of the first seizure by prophylactic antiepileptic treatment aims at avoiding these severe developments (67). The seizures decrease strongly after puberty. Ocular follow-up is also mandatory because of the risk of choroidal vascular anomaly and of glaucoma. The PWS can be treated with the PDL after pharmacological control of epilepsy is obtained. Surgical treatment (callosotomy, hemispherotomy, hemispherectomy) is performed in patients with seizures that are intractable to medication, first to end seizures, and hopefully to improve function secondarily (37).

III.A.3.2 KLIPPEL–TRENAUNAY SYNDROME AND RELATED SYNDROMES

At the limb and trunk level CM/PWSs occur in various clinical situations including:

1. diffuse CMs scattered over an extremity and adjacent trunk with apparently unsystematic spreading and no associated abnormality;

Table 13 Clinical characteristics of two different limb complex-combined vascular malformations with progressive overgrowth of the affected extremity.

Characteristics	*Klippel–Trenaunay syndrome*	*Parkes Weber syndrome*
Hemodynamics	Slow-flow	Fast-flow
Type of vascular anomaly	CM (geographic or not), VM (varicose veins), LM (lymphedema, lymphatic vesicles)	Multiple AVFs/AVM, pseudo-CM on skin (stage I dormant AVM), lymphedema
Skin temperature	Normal	Increased
Progressive overgrowth in length and girth	+	+
Visceral involvement	Possibly: GI tract, urinary, genitalia	Rare: AVM (pelvic), Cobb syndrome
Chronic coagulopathy with high D-dimers and low fibrinogen	+	–
Increased cardiac output and possibly congestive cardiac failure	–	+
Deep vein thrombosis, risk of pulmonary embolism	+	–
Venous stasis skin alteration, ulcers	+	–
Pseudo Kaposi, skin ischemic changes, ulcers	–	+

CM=capillary malformation; VM= venous malformation; LM= lymphatic malformation; AVM=arteriovenous malformation; AVF=arteriovenous fistula.

2. PWS fully covering a limb with congenital hypertrophy of the same extremity, with proportionate growth over the years;
3. a slow-flow combined and complex vascular malformation with CM, varicose veins, very often LM manifesting as either lymphedema or lymphatic vesicles or both, and progressive overgrowth in length and girth of the affected limb: this is Klippel–Trenaunay syndrome (KTS) (7) (Table 13).

KTS is associated with SWS in some patients. It may occur in Proteus syndrome. In infants a geographic skin stain on the external aspect of the thigh and knee, rapidly colonized by clear and purple lymphatic vesicles, is predictive of complicated KTS, with lymphatic anomalies increasing over the years and a usually severe progressive discrepancy in limb growth (44).

The work-up for young patients with KTS should not be invasive: we rarely need angiographic or lymphoscintigraphic data for their management, and an US/Doppler duplex scan, sometimes coupled with MRI, gives adequate data on the vascular anomalies, extent of lesions, and possible associated intestinal and urinary vascular anomalies. Patients with KTS and limb hypertrophy are not at higher risk of Wilms tumor than the general population and thus they do not need routine Wilms tumor screening (24). Another study based on a literature review found only one report of hemihypertrophy, Wilms tumor, and KTS (a picture confirms the diagnosis) in 58 cases, and it concludes that routine screening for Wilms tumor in patients with KTS is unnecessary, unless the patient has generalized hemihypertrophy (39).

The mainstay of management of KTS in pediatric patients with KTS is orthopedic assessment once a year, and wearing elastic garments on a lifelong basis. Laser (FPDL or other) treatments are rarely very useful and adverse effects are more frequent than at other sites. Epiphyseodesis is considered at around 10 to 13 years of age, depending on the growth curve of the child, when leg discrepancy is important (if more than 2 or 3 cm). Surgical treatment of varicose veins is not considered before puberty, except for very enlarged marginal veins in the thigh.

III.A.3.3 PROTEUS SYNDROME AND PROTEIFORM SYNDROMES

Proteus syndrome is a complex syndrome (34, 69). It combines asymmetric growth of bones in a haphazard distribution, mainly in the distal extremities (macrodactyly in digits of the hands or feet), spinal cord (creating scoliosis), and skull (with exostoses). Subcutaneous benign tumors such as lipoma, fibroma, and plantar collagenoma (this connective tissue nevus gives to the sole of foot, and sometimes the palm of hand, a cerebriform aspect, and is considered as an absolute criterion for a diagnosis of Proteus syndrome (Table 14) (8, 9)). Epidermal nevus and vascular anomalies are also present. Hyperplasia is the most obvious presentation of Proteus lesions, but hypoplasia is also observed: either global hypoplasia, e.g. of an extremity, or patchy dermal hypoplasia (31). The vascular anomalies in Proteus syndrome have been underappraised until recently: Hoeger et al. (33) stressed the fact that they are present in 100% of patients with Proteus syndrome and that more than one type is often identified in a single patient. Extensive PWSs of a crimson red color at birth, macrocystic LM that may develop suddenly and quickly, varicose veins, and complex combined slow-flow vascular malformations of the KTS type, are all very common in Proteus syndrome. SWS is rarely present: it may occur in a patient whose PWS is in the V1 area, in the context of Proteus syndrome (unpublished personal data). Also, in our experience, no fast-flow anomaly with arteriovenous shunting (either localized or of the Parkes Weber syndrome type) is observed in Proteus syndrome, all the associated vascular anomalies being of the slow-flow type. Other reported findings are visceral anomalies. Hemimegalencephaly and migrational disorders seem to be the most common demonstrated brain anomaly, among a range of other situations, but seizures and intellectual impairment have rarely been reported (14). Benign and malignant neoplasias may affect the ovaries, testes, and central nervous system. In the most severe cases abnormalities tend to expand earlier in life.

Table 14 Revised diagnostic criteria for Proteus syndrome.

General criteria	*Specific criteria*
All of the following:	Either:
Mosaic distribution of lesions	Category A or,
Sporadic occurrence	Two from category B or,
Progressive course	Three from category C
Specific criteria categories	
A. 1. Cerebriform connective tissue nevus[a]	C. 1. Dysregulated adipose tissue
	Either one:
B. 1. Linear epidermal nevus	a. Lipomas
2. Asymmetric, disproportionate overgrowth[b]	b. Regional absence of fat
One or more:	2. Vascular malformations
a. Limbs:	One or more:
Arms/legs	a. Capillary malformation
Hands/feet/digits	b. Venous malformation
Extremities	c. Lymphatic malformation
b. Hyperostoses of the skull	3. Lung cysts
c. External auditory meatus	4. Facial phenotype[c]
d. Megaspondylodysplasia	All:
e. Viscera:	a. Dolichocephaly
Spleen/thymus	b. Long face
3. Specific tumors before 2nd decade	c. Down slanting palpebral fissures and/or minor ptosis
One of the following:	d. Low nasal bridge
a. Ovarian cystadenoma	e. Wide or anteverted nares
b. Parotid monomorphic adenoma	f. Open mouth at rest

To make a diagnosis of Proteus syndrome, one must have *all* the general criteria, and various specific criteria.

[a]Cerebriform connective tissue nevi are skin lesions characterized by deep grooves and gyration as seen on the surface of the brain.

[b]Asymmetric, disproportionate overgrowth should be carefully distinguished from asymmetric, proportionate overgrowth (see Discussion for recommended methods of distinction).

[c]The facial phenotype has been found, to date, only in PS in patients who have mental deficiency, and, in some cases, seizures and/or brain malformations.

Reproduced with permission from: Turner JT, Cohen MM, Biesecker LG. Reassessment of the Proteus syndrome literature. *Am J Med Genet* 2004; **130A**: 111–22. (Table III).

The disease is sporadic. Lesions are distributed in a mosaic state (8, 66). Mutations of *PTEN*, once considered as the cause of the disorder, were then considered not to be implicated in Proteus syndrome (66). Management is based on a palliative symptomatic approach, depending on the signs and symptoms, but orthopedic management is mandatory in all patients from infancy.

Criteria for diagnosing Proteus syndrome have been established (see Table 14). "Proteiform" syndromes exist with similar, predominant vascular anomalies, and a milder degree of orthopedic abnormalities and complications, often a moderately progressive hemi-hypertrophy and macrodactyly.

III.A.4 Telangiectasia and Syndromes with Telangiectasia

III.A.4.1 CUTIS MARMORATA TELANGIECTATICA CONGENITA

Also known as Van Lohuizen syndrome (19, 22) cutis marmorata telangiectatica congenita (CMTC) is mainly a sporadic idiopathic disease. Rare familial cases have been reported but these diagnoses are not fully convincing. A predilection for females is mentioned in some series (15, 52). The main vascular feature is telangiectasia. Skin is marbled: a more or less purple vascular reticulated network differs from common livedo in that there are associated telangiectases and focal linear atrophy in the center of some purple bands and meshes. Some thin branching telangiectatic edges of the strips are reminiscent of livedo racemosa. Atrophy can be prominent over the joints: these scarlet, atrophic, sometimes slightly hyperkeratotic lesions tend to ulcerate and end in bad scars. Some patients have associated blotchy, often pale PWSs. With time, lesions of CMTC tend to fade. However, if some CMTC may disappear, many patients, in our experience, remain with a residual violet telangiectatic more or less conspicuous vascular network throughout life (17). Ulcerations leave scars, usually over the knee or elbow. Some phlebectasia may be visible in late lesions. CMTC is either widespread or more frequently localized to one or more limbs and the trunk, or only part of an extremity. De Villers et al. (15) beautifully illustrated the various patterns of extent and distribution of CMTC in their 35 patients. CMTC is a benign vascular disease in a majority of infants. Many cases are limited to the skin (52). The most common associated feature is hypotrophy of the involved limb, or hemiatrophy if two limbs are affected. This discrepancy is obvious in infants with partial segmental CMTC, the most common situation: 65% of the 85 cases reported by Ben Amitai (6) had a localized CMTC. Hypotrophy mainly affects the circumference of the involved arm or leg, and predominantly concerns the subcutaneous fat; it does not get worse over the years of growth of the child. Diffuse CMTC is rare but it tends to have more severe associated abnormalities: beside orthopedic anomalies, as already described, ocular anomalies (glaucoma) and various neurological abnormalities are the most frequently reported associations. For the treatment of residual CMTC, laser treatment with PDL should be used with caution because these lesions tend to ulcerate and make crusts, even with low fluence, and scars are easily left (17).

III.A.4.2 ADAMS–OLIVER SYNDROME

This syndrome is described as the association of CMTC, scalp aplasia cutis, and transverse limb defects (16).

III.A.4.3 MACROCEPHALY – CUTIS MARMORATA SYNDROME

This syndrome combines macrocephaly, with or without intellectual impairment and brain anomalies, ocular anomalies, a midfacial CM, staining the glabellum, nose and lip philtrum, a diffusely marbled skin (in fact a marbled skin – cutis marmorata – but not a classic CMTC) and orthopedic anomalies (56).

III.A.4.4 RETICULATE DIFFUSE CM

A diffuse reticulate capillary malformation, giving the skin a marbled livedoid pattern, without the telangiectasia and depressed lines seen in typical CMTC, is rarely present in an infant. This appearance, fixed throughout life, carries a high risk of associated internal vascular abnormalities, including transient brain ischemic attacks and visceral vascular anomalies (pulmonary, renal, and ocular) (17).

III.A.4.5 RENDU–OSLER–WEBER DISEASE OR HEREDITARY HEMORRHAGIC TELANGIECTASIA

This autosomal-dominant disorder is inherited with varying penetrance and expressivity, and there are a wide variety of phenotypes (5). It is characterized by skin and mucosal telangiectasia, particularly nasal telangiectasia accountable for recurrent prolonged epistaxis. Nasal telangiectasia are mainly located in the anterior nasal cavity and on the middle turbinates (22). Telangiectasia can also affect the stomach and GI tract and can create severe visceral hemorrhages. Anemia requires iron supplementation. Arteriovenous malformations (AVM) and arteriovenous fistulas (AVF) are also observed in some hereditary hemorrhagic telangiectasia (HHT) patients: pulmonary, cerebral, spinal and liver fast-flow lesions can develop.

Two genotypes of HHT are currently known: HHT1 is linked to *endoglin (ENG)* mutations (chromosome 9q33) and HHT2 is linked to *ALK1* mutations (chromosome 12q13). A third locus has been localized: HHT3 maps to 5q31.5–32

(13), but the mutated gene is unknown. According to Kuehl et al. (38) AVMs occur more frequently in patients with *ALK1* mutations than in patients with *ENG* mutations. DNA testing for HHT1 and HHT2 is now available and it will enable us to detect asymptomatic patients in a given family, even during infancy, and screen them for their risk of AVM, as AVM of lungs and brain may be controlled by endovascular embolization (13). Pulmonary AVMs place the patient at risk of brain abscess due to the loss of the pulmonary filter, and prophylactic antibiotic treatment is advised. Molecular diagnosis also permits avoidance of unnecessary radiological imaging in nonaffected relatives (4).

III.A.4.6 ATAXIA TELANGIECTASIA

Ataxia telangiectasia (AT) is a rare autosomal recessive disease that combines ocular and cutaneous telangiectasia, progressive cerebellar ataxia and humoral immune deficiency (mainly IgA deficiency, but also IgG deficiency, and B and T lymphocytes altered response) responsible for recurrent sinopulmonary infections. Gait abnormalities tend to appear before telangiectasia (10). These patients also have a predisposition to cancer and a sensitivity to ionizing radiation. Alpha-fetoprotein levels are elevated (26). The disease is linked to mutations of *ATM* gene mapping to chromosome 11q22–23. Heterozygous carriers of germline ATM mutations are also at higher risk of malignancy (breast cancer) (32).

III.A.5 Angiokeratomas

Angiokeratoma defines the combination of ectatic capillaries of the dermis and hyperkeratotic epidermis giving the lesion both a dark-red hue and a scaly or warty central surface (55).

Various presentations exist, from solitary lesions to diffusely scattered plaques with always a distinctive dark-red color and a more or less obvious hyperkeratosis (60). "Fordyce angiokeratomas" occur as red to dark, 2 to 4 mm papules on the genitalia of males (mainly on the scrotum) and females (on the vulva) in late adulthood (55). "Angiokeratomas of Mibelli" appear on the fingers and toes and they may ulcerate and bleed easily. These acral tiny angiokeratomas sometimes involve other sites than hands and feet (63) and familial forms have been reported. "Solitary angiokeratoma" may mimic melanoma. "Angiokeratoma circumscriptum" develops as one or few large warty purple plaques or in a metameric linear distribution over an entire limb. "Hutchinson angioma serpiginosum" is made up of tiny papules of a bright dark red color. This metameric sporadic and idiopathic lesion is also known as Fabry II disease. It occurs on the limbs and corresponding trunk, and should be differentiated from "unilateral nevoid telangiectasia" developed around puberty and in young adults on the trunk, neck, and upper extremities. "Angiokeratoma corporis diffusum" is often indicative of an hereditary enzymatic disease.

Angiokeratoma corporis diffusum and Anderson–Fabry disease

This is an X-linked hereditary lysosomal storage disorder (OMIM # 301 500) caused by an absence or a deficit in the enzyme alpha galactosidase A (α-gal A), leading to lysosomal neutral glycosphingolipids (globotriaosylceramides) accumulation in various cellular types (in nearly all tissues). The mutated gene maps to Xq22. A large number of mutations have been reported but no genotype-phenotype correlation has been established. Hemizygous men are predominantly affected and in the past the disease was lethal at around 40 years of age. Carrier females may develop a milder form of the disease and 30% of them have angiokeratomas (40). In men, symptoms developing in childhood include angiokeratoma corporis diffusum (a majority of the tiny dark-red palpable lesions being in the buttocks and thigh, but they may also cover the elbows, feet, hands and navel (40); hyperkeratosis may be clinically inconspicuous), acroparesthesia (a burning and tingling pain of hands and feet that spreads to more proximal sites), hypohidrosis or anhidrosis, cornea verticillata. Visceral lesions appear in young adults: cardiac and pulmonary symptoms, transient ischemic brain attacks, stroke, and renal failure. The biopsy of an angiokeratoma shows lysosomal fine lamellar inclusions on electron microscopy. The diagnosis relies on the detection of α-gal A deficit in leucocytes and plasma. To avoid misinterpretation of inclusion bodies in cells in a biopsy of a skin lesion, the diagnosis requires biochemical confirmation (enzymatic analysis) and DNA mutation analysis (23, 42). Now-available enzyme replacement therapy with recombinant human alpha-galactosidase A (rh-alpha GalA = agalsidase alfa®) is a major step in the management of Fabry disease and the safety of the treatment has been reported in a multicenter phase 3 trial (70). It stabilizes, limits or prevents visceral lesions and it should improve not only the quality of life but also the prognosis, particularly the kidney and myocardial function in patients diagnosed early before the development of visceral complications (23).

Angiokeratoma corporis diffusum may also be the vascular skin marker of other lysosomal enzyme deficit and lysosomal storage disorders (β mannosidase deficiency, α fucosidase deficiency, α NAGA deficiency, sialidase deficiency, etc.), or may occur without any currently detectable inborn error of metabolism.

Figures

CAPILLARY MALFORMATIONS
Pathology

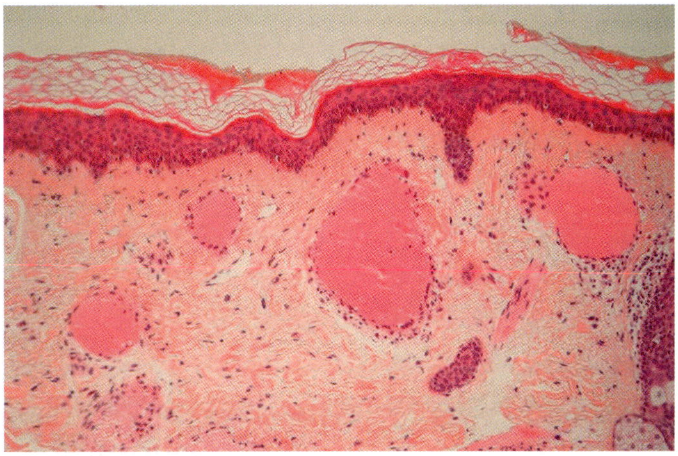

In young patients CMs are made of dilated capillaries, situated in the superficial reticular dermis. Their number is considered normal but their diameter is increased.

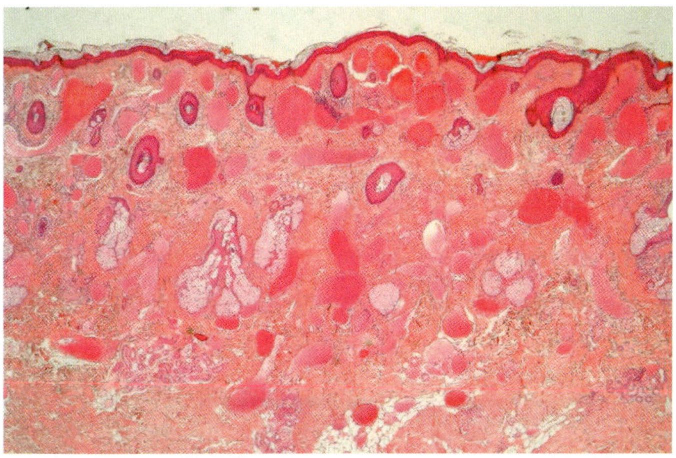

In adults the numbers of vessel sections appear increased on histological sections, and dilated vessels are found also in the deep reticular dermis. Their wall tends to thicken, resembling a venule.

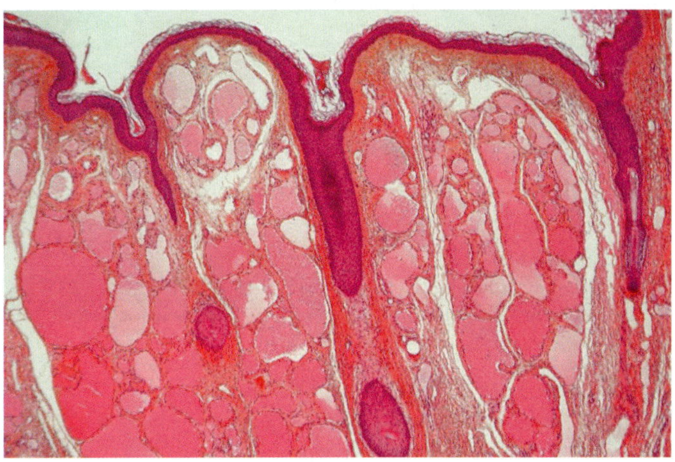

In hypertrophic CM the capillaries are more numerous and large, filling the dermis. The capillary sections tend to be grouped, each group probably representing multiple sections of the same tortuous vessel.

Pathology

In hypertrophic CM some groups of capillaries form well-delineated nodules of closely packed vessels, reminiscent of some nodular venous malformations.

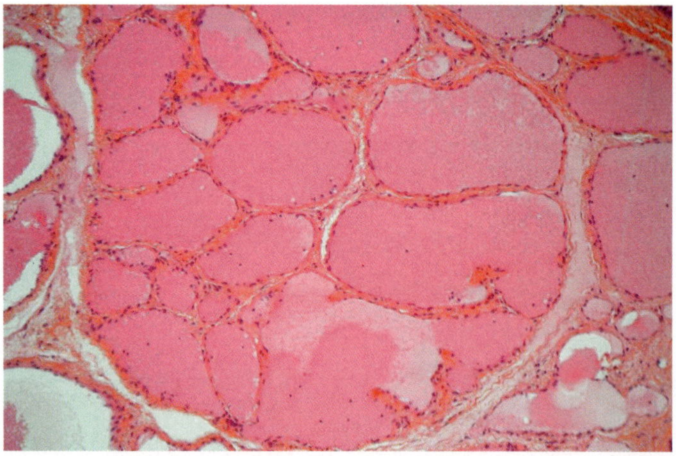

The deep part of hypertrophic CM often contains aggregates of coiled veins in the hypodermis.

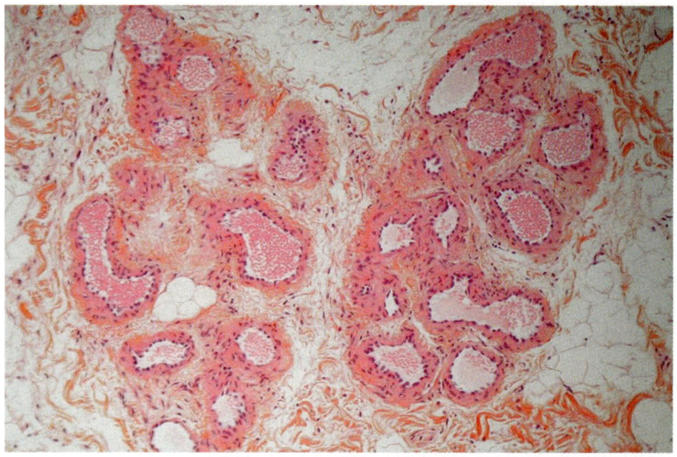

The nodules that are present on hypertrophic CM, may be either pyogenic granuloma (a reactive proliferation of capillaries mimicking a capillary hemangioma) or contain aggregates of dilated capillaries/venules.

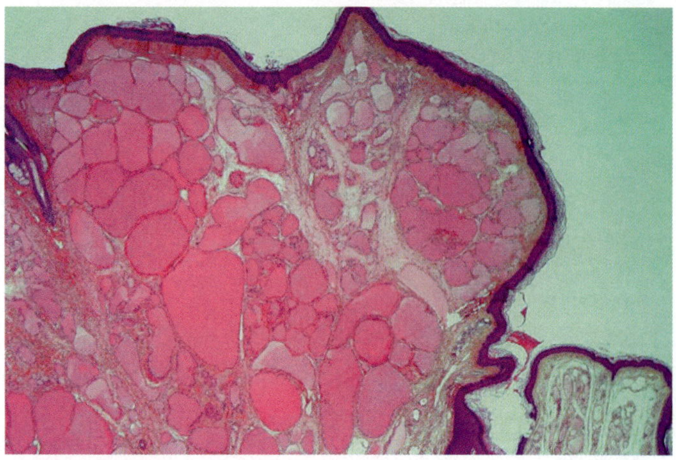

Pathology

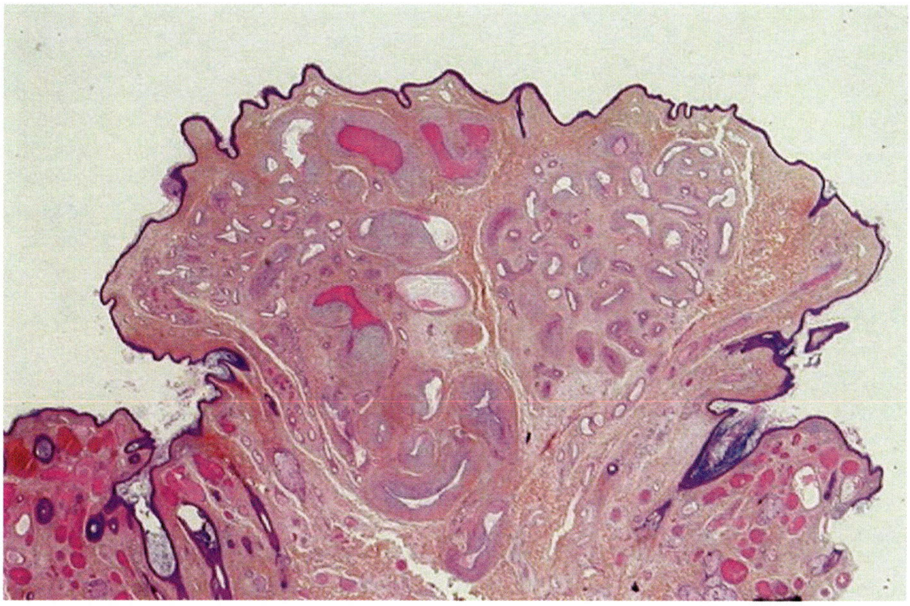

In some hypertrophic nodules, the wall of the vessels is considerably thickened and fibrous

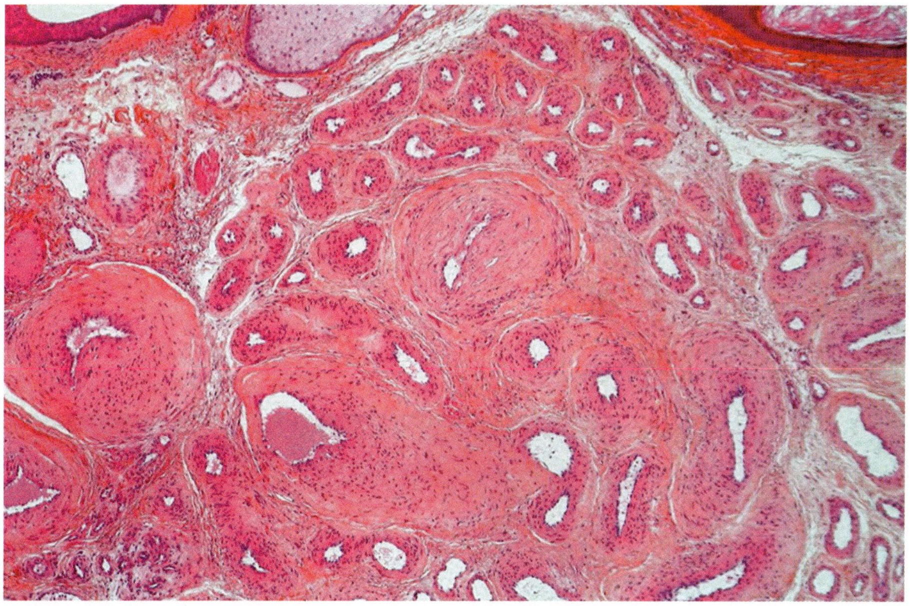

This type of lesion may be histologically misdiagnosed as AVM if the pathologist is unaware of its situation on a hypertrophic CM.

Clinical Aspects

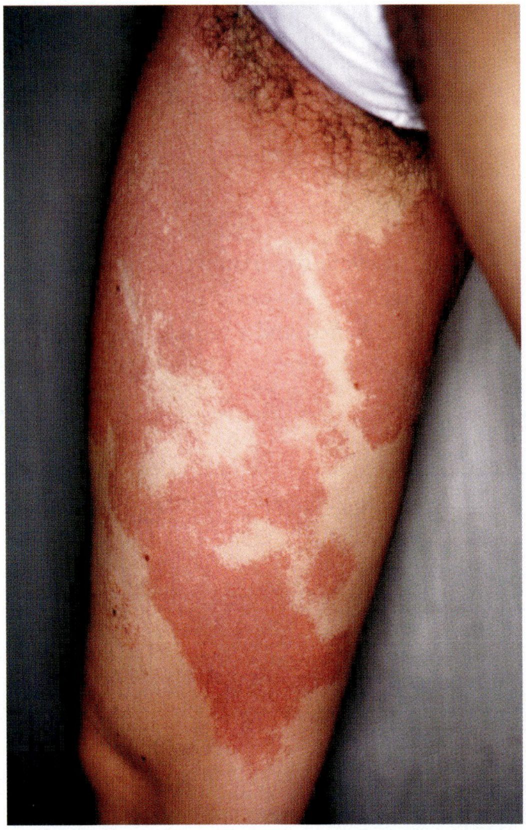

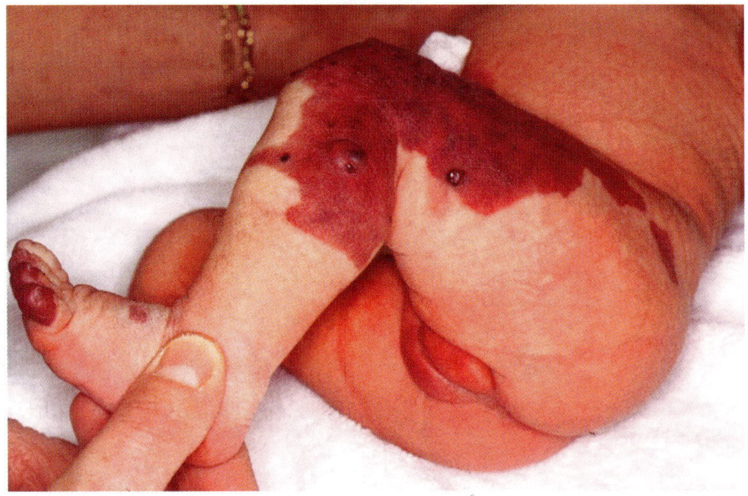

A geographic limb PWS at birth is more predictive of a complicated course than a spotted, blotchy PWS (44). The redness of the skin at birth is linked to increased hemoglobin at birth, and it will not persist. Thus, as the infant skin becomes paler after three or four weeks, the PWS also loses some of its often intense neonatal color: this often gives the parents strong but erroneous hope of spontaneous regression.

Spotted and blotchy pure capillary malformation of the thigh, not included in a syndrome: the PWS is flat, the color has not changed over

Evanescent or fading macule is also known as salmon patch, stork bite in the nape, aigrette or angel kiss in the glabellum. It was described by Unna in 1884 and it is sometimes called nevus of Unna. This red CM tints the mid-forehead and glabellum, extending frequently to the upper eyelids, tip of the nose and upper lip; in the posterior cephalic area salmon patches occupy the mid-nape and mid-occipital scalp. On the face they usually fade spontaneously and disappear before 5 years of age. Leung et al. (41) examined 808 caucasian newborns and 1575 caucasian children and found salmon patches in nearly half of the infantile population, equally in females and males. Black infants appeared less affected (27%) and oriental infants seemed rarely affected (4%) in another study (49).

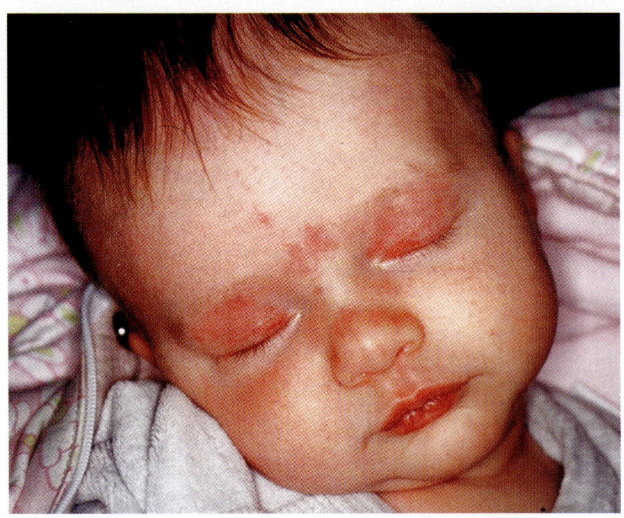

Clinical Aspects

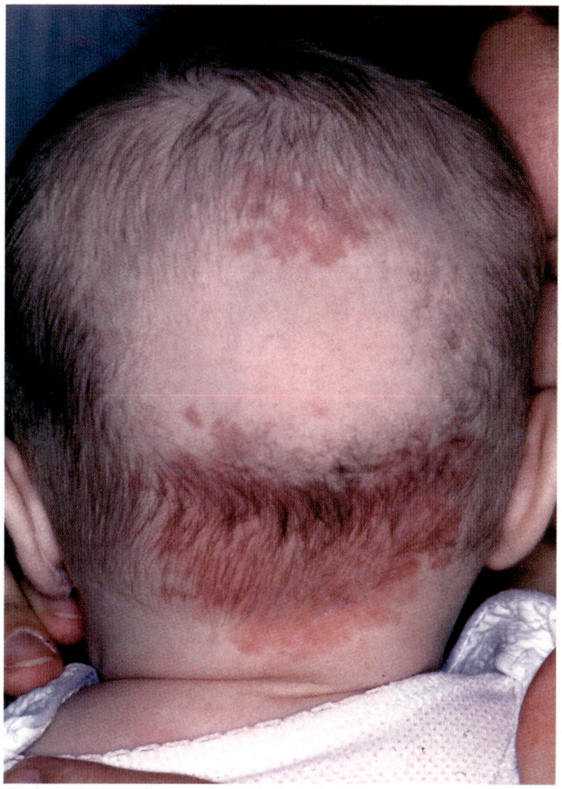

The same stain in the middle of the nape and occipital scalp tends to persist. In a series of 1340 children, aged 7–11 years, about 30% had a persisting salmon patch on the nape of the neck (45).

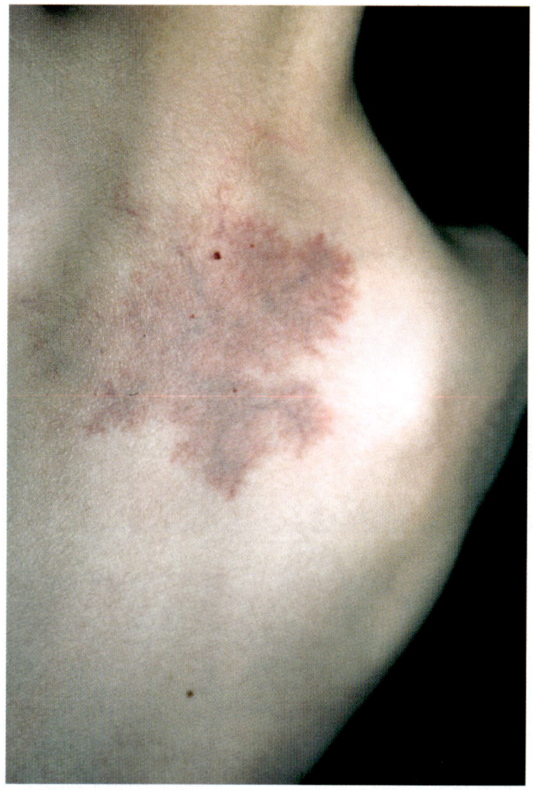

The butterfly-shaped mark was described in the lumbar and sacral area, as an isolated stain, not a marker of occult spinal dysraphism (47). This salmon patch was also described as sacral medial telangiectatic vascular nevus and it was suggested that it was more common in children with mental retardation (50, 59).
It can occur in the upper back; this adolescent boy had no associated anomaly (no spinal dysraphism, no mental retardation).

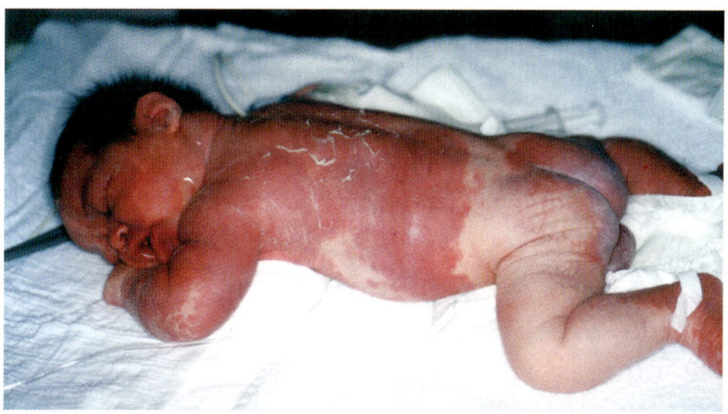

PWS may disseminate all over the body: this infant had left facial PWS, left arm, trunk and right leg PWSs. He died at 3 months of age of uncontrolled seizures linked to Sturge–Weber syndrome. His brain was profoundly damaged at birth on CT evaluation, with severe left hemiatrophy and calcifications, findings rarely present so early in life.

Clinical Aspects

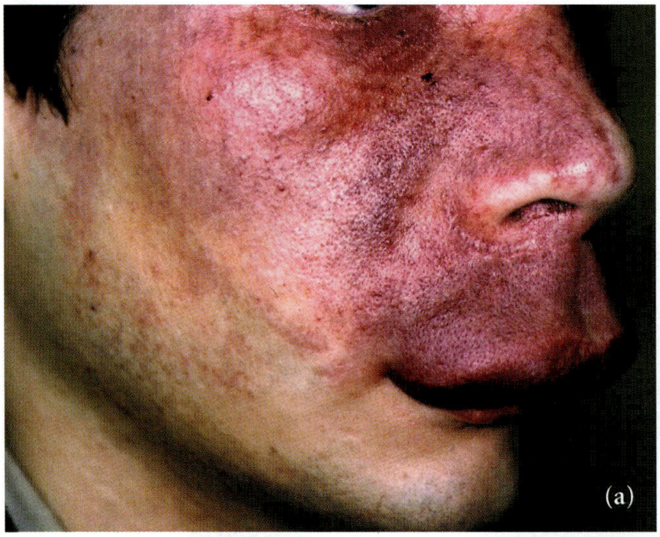

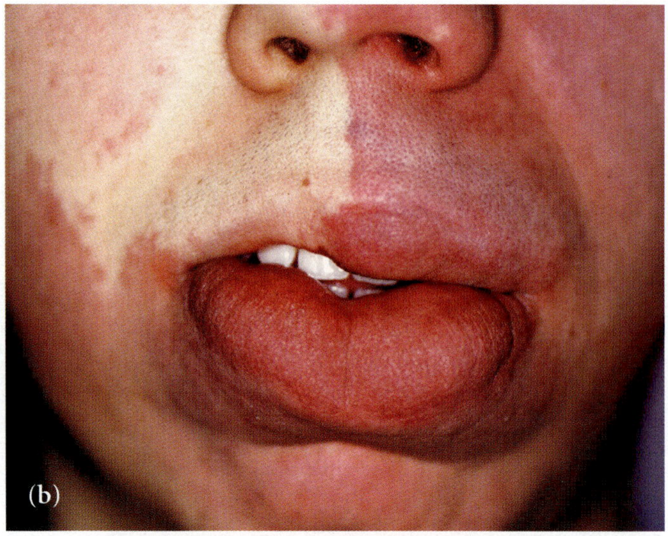

The young man has a bilateral V2 PWS: the involved upper lip progressively enlarged and thickened to end in this macrocheily at the end of puberty (a). The woman has three-quarters of her lips affected with PWS and only these areas ended in macrocheily (b). Surgical repair can be considered in both patients. Gingival hypertrophy (c) also complicates CM of the gums.

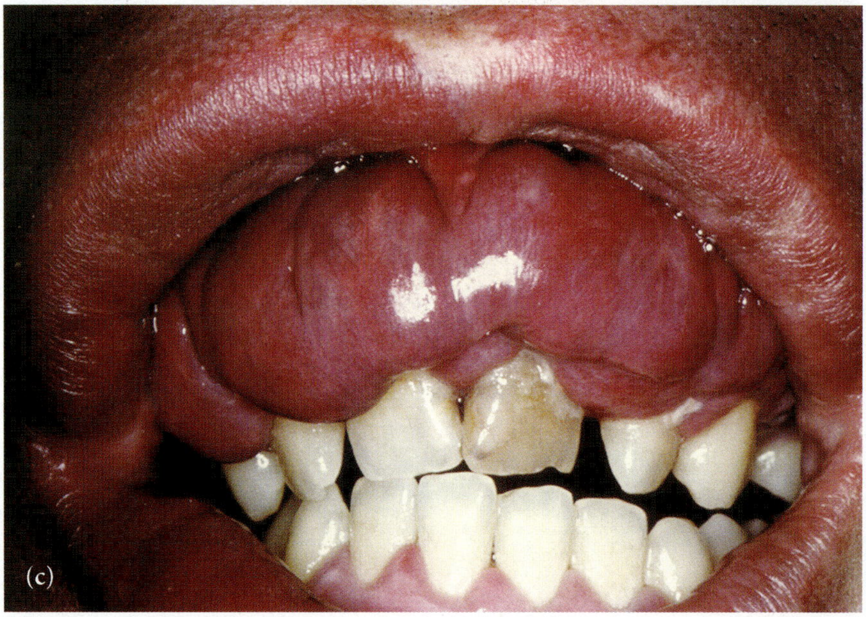

Clinical Aspects

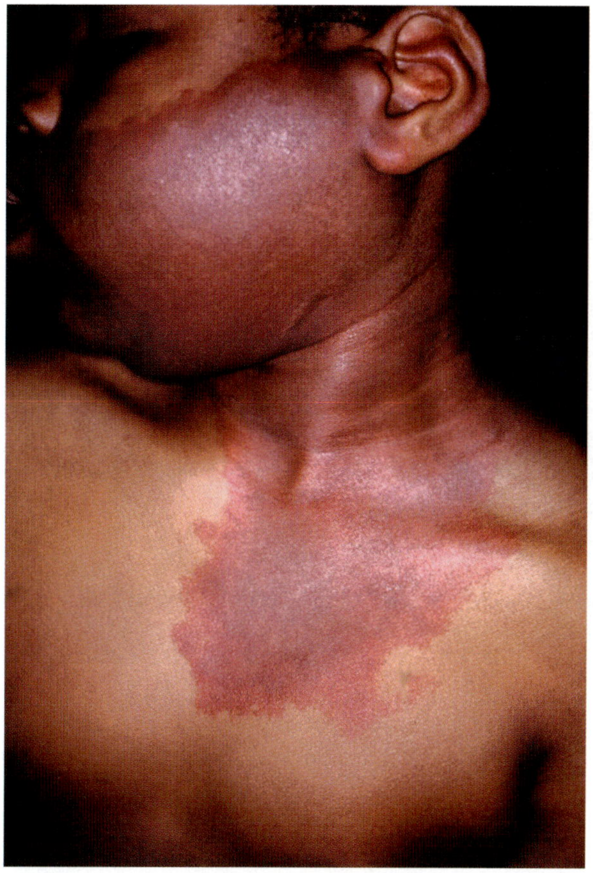

This boy of African descent underwent an evenly distributed hyperplasia of the facial part of his PWS, while the neck and trunk PWS remained flat. Tissular hyperplasia occupied not only the V2–V3 skin but also the underlying soft tissues and bone.

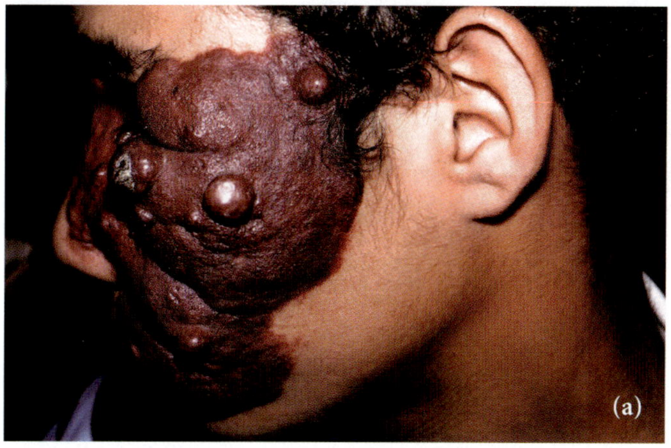

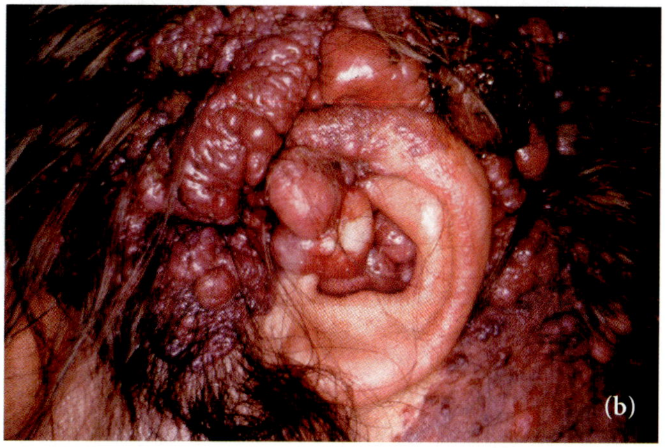

Nodular hyperplasia is quite common with V2 PWS. It begins by adolescence (a). In a group of 173 patients, 11% had a thickened PWS, nodularity was present in one fourth, and both types of hyperplastic skin changes occurred in 6% (36). Nodularity is sometimes misdiagnosed as AVM but there are no clinical fast-flow signs (no bruit, no thrill) and no arteriovenous fistulae are detected by US/Doppler examination. The nodular growths are particularly impressive around and inside the external ear of this man (b); this should not be mistaken for angiolymphoid hyperplasia with eosinophils (a biopsy may be useful).

Clinical Aspects

Contrary to what regularly happens with facial PWS, tissular hyperplasia rarely happens with trunk and limb PWS, as occurred on the palm and tips of fingers of this man who has CM of roughly an entire hand. The red color of a CM affecting a limb is commonly darker on the distal extremity than on the upper part of the affected limb.

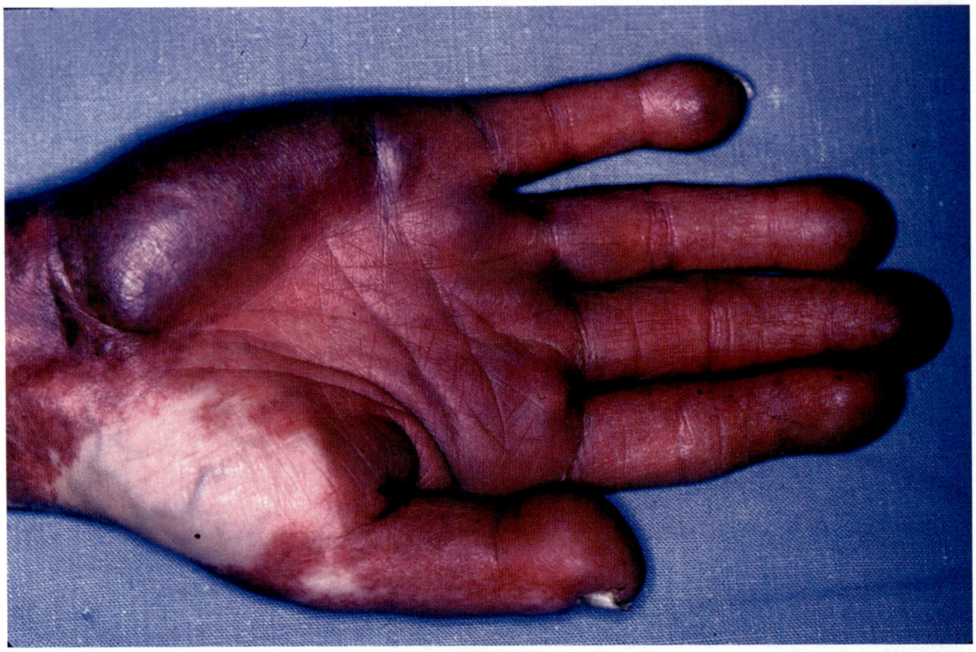

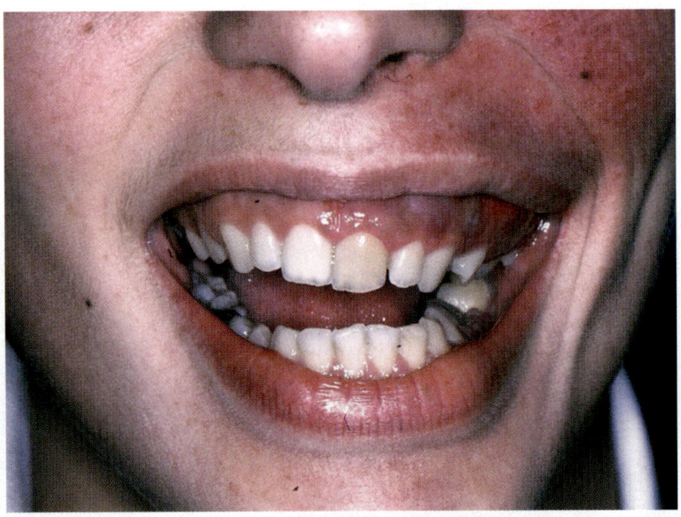

Enlarged maxilla with a V2 PWS creates diastema and dental malocclusion. After radiographically evaluating this bony growth, management consists of orthodontic treatment and sometimes subsequent orthognathic surgery, after the eruption of the secondary teeth.

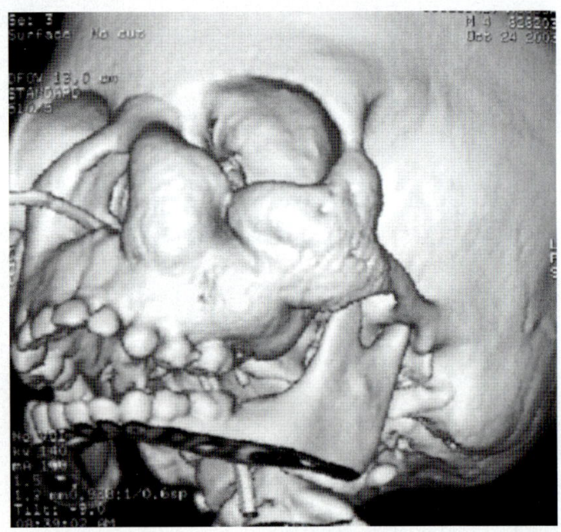

In this 10-year-old with an asymmetric face, due to V2 PWS on the left, the 3-D CT scan shows the thick left maxillary bone which has enlarged in the three planes.

Clinical Aspects

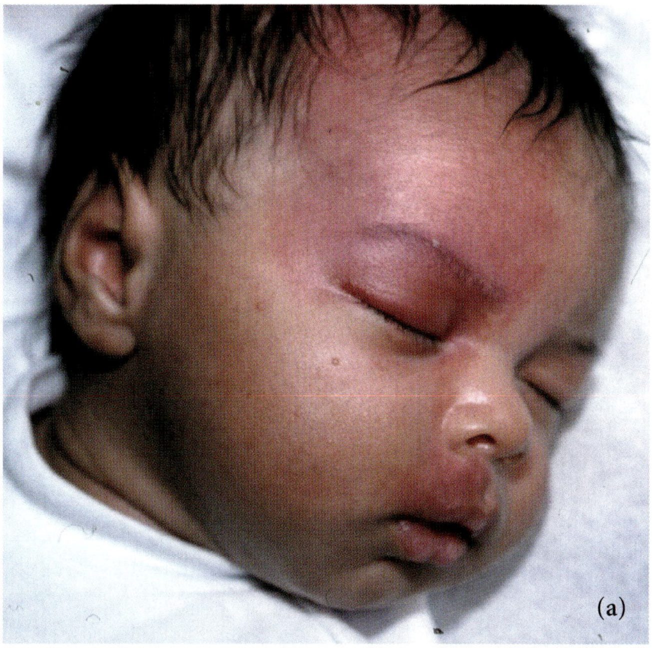

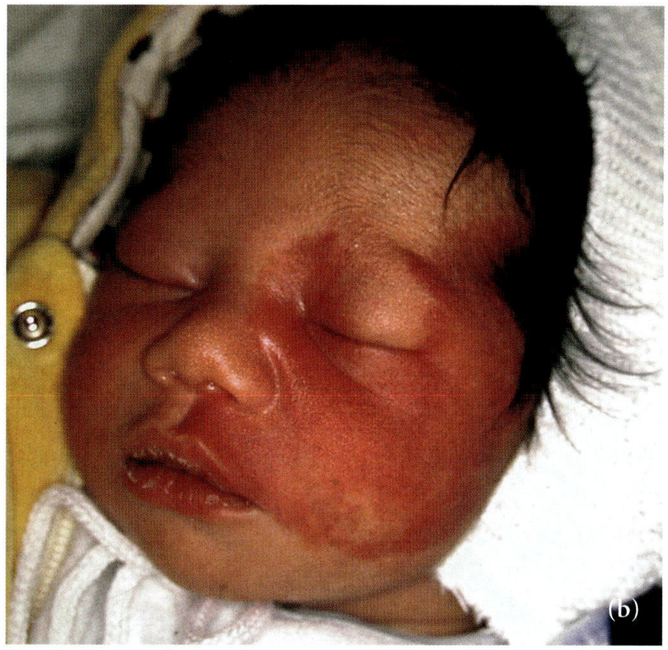

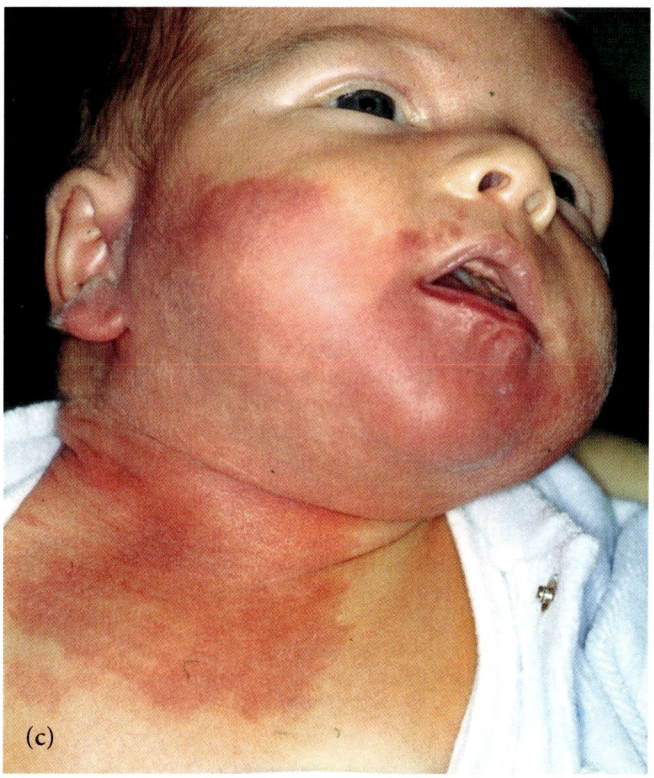

Three infants with the three types of facial PWS: the so-called V1 (a) or forehead and upper eyelid, V2 (b) or maxillary skin, and V3 (c) or mandibular area.

Clinical Aspects

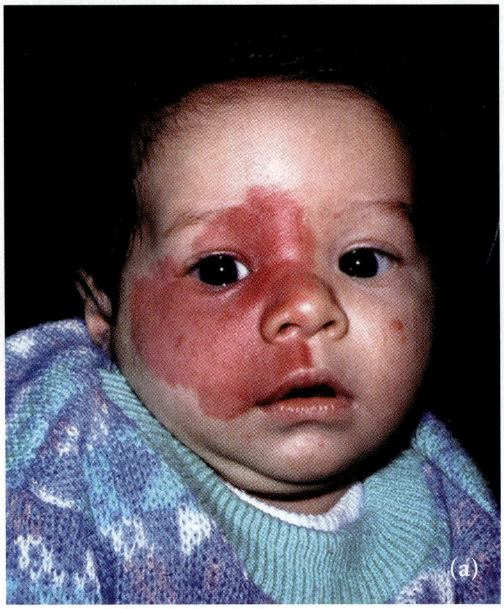

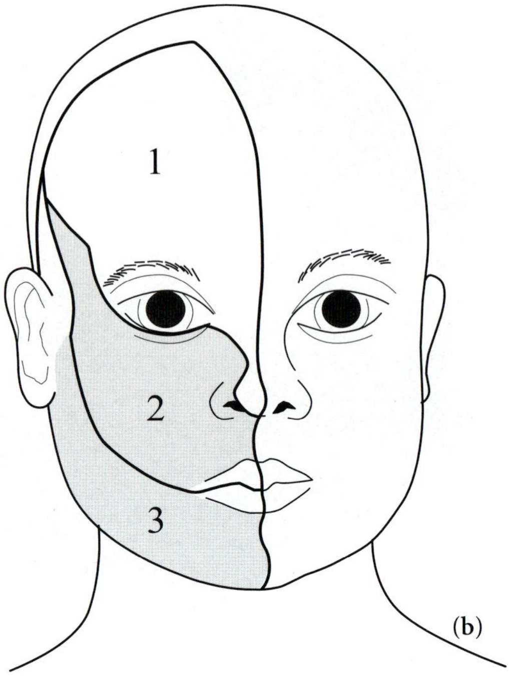

The picture (a) and the drawing (b, c) show the controversial watersheds of V1–V2. In most cases this type of involvement in (a) is not an association of V2 and V1 CM, but a pure V2 PWS reaching the external and/or internal part of the upper eyelid, with no risk of SWS (a). The dermis of these territories is made of mesoderm-derived endothelial cells ensheathed with pericytes and smooth muscle cells originating from the cephalic neural crest (CNC) (20). The boundaries, between these inflows of cells originating from the CNC, are not strictly defined. This explains the overlap of V1 and V2. In a large facial PWS, the risk of SWS is connected with the V1 location of PWS (10% of infants with such skin involvement are at risk). The variable watersheds between V1 and V2 may be puzzling for those taking the decision to screen the infant neuroradiologically or not.

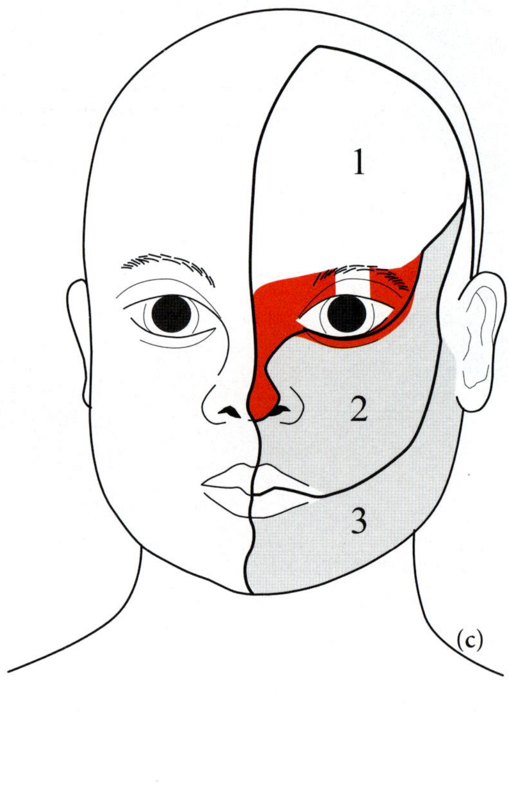

Clinical Aspects

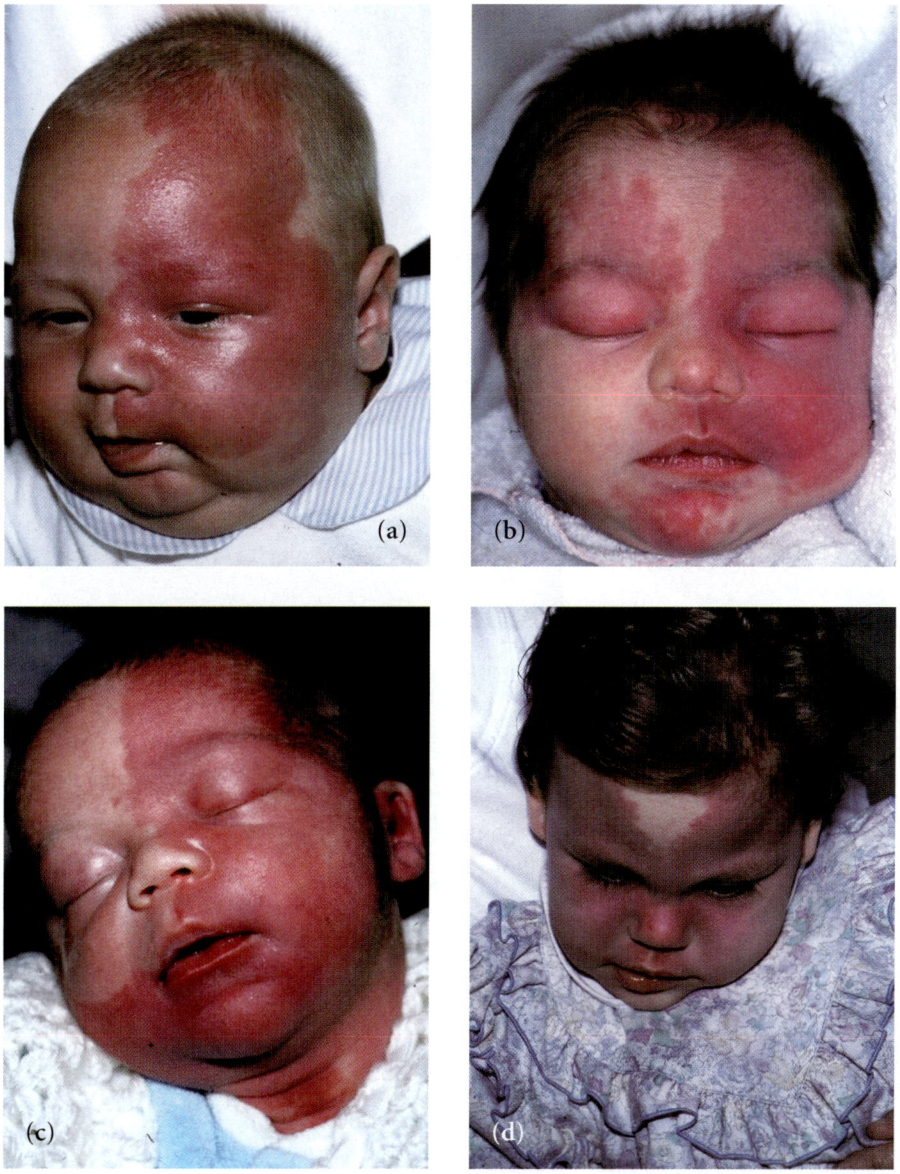

Facial PWSs can affect one, two, three or more "trigeminal areas" (V1, V2, V3) uni- or bilaterally, being easily identifiable even in extensive lesions. It seems that there is a higher risk of SWS when there is bilateral involvement of the face, including the two V1 areas. When the whole face is involved there is often a minor preserved white line or area in the middle of the face (d).

Clinical Aspects

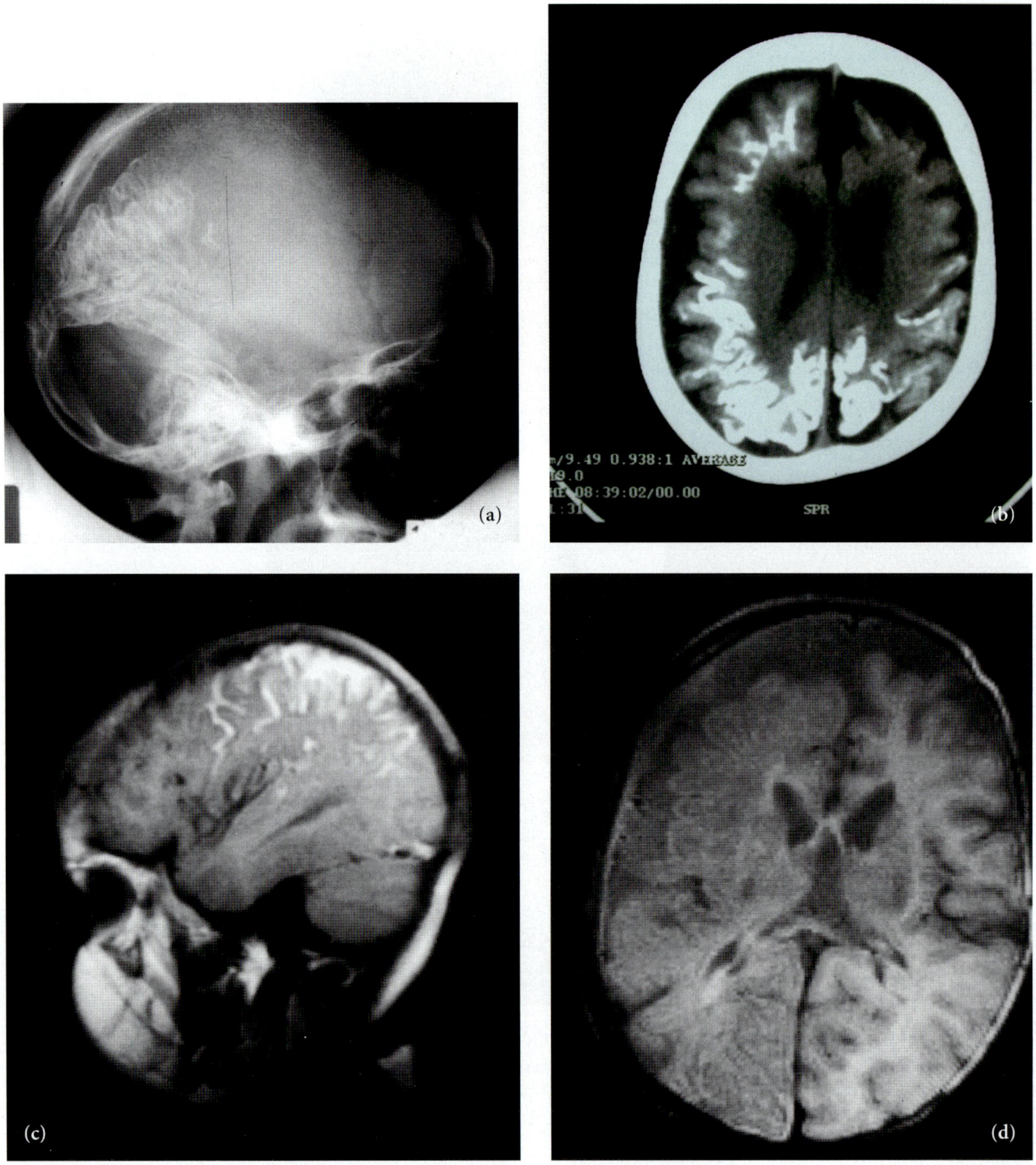

The neuroradiological evaluation of SWS brain anomalies depends on the age of the patient. Plain radiographs (a) show the calcifications molding the cortex, but this is rarely an early finding. Early CT scans with iodinated contrast can show the pial vascular anomaly and localized cerebral atrophy, later they demonstrate gyriform dense calcifications hiding most of the vascular meningeal lesion (b). MRI is the best early diagnostic imaging tool in an at-risk infant with V1 PWS: T1-weighted sequences after gadolinium enhancement demonstrate the pial vascular malformation (c); other anomalies include cerebral atrophy, enlarged choroid plexus, and, in infants less than 6 months old, accelerated myelination in the affected hemisphere (d) (2, 35).

Clinical Aspects

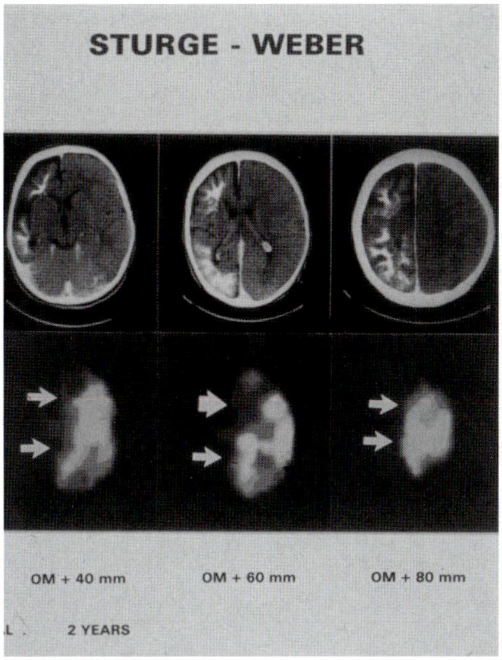

SPECT scans (Single Photon Emission Computed Tomography) with Xe-133 (courtesy of Dr. C. Chiron, Hôpital Necker-Enfants Malades, Paris, France) permit the study of the regional cerebral blood flow (rCBF). In infants it gives a good indication of the extent of the involvement: the picture shows that the decrease of rCBF is usually wider than the lesion evidenced by CT scan. This functional cerebral imaging shows a decreased rCBF after the first seizures in the area of the pial vascular anomaly, whereas rCBF is temporarily increased, before the first seizure (11, 53). The more extensive the pial vascular lesion is, the more severe the course of the neurological symptoms will be. According to Ville et al. (67) motor functions are affected by ischemic events whereas the cognitive function alteration is likely linked to epilepsy. PET scans (Positron Emission Tomography) study the cerebral glucose metabolism; results are comparable to data obtained with SPECT scans in SWS (12).

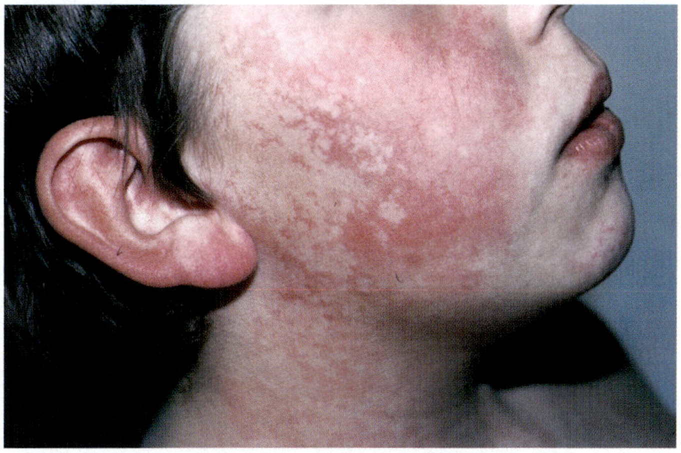

Above: Nevus anemicus is often intermingled with CM, in both facial or trunk and limb lesions, as a twin-spotting phenomenon (29). These pale blanching macules do not redden when the skin is rubbed, in contrast to the surrounding CM and normal skin.

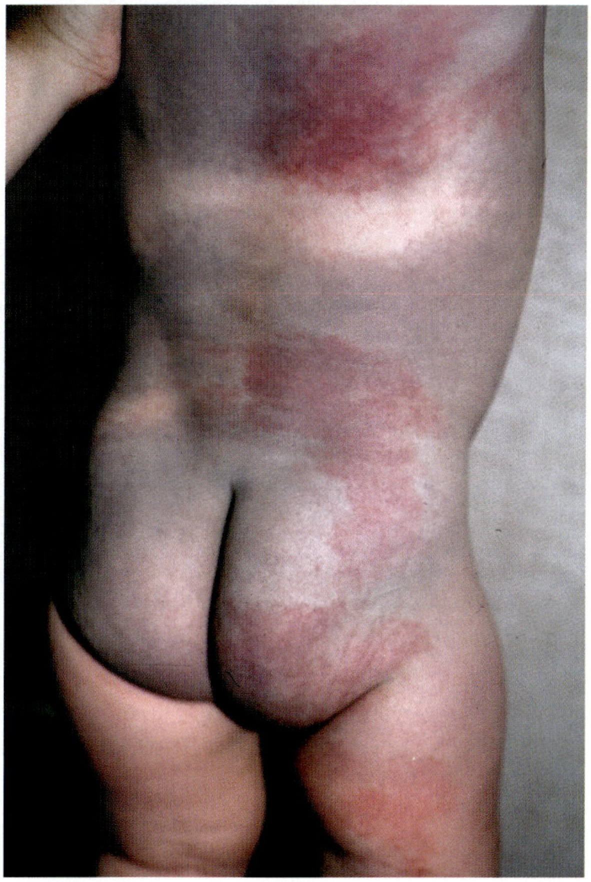

Right: Phakomatosis pigmentovascularis (PPV) type II a in a girl at 1 year. Spontaneous fading of both the Mongolian spots and PWS is likely to occur after a few years. Type II is the most common type of PPV, and it seems particularly frequent in infants of Asian or African ancestry.

Clinical Aspects

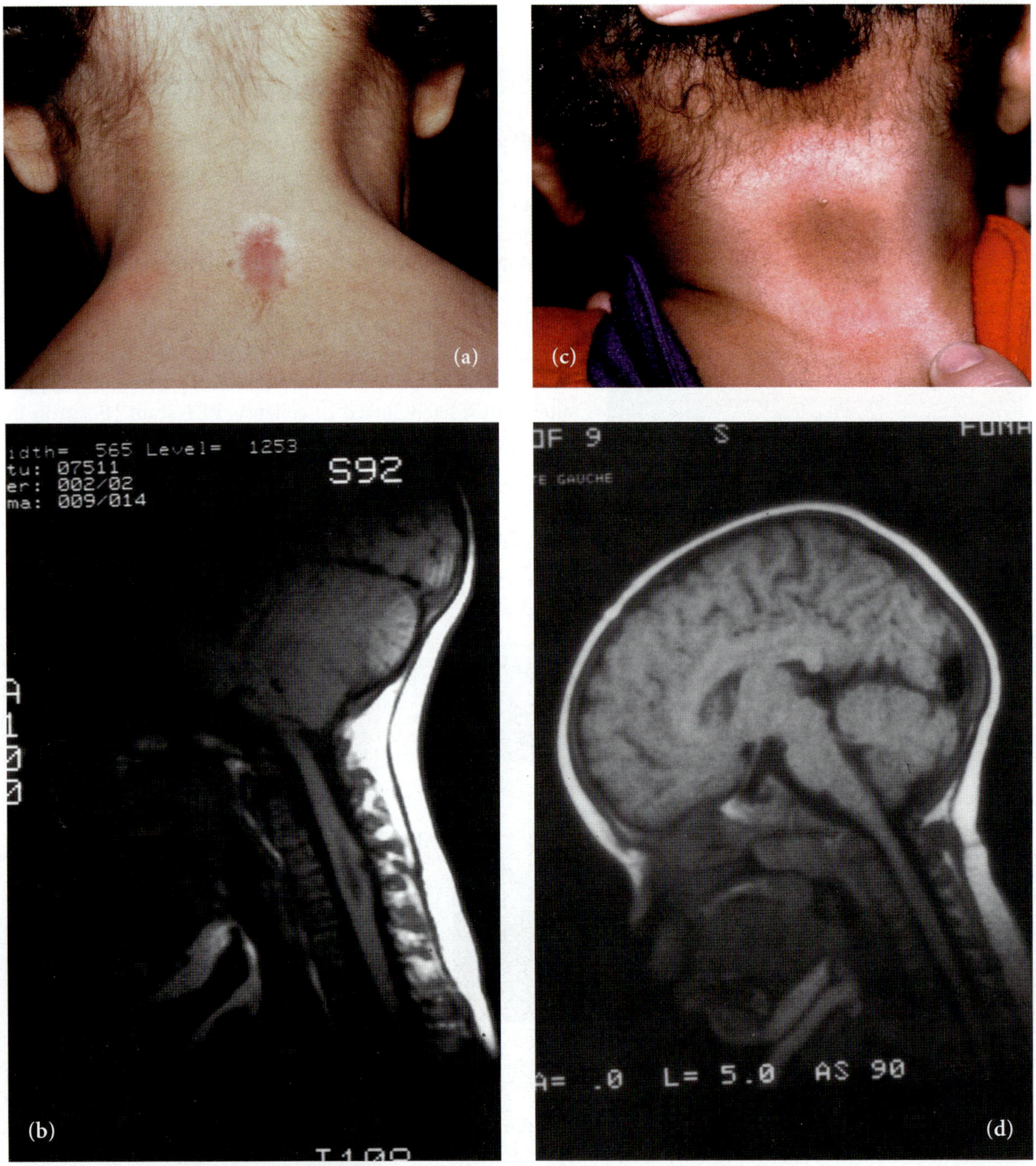

This girl had a red stain with a pale halo, a sinus tract and a thin tuft of hair in the middle of the nape (a). Because of these associated cutaneous signs MRI investigation was performed and found an attached cervical spinal cord and syringomyelia (b). After surgical treatment to set free the cord, the syringomyelia disappeared. The other infant had a CM and a fistula also in the middle of the nape (c); MRI revealed a cyst (d) connecting the sinus tract and the cord; the cyst, an epidermoïd cyst, was surgically removed with a good outcome.

Clinical Aspects

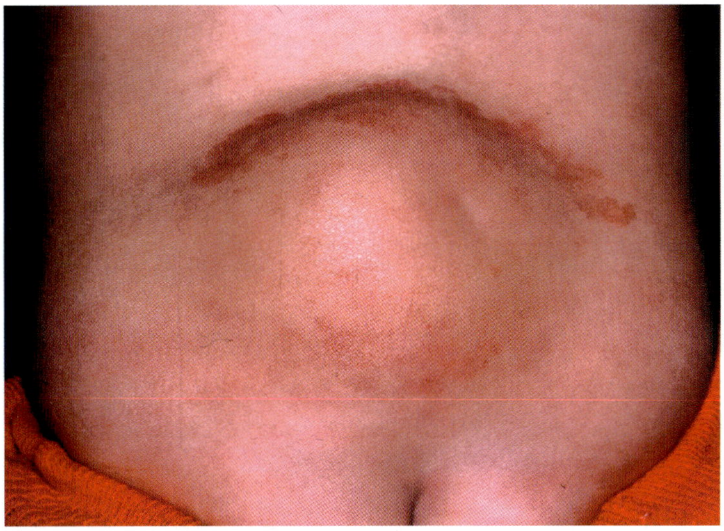

This child has a minor midline lumbar CM, a congenital bump (lipoma) and a dimple: the combination of markers in the midline requires neuroradiologic evaluation. MRI found a spina-lipoma and attached cord. Guggisberg et al. (25) confirmed the work of Tavafoghi (64): in a series of 54 children with midline lumbosacral lesions, they demonstrated that a single vascular marker, either CM or hemangioma, is not an indicator of occult spinal dysraphism; but, when there are other markers associated with the vascular one, the risk of having occult spinal dysraphism is high. These markers include: pit, dimple, sinus tract, tail-like fibroma, hypertrichosis, lipoma, deviated gluteal cleft, melanocytic nevus and congenital scar.

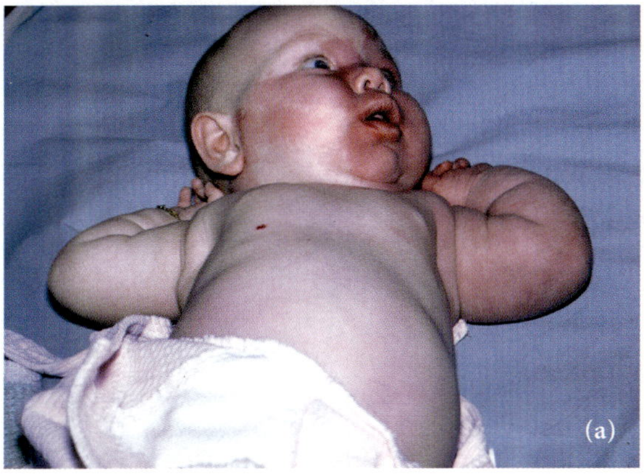

(a)

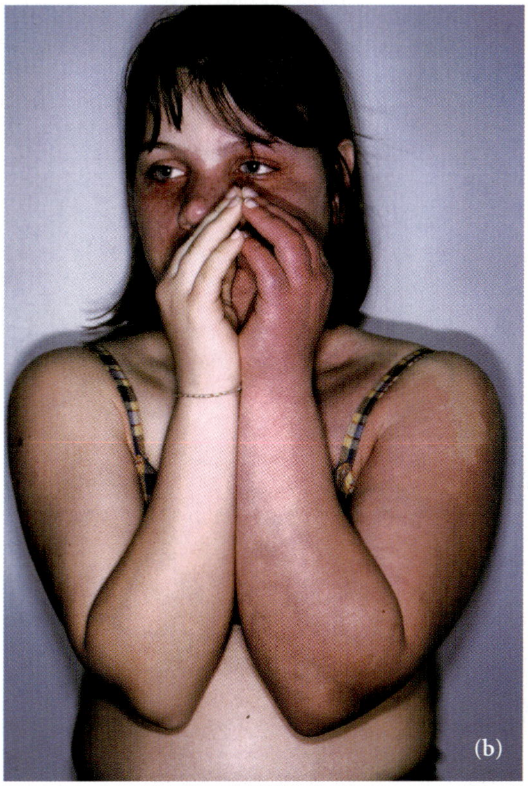

(b)

The left hemifacial PWS is combined with a complete involvement of the left arm by a CM, and there is congenital hypertrophy of this arm (a). The girl did not develop SWS and is doing quite well. The congenital overgrowth of the arm did not worsen (there was proportionate growth to the end of adolescence) and she did not develop varicose veins (b): this syndrome differs from KTS.

Clinical Aspects

A geographic stain in the lateral aspect of the thigh and knee suggests a complex combined slow-flow vascular malformation (KTS) and a high risk of further lymphatic abnormalities (44). In this child LM is already evident due to the presence of some clear vesicles; there is an associated diffuse lipomatosis.

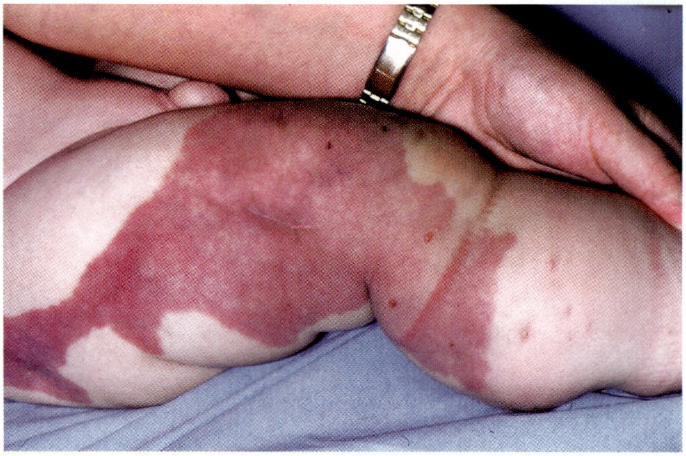

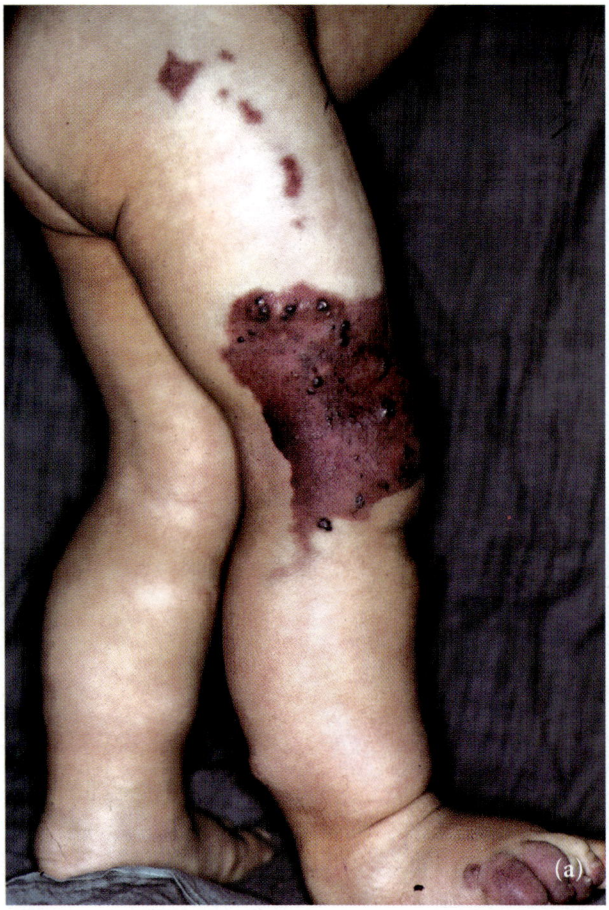

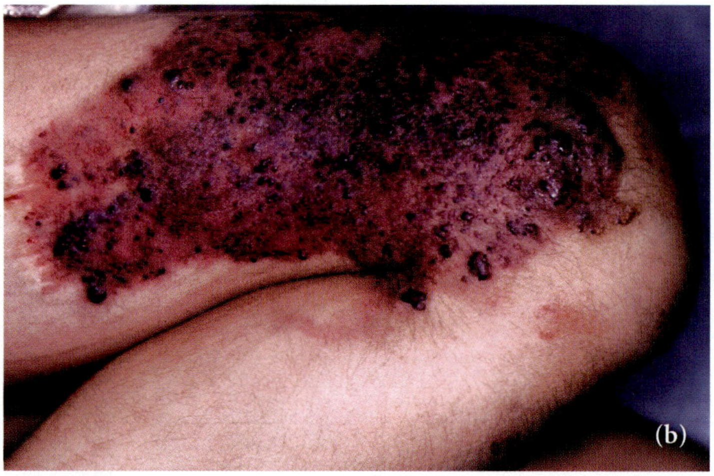

These two photographs show the worsening of the lymphatic component over the thigh's geographic stain between 1 year (a) and 7 years of age (b) in a boy with KTS affecting both legs and extending to the GI tract and urinary tract. In this child a chronic intravascular coagulopathy caused visceral, intestinal and urinary bleeding episodes, controlled with low-molecular-weight heparin treatment.

Clinical Aspects

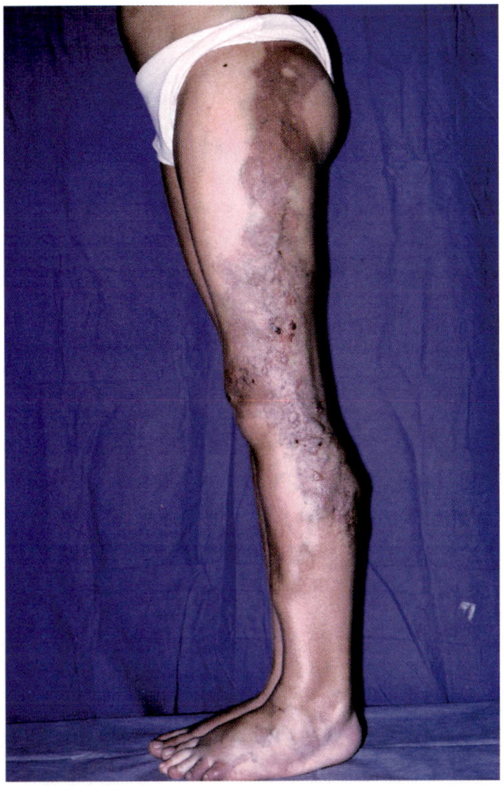

A very disabling KTS. The hemorrhagic vesicles, oozing and bleeding, complicate conservative management with elastic garments. Large varicose veins are visible along the leg and the patient experiences heaviness of the limb when standing without elastic stockings. The quality of her life is severely impaired. This sometimes leads to consideration of resection of the geographic stain with the lymphatic anomalies, totally or partially, after cutaneous expansion, and surgical treatment of the varicose veins when the deep venous system is normal. However, extensive surgical treatments bring complications. Untoward side-effects include infection, lymphedema, increased superficial varicosities and function-altering fibrosis. Aggressive surgical approaches resulting in severe complications sometimes end in amputation.

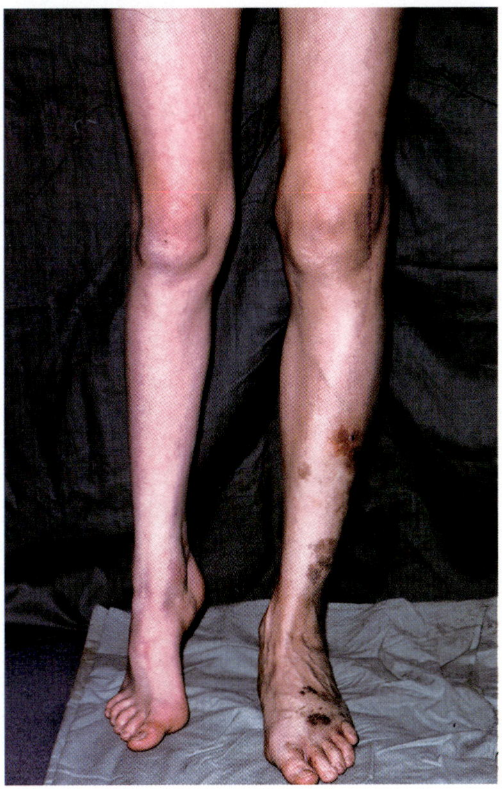

KTS does not always occur with a geographic CM of the external aspect of the thigh, and lymphatic anomalies. This patient has some blotchy PWSs scattered over the lower limb, a marginal vein on the external part of the thigh and dilated veins on the foot; he has developed a leg length discrepancy of 8 cm, which unfortunately was not controlled by stapling epiphyseodesis performed too late before the end of his growth (18).

Clinical Aspects

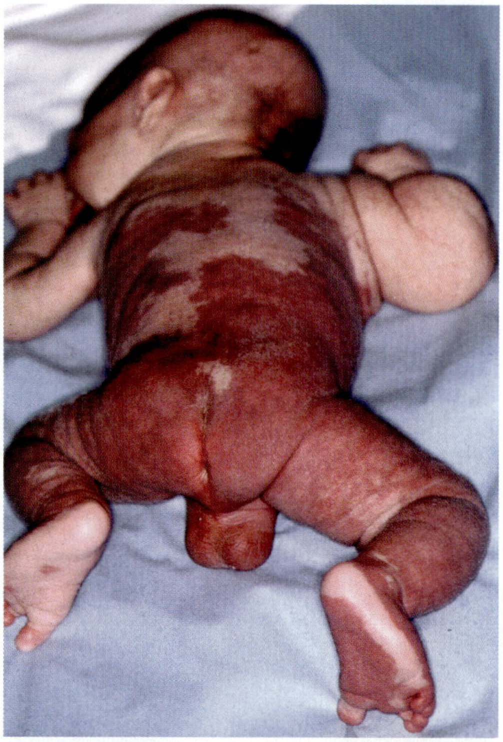

Diffusely scattered PWSs, over the trunk and limbs, are a common finding in infants with Proteus or Proteiform syndromes. Their bright red tint, at birth, as a rule significantly lightens after a few years; thus it is not worth undertaking extensive pulsed dye laser treatment: laser will be used only for CMs of visible areas (the face). This infant has right hemihypertrophy affecting one vascular extremity (leg) and one nonvascular one (arm).

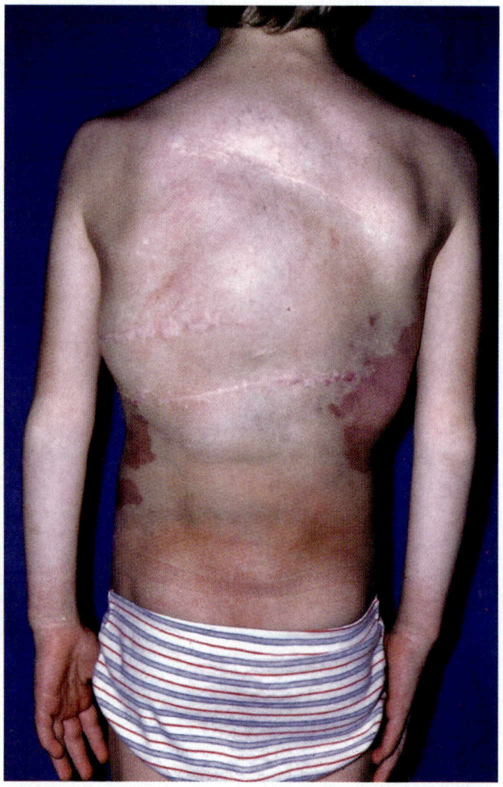

Patients with Proteus syndrome develop large lipomas (particularly on the back and abdomen), recurring after excision (see the large scars on the back, evidence of the previous resection). Some lipomas have intra-abdominal extension. This young man also has a slow-flow vascular malformation combining large CM of the trunk and underlying dilated veins.

Clinical Aspects

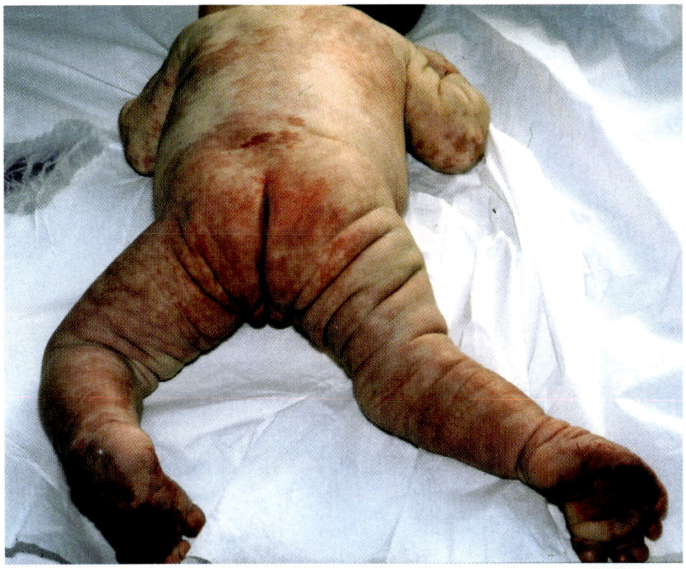

This girl with Proteus syndrome had severe orthopedic anomalies at birth (of the knees and feet) and a diffuse connective tissue nevus of the posterior part of the legs creating a firm folded skin. She had syndactyly on both feet and lipoma in the lumbar skin. She then developed overgrowth of some toes and fingers, plantar thickening, lipoma in the back, and hemifacial hypertrophy. On the other hand, the diffuse CMs spontaneously lightened with time.

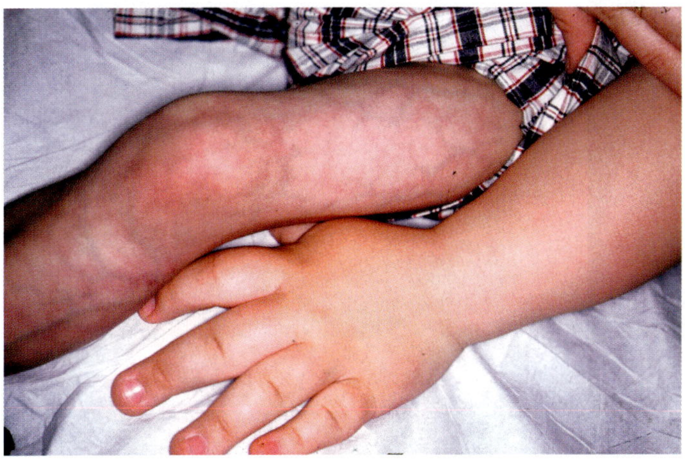

From birth this boy had anomalies suggestive of Proteus syndrome. Vascular anomalies, including CM and dilated varicose veins, were located on the lower extremities, whereas limb overgrowth affected only the upper part of the body: the picture shows the striking overgrowth of the left hand and arm at 2 years, compared to the thin vascular leg; the same clinical findings exist on the right side. This association of overgrowth and deficient growth (the "plus/minus phenomenon") was stressed by Happle (29).

Clinical Aspects

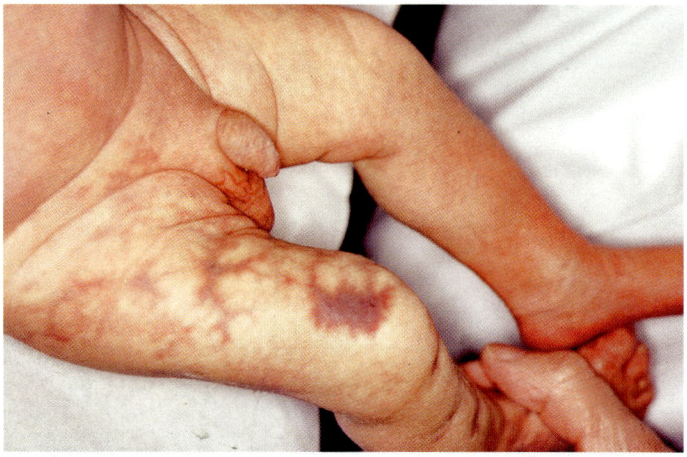

Monomelic CMTC at birth with the typically branching out streaks and bands, fragile lesion of the knee and atrophic linear lesions in the distal part of the leg.

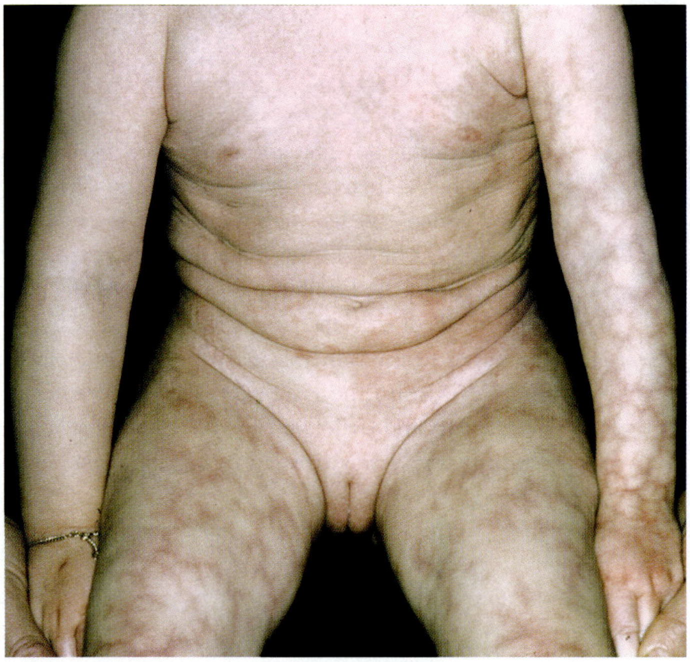

CMTC persisting in a child and involving three limbs and the trunk. Hypotrophy of the involved left arm is evident, compared to the non-vascular right arm.

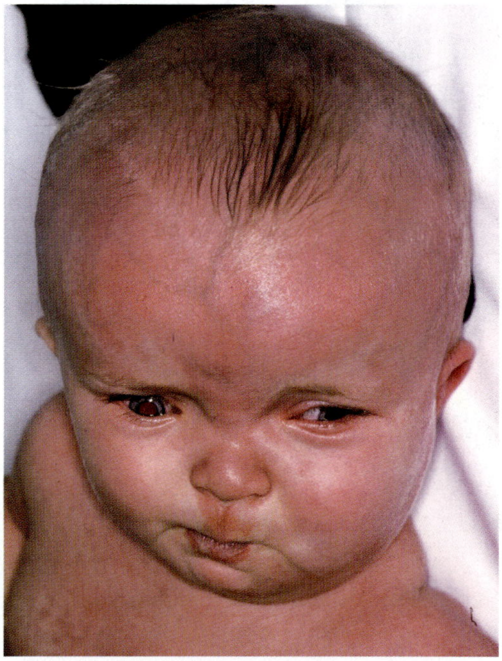

Macrocephaly–cutis marmorata syndrome: this child has a striking CM in a triangular shape on the mid-forehead, just avoiding the eyebrow areas; there are also mid-face CMs staining the nose, upper, and lower lip, a diffusely marbled skin on the body, and strabismus.

Clinical Aspects

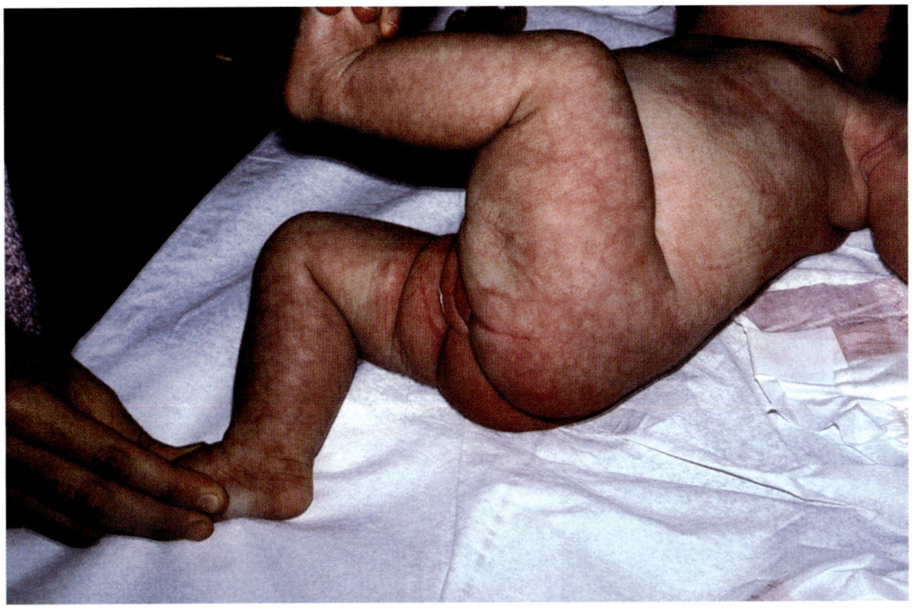

This diffuse reticulate CMs persisted (it was not a physiological neonatal transient livedo) and the girl experienced transient ischemic brain attacks and blindness.

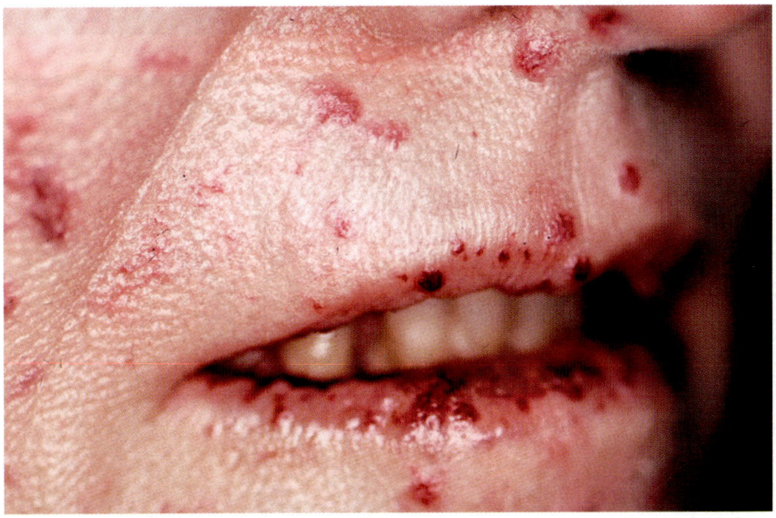

HHT in an elderly woman. HHT may not manifest until late in life. Telangiectasia in HHT are multiple and common sites are the lips and mouth, as well as the fingers. According to Begbie et al. (5) 90% of patients with HHT have nose bleeds and 80% have skin and mouth telangiectasia. Nasal telangiectasia has various morphologies, ranging from spots and loops to clusters of capillaries, and as the bulk of telangiectasia increases with age, hemorrhages create anemia requiring iron supplementation. Some patients experiencing massive hemorrhages require blood transfusions. Too frequent cauterization of nasal telangiectasia damages the nasal mucosa and may generate nasal septum perforation. Direct puncture and micro-sclerotherapy of the nasal telangiectasia with Ethibloc® is a good therapeutic option for such epistaxis.

Clinical Aspects

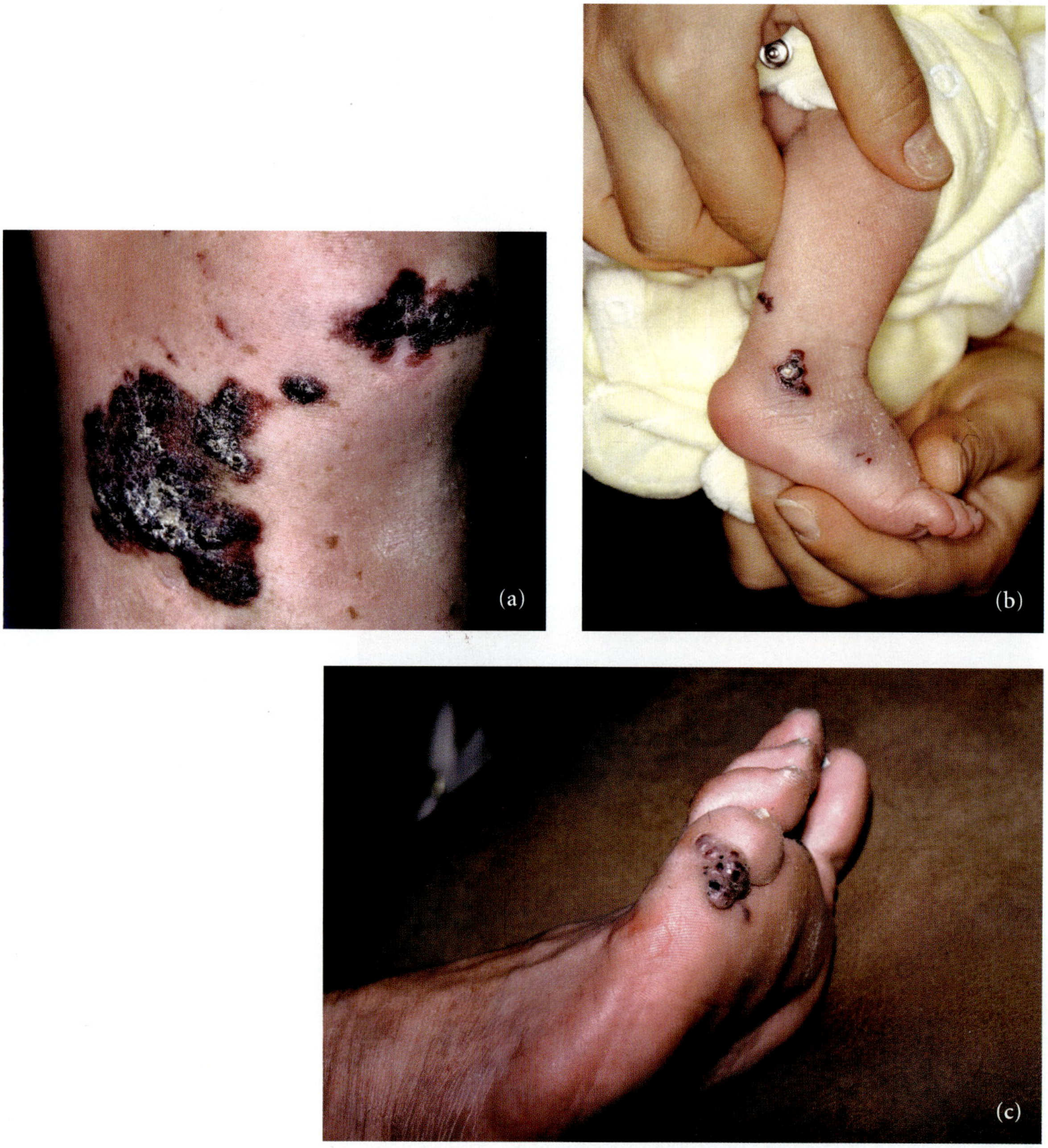

Angiokeratoma circumscriptum (AKC): the plaque-type lesion is obviously hyperkeratotic and in this knee area (a), barely protected from trauma in an active child, bleeding is problematic. Epidermal hyperkeratosis increases over the years and this allows the lesion to bleed with minor trauma. Often an underlying capillary-venous malformation gives the skin around the AKC a bluish color: in this newborn (b) this allows us to predict a further worsening of the AKC. AKC of toes or fingers are usually called AK of Mibelli (c). Excision is the only effective treatment for AKC. However, in very large lesions surgical treatment is not realistic, even after cutaneous expansion. Then, CO2 laser or 1064 nm Nd-YAG laser resurfacing treatment, sometimes combined with pulsed dye laser, can be considered to achieve a smoother surface and decrease the color, but it is seldom possible to eradicate the angiokeratoma.

Clinical Aspects

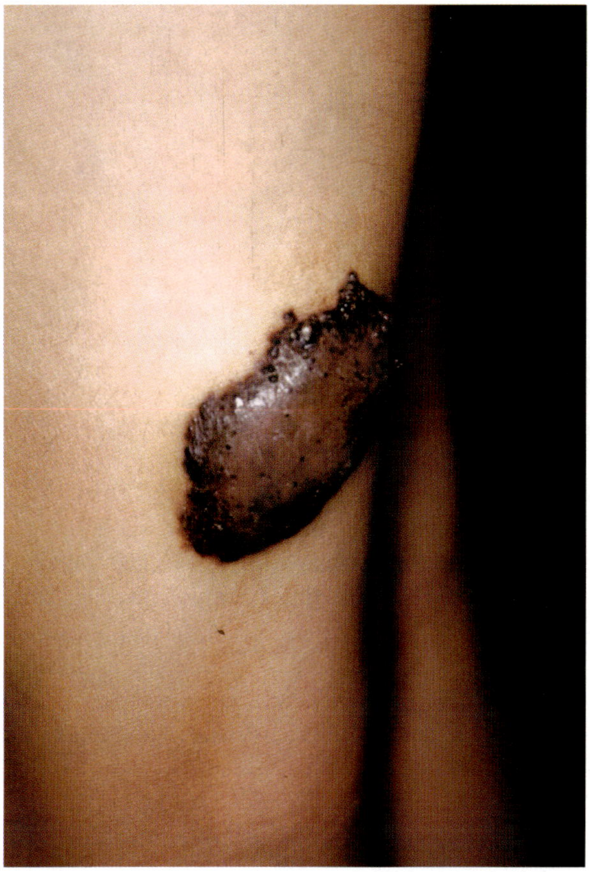

This large solitary angiokeratoma circumscriptum of the thigh of a 15-year-old girl, which had recently thickened and darkened, was misdiagnosed as melanoma before she had a biopsy.

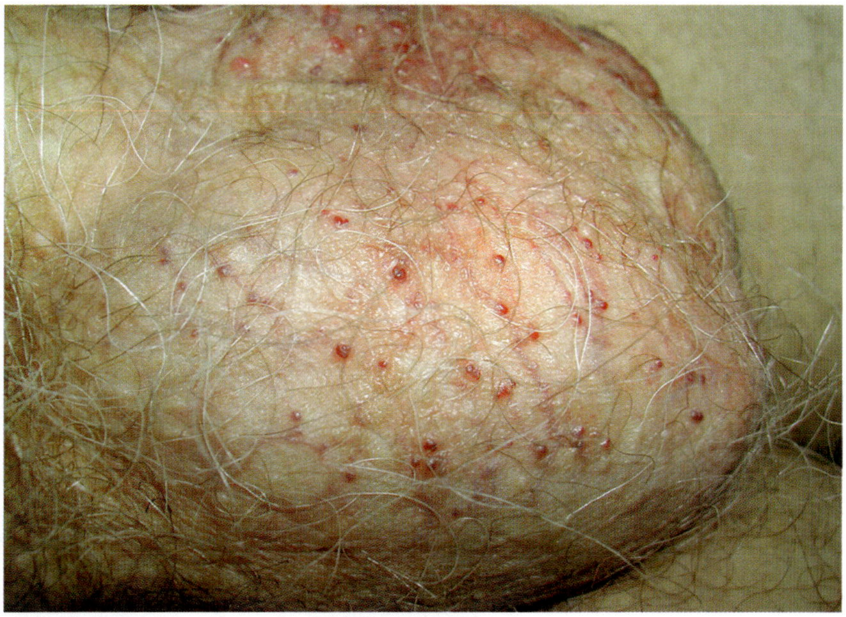

Fordyce angiokeratomas speckled on the scrotum often have a smooth surface and are associated with symptoms of local venous hypertension (varicose veins, varicocele). In this patient lesions were improved with 3% polidocanol intralesional injections.

Clinical Aspects

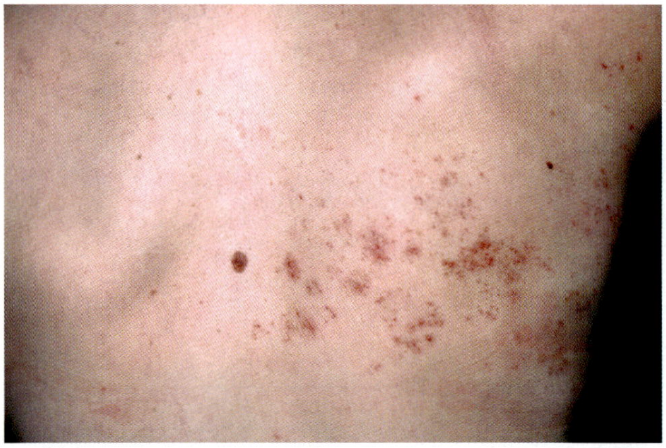

Angioma serpiginosum of Hutchinson comprise minor punctate red or violet papules, usually grouped on top of small capillary pink macules. These red tiny dots have minor hyperkeratosis and they form whorled and annular figures on a limb (mostly the lower extremity) and the corresponding trunk. During adolescence they slowly progress, unilaterally, in a metameric distribution, to stabilize in adulthood. A case reported by Al Hawsawi et al. (3) suggested a Blaschko-linear distribution in arm involvement. Pathology shows thick-walled dilated capillaries and a slight epidermal hyperkeratosis, and these lesions were considered in to be angiokeratomas.

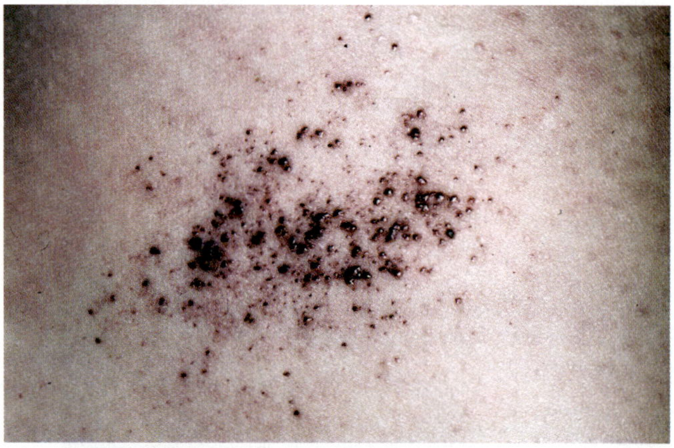

Diffusely spreading, punctate and red papules constitute angiokeratoma corporis diffusum. Hyperkeratosis is not evident clinically. In this patient red papules had increased by adolescence and he had painful acroparesthesias. The biopsy of a tiny vascular spot indicated striated lysosomes on electron microscopy, with electron-dense lipid deposits with a distinctive lamellar structure; there was an important galactosidase A deficiency and genotyping confirmed Fabry disease.

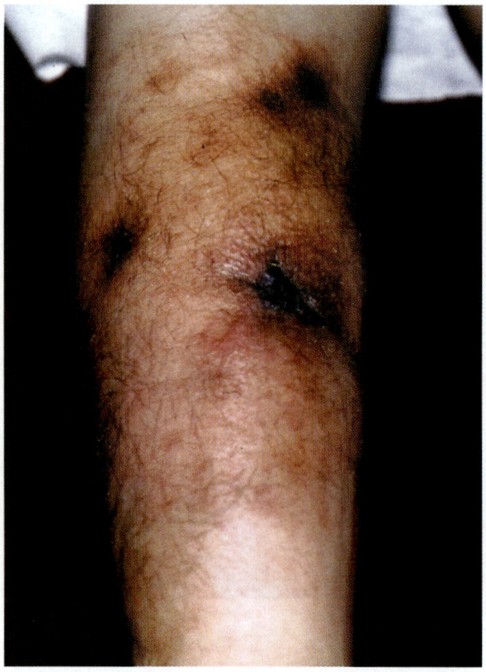

Eccrine angiomatous hamartoma in a boy who has Noonan syndrome. The lesion is extensive and not well-defined, covering the anterior aspect of the leg. It hurts on palpation and sudden contact. The brownish color is associated with prominent hypertrichosis and intermittent sweating. The size of the lesion does not allow surgical excision.

Clinical Aspects

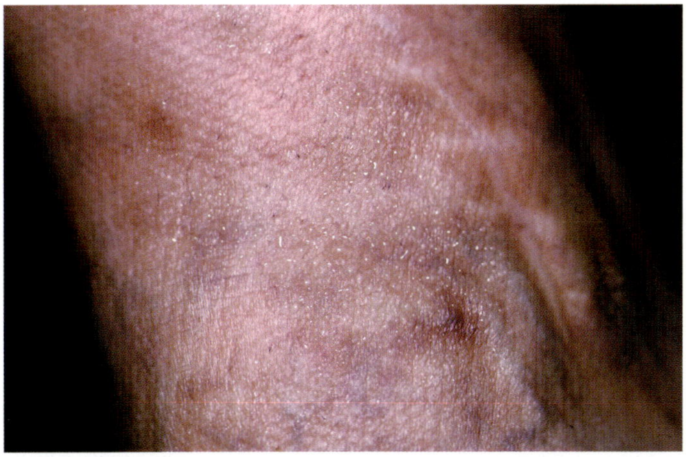

This eccrine angiomatous hamartoma creates ill-defined infiltration of the leg and blotchy pink areas. Some dilated venous-like channels are visible as bluish streaks. Sweating became obvious in this anxious patient during examination, and droplets of sweat emerged only in this area of the skin. With his pain increasing, this patient is looking for a treatment but excision is difficult due to the site and size.

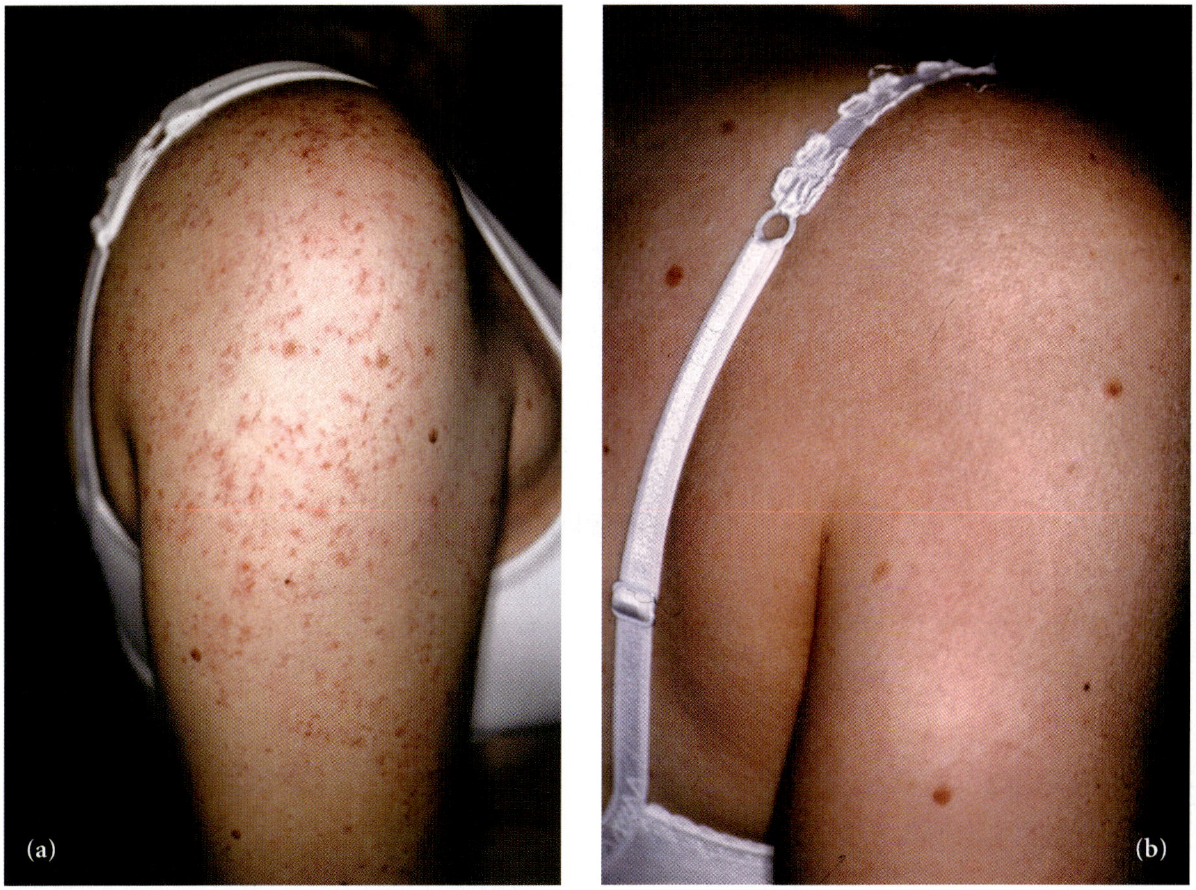

(a) (b)

During pregnancy diffuse telangiectasia sometimes appear, as on the arms and trunk of this young woman (a); 6 months after the birth of her baby the telangiectasia had completely disappeared (b). This patient also had an arteriovenous malformation of one hand, known from childhood, which did not change during and after her pregnancy.

Clinical Aspects

Association of vascular malformation and vascular tumor (or overlapping lesions) can be observed: the growth of multiple pyogenic granulomas on a CM is not rare.

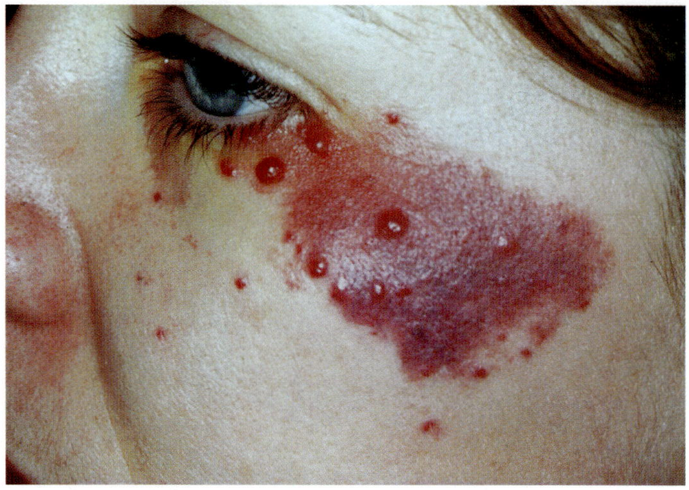

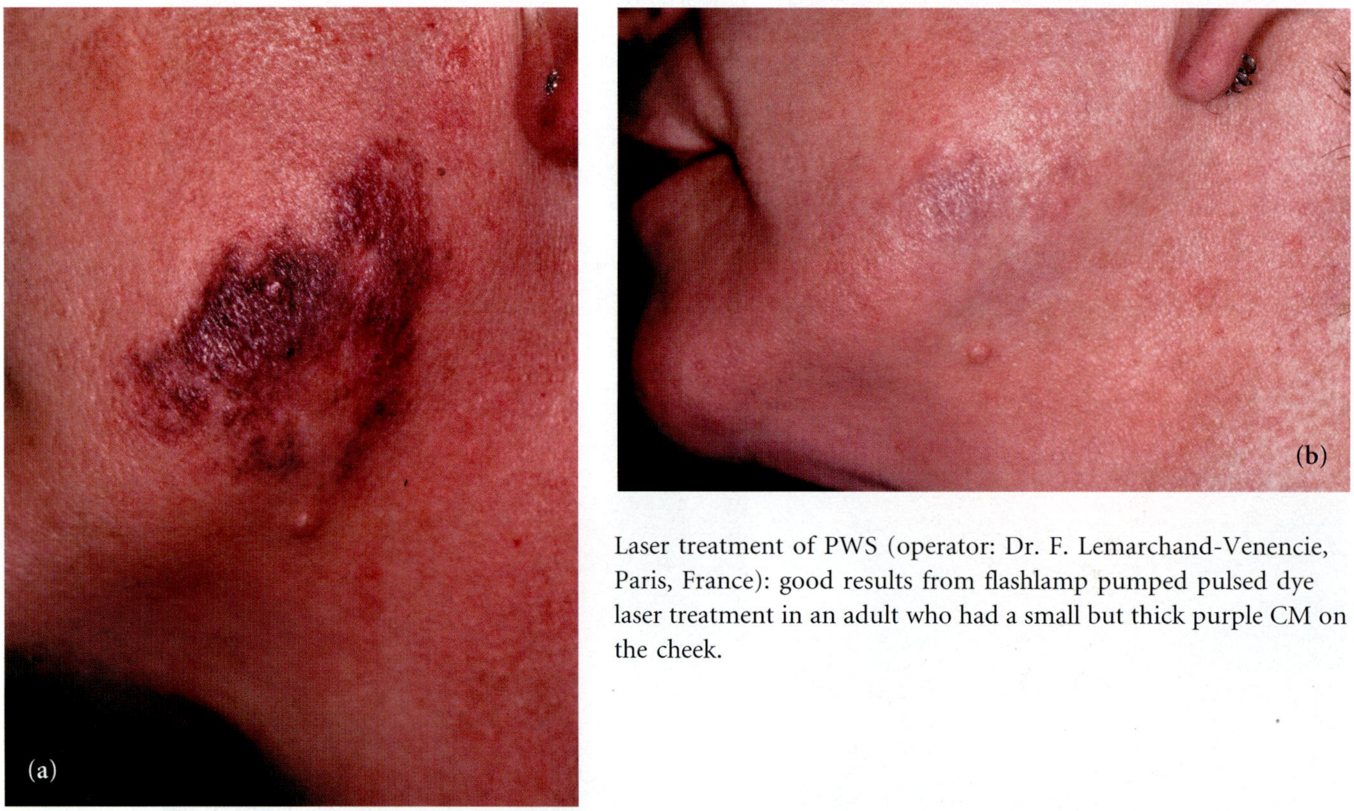

Laser treatment of PWS (operator: Dr. F. Lemarchand-Venencie, Paris, France): good results from flashlamp pumped pulsed dye laser treatment in an adult who had a small but thick purple CM on the cheek.

Clinical Aspects

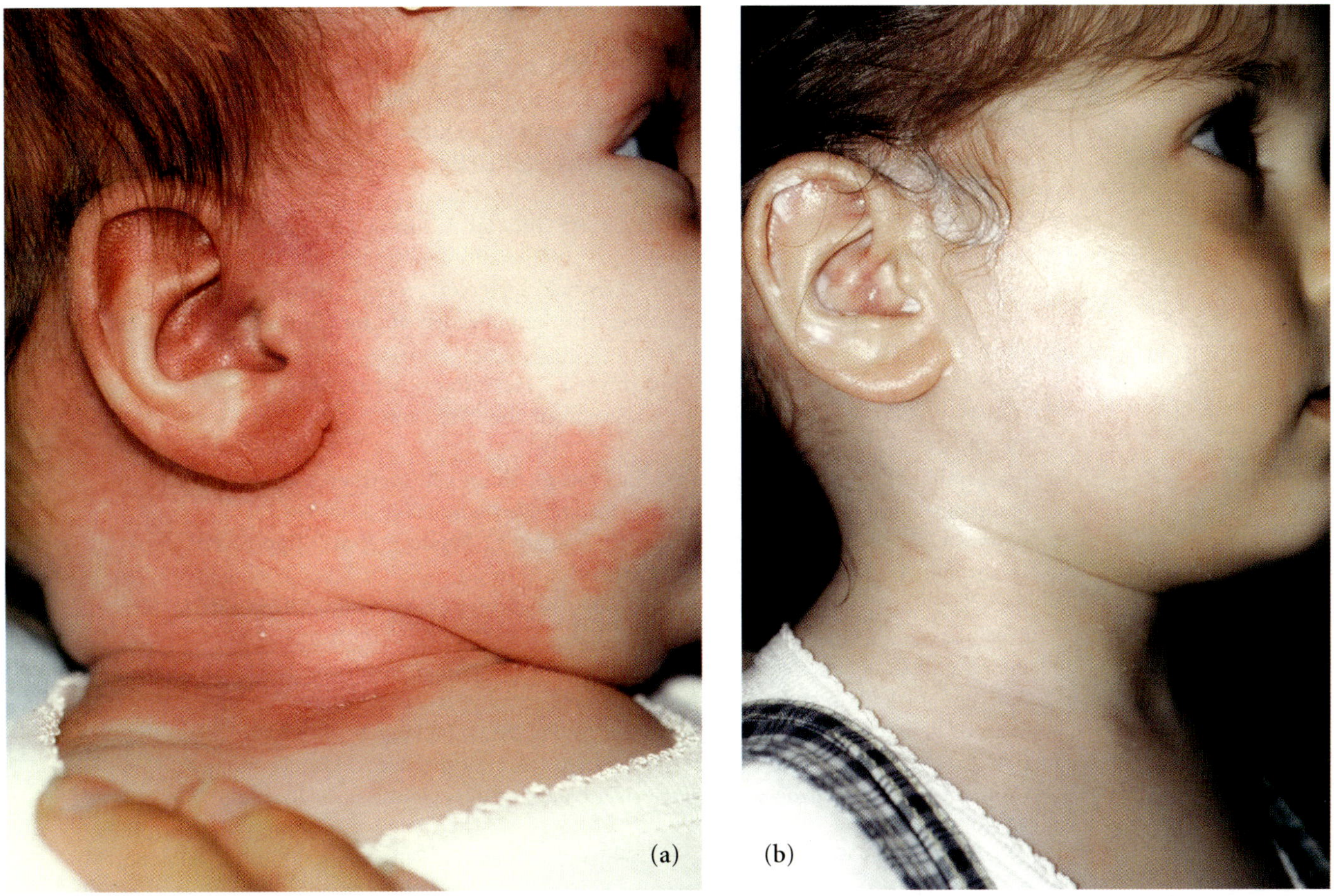

This girl with CM of the neck, ear, cheek, and temporal area as seen at 2 months of age, before the first flashlamp pumped pulsed dye laser treatment (FPDL) (a), and at 4 years of age (b) after seven sessions on the whole CM surface, five with the 585 nm and two with the 595 nm FPDL. Treatments were performed under local anesthesia with Emla® cream (operator: Dr. Virginie Fayard, Paris, France).

References

1 Adams BB, Lucky AW. Acquired port-wine stains and antecedent trauma: case report and review of the literature. *Arch Dermatol* 2000; **136**: 897–9.

2 Adamsbaum C, Pinton F, Rolland Y, Chiron C, Dulac O, Kalifa G. Accelerated myelination in early Sturge–Weber syndrome: MRI-SPECT correlations. *Pediatr Radiol* 1996; **26**: 759–62.

3 Al Hawsawi K, Al Aboud K, Al Aboud D, Al Githami A. Linear angioma serpiginosum. *Pediatr Dermatol* 2003; **20**: 167–8.

4 Bayrak-Toydemir P, Mao R, Lewin S, McDonald J. Hereditary hemorrhagic telangiectasia: an overview of diagnosis and management in the molecular era for clinicians. *Genet Med* 2004; **6**: 175–91.

5 Begbie ME, Wallace GM, and Shovlin CL. Hereditary haemorrhagic telangiectasia (Osler–Weber–Rendu syndrome): a view from the 21st century. *Postgrad Med J* 2003; **79**: 18–24.

6 Ben-Amitai D, Davidson S, Schwartz M, Prais D, Shamir R, Metzker A et al. Sacral nevus flammeus simplex: the role of imaging. *Pediatr Dermatol* 2000; **17**: 469–71.

7 Berry SA, Peterson C, Mize W, Bloom K, Zachary C, Blasco P et al. Klippel–Trenaunay syndrome. *Am J Med Genet* 1998; **79**: 319–26.

8 Biesecker LG. The multifaceted challenges of Proteus syndrome. *JAMA* 2001; **285**: 2240–3.

9 Biesecker LG, Peters KF, Darling TN, Choyke P, Hill S, Schimke N et al. Clinical differentiation between Proteus syndrome and hemihyperplasia: description of a distinct form of hemihyperplasia. *Am J Med Genet* 1998; **79**: 311–18.

10 Cabana MD, Crawford TO, Winkelstein JA, Christensen JR, Lederman HM. Consequences of the delayed diagnosis of ataxia–telangiectasia. *Pediatrics* 1998; **102**: 98–100.

11 Chiron C, Raynaud C, Tzourio N, Diebler C, Dulac O, Zilbovicius M et al. Regional cerebral blood flow by SPECT imaging in Sturge–Weber disease: an aid for diagnosis. *J Neurol Neurosurg Psychiatry* 1989; **52**: 1402–9.

12 Chugani HT. The role of PET in childhood epilepsy. *J Child Neurol* 1994; **9** Suppl 1: S82–8.

13 Cole SG, Begbie ME, Wallace GM, Shovlin CL. A new locus for Hereditary Haemorrhagic Telangiectasia (HHT3) maps to chromosome 5. *J Med Genet* 2005; **42**: 577–82.

14 DeLone DR, Brown WD, Gentry LR. Proteus syndrome: craniofacial and cerebral MRI. *Neuroradiology* 1999; **41**: 840–3.

15 Devillers AC, de Waard-van der Spek FB, Oranje A P. Cutis marmorata telangiectatica congenita: clinical features in 35 cases. *Arch Dermatol* 1999; **135**: 34–8.

16 Dyall-Smith D, Ramsden A, Laurie S. Adams–Oliver syndrome: aplasia cutis congenita, terminal transverse limb defects and cutis marmorata telangiectatica congenita. *Australas J Dermatol.* 1994; **35**: 19–22.

17 Enjolras O. Cutis marmorata telangiectatica congenita. *Ann Dermatol Venereol* 2001; **128**: 161–6.

18 Enjolras O, Chapot R, Merland JJ. Vascular anomalies and the growth of limbs: a review. *J Pediatr Orthop B* 2004; **13**: 349–57.

19 Enjolras O, Riché MC, Mulliken JB, Merland JJ, *Hémangiomes et Malformations Vasculaires. Atlas.* Paris: Medsi/McGraw Hill, 1990,.

20 Etchevers HC, Vincent C, Le Douarin NM, Couly GF. The cephalic neural crest provides pericytes and smooth muscle cells to all blood vessels of the face and forebrain. *Development* 2001; **128**: 1059–68.

21 Eubanks LE, McBurney EI. Videomicroscopy of port-wine stains: correlation of location and depth of lesion. *J Am Acad Dermatol* 2001; **44**: 948–51

22 Folz BJ, Wollstein AC, Lippert BM, Werner JA. Morphology and distribution of nasal telangiectasia in HHT-patients with epistaxis. *Am J Rhinol* 2005; **19**: 65–70.

23 Germain DP. Fabry disease in 2004. *Rev Prat* 2003; **53**: 2215–20.

24 Greene AK, Kieran M, Burrows PE, Mulliken JB, Kasser J, Fishman SJ. Wilms tumor screening is unnecessary in Klippel–Trenaunay syndrome. *Pediatrics* 2004; **113**: e326–9.

25 Guggisberg D, Hadj-Rabia S, Viney C, Bodemer C, Brunelle F, Zerah M et al. Skin markers of occult spinal dysraphism in children: a review of 54 cases. *Arch Dermatol* 2004; **140**: 1109–15.

26 Gungor T, Buhring I, Cremer R, Gartenschlager M, Zielen S. Pathogenesis, diagnosis, clinical and therapeutic aspects of ataxia telangiectasia. *Klin Padiatr* 1997; **209**: 328–35.

27 Hagiwara K, Uezato H, Nonaka S. Phacomatosis pigmentovascularis type IIb associated with Sturge–Weber syndrome and pyogenic granuloma. *J Dermatol* 1998; **25**: 721–9.

28 Hansen K, Kreiter CD, Rosenbaum M, Whitaker DC, Arpey CJ. Long-term psychological impact and perceived efficacy of pulsed-dye laser therapy for patients with port-wine stains. *Dermatol Surg* 2003; **29**: 49–55.

29 Happle R. Loss of heterozygosity in human skin. *J Am Acad Dermatol* 1999; **41**: 143–64.

30 Happle R, Steijlen PM. Phacomatosis pigmentovascularis interpreted as a phenomenon of twin spots. *Hautarzt* 1989; **40**: 721–4.

31 Happle R, Steijlen PM, Theile U, Karitzky D, Tinschert S, Albrecht-Nebe H et al. Patchy dermal hypoplasia as a characteristic feature of Proteus syndrome. *Arch Dermatol* 1997; **133**: 77–80.

32 Heikkinen K, Rapakko K, Karppinen SM, Erkko H, Nieminen P, Winqvist R. Association of common ATM polymorphism with bilateral breast cancer. *Int J Cancer* 2005; **116**: 69–72.

33 Hoeger PH, Martinez A, Maerker J, Harper JI. Vascular anomalies in Proteus syndrome. *Clin Exp Dermatol* 2004; **29**: 222–30.

34 Hotamisligil GS, Ertogan F. The Proteus syndrome: association with nephrogenic diabetes insipidus. *Clin Genet* 1990; **38**: 139–44.

35 Jacoby CG, Yuh WT, Afifi AK, Bell WE, Schelper RL, Sato Y. Accelerated myelination in early Sturge–Weber syndrome demonstrated by MR imaging. *J Comput Assist Tomogr* 1987; **11**: 226–31.

36 Klapman MH, Yao JF. Thickening and nodules in port-wine stains. *J Am Acad Dermatol* 2001; **44**: 300–2.

37 Kossoff EH, Buck C, Freeman JM. Outcomes of 32 hemispherectomies for Sturge–Weber syndrome worldwide. *Neurology* 2002; **59**: 1735–8.

38 Kuehl HK, Caselitz M, Hasenkamp S, Wagner S, El-Harith el HA, Manns MP et al. Hepatic manifestation is associated with ALK1 in hereditary hemorrhagic telangiectasia: identification of five novel ALK1 and one novel ENG mutations. *Hum Mutat* 2005; **25**: 320.

39 Kundu RV, Frieden IJ. Presence of vascular anomalies with congenital hemihypertrophy and Wilms tumor: an evidence-based evaluation. *Pediatr Dermatol* 2003; **20**: 199–206.

40 Larralde M, Boggio P, Amartino H, Chamoles N. Fabry disease: a study of 6 hemizygous men and 5 heterozygous females with emphasis on dermatologic manifestations. *Arch Dermatol* 2004; **140**: 1440–6.

41 Leung AK, Telmesani AM. Salmon patches in Caucasian children. *Pediatr Dermatol* 1989; **6**: 185–7.

42 Linthorst GE, De Rie MA, Tjiam KH, Aerts JM, Dingemans KP, Hollak CE. Misdiagnosis of Fabry disease: importance of biochemical confirmation of clinical or pathological suspicion. *Br J Dermatol* 2004; **150**: 575–7.

43 Loo WJ, Lanigan SW. Recent advances in laser therapy for the treatment of cutaneous vascular disorders. *Lasers Med Sci* 2002; **17**: 9–12.

44 Maari C, Frieden IJ. Klippel–Trenaunay syndrome: the importance of "geographic stains" in identifying lymphatic disease and risk of complications. *J Am Acad Dermatol* 2004; **51**: 391–8.

45 Maniscalco M, Guareschi E, Noto G, Patrizi A. Midline telangiectatic nevus (salmon patch) of the nape of the neck. *Eur J Pediatr Dermatol* 2003; **13**: 81–4.

46 Martinelli PT, Tschen JA. Eccrine angiomatous hamartoma: a case report and review of the literature. *Cutis* 2003; **71**: 449–55.

47 Metzker A, Shamir R. Butterfly-shaped mark: a variant form of nevus flammeus simplex. *Pediatrics* 1990; **85**: 1069–71.

48 Nagore E, Requena C, Sevila A, Coll J, Costa D, Botella-Estrada R et al. Thickness of healthy and affected skin of children with port wine stains: potential repercussions on response to pulsed dye laser treatment. *Dermatol Surg* 2004; **30**: 1457–61.

49 Osburn K, Schosser RH, Everett MA. Congenital pigmented and vascular lesions in newborn infants. *J Am Acad Dermatol* 1987; **16**: 788–92.

50 Patrizi A, Neri I, Orlandi C, Marini R. Sacral medial telangiectatic vascular nevus: a study of 43 children. *Dermatology* 1996; **192**: 301–6.

51 Piaserico S, Belloni Fortina A. Posttraumatic port-wine stain in a 4-year-old girl: Fegeler syndrome. *Pediatr Dermatol* 2004; **21**: 131–3.

52 Picascia DD, Esterly NB. Cutis marmorata telangiectatica congenita: report of 22 cases. *J Am Acad Dermatol* 1989; **20**: 1098–104.

53 Pinton F, Chiron C, Enjolras O, Motte J, Syrota A, Dulac O. Early single photon emission computed tomography in Sturge–Weber syndrome. *J Neurol Neurosurg Psychiatry* 1997; **63**: 616–21.

54 Prigent F, Kahn A, Martinet C, Saigot T. Pigmented-vascular phakomatosis type IIIa. *Ann Dermatol Venereol* 1991; **118**: 531–3.

55 Requena L, Sangueza OP. Cutaneous vascular anomalies. Part I. Hamartomas, malformations, and dilation of preexisting vessels. *J Am Acad Dermatol* 1997; **37**: 523–49; quiz 549–52.

56 Robertson SP, Gattas M, Rogers M, Ades LC. Macrocephaly–cutis marmorata telangiectatica congenita: report of five patients and a review of the literature. *Clin Dysmorphol* 2000; **9**: 1–9.

57 Ruiz-Maldonado R, Tamayo L, Laterza AM, Brawn G, Lopez A. Phacomatosis pigmentovascularis: a new syndrome? Report of four cases. *Pediatr Dermatol* 1987; **4**: 189–96.

58 Sanchez-Carpintero I, Mihm MC, Mizeracki A, Waner M, North PE. Epithelial and mesenchymal hamartomatous changes in a mature port-wine stain: Morphologic evidence for a multiple germ layer field defect. *J Am Acad Dermatol* 2004; **50**: 608–12.

59 Schepis C, Greco D, Failla P, Siragusa M, Romano C, Scaffidi M et al. Medial telangiectatic sacral nevi and MCA/MR syndromes. *Pediatr Dermatol* 2003; **20**: 370–1.

60 Schiller PI, Itin PH, Angiokeratomas: an update. *Dermatology* 1996; **193**: 275–82.

61 Selim MM, Kelly KM, Nelson JS, Wendelschafer-Crabb G, Kennedy WR, Zelickson BD. Confocal microscopy study of nerves and blood vessels in untreated and treated port wine stains: preliminary observations. *Dermatol Surg* 2004; **30**: 892–7.

62 Smoller BR, Rosen S. Port-wine stains. A disease of altered neural modulation of blood vessels? *Arch Dermatol* 1986; **122**: 177–9.

63 Sommer S, Merchant WJ, Sheehan-Dare R. Severe predominantly acral variant of angiokeratoma of Mibelli: response to long-pulse Nd:YAG (1064 nm) laser treatment. *J Am Acad Dermatol* 2001; **45**: 764–6.

64 Tavafoghi V, Ghandchi A, Hambrick GW Jr, Udverhelyi GB. Cutaneous signs of spinal dysraphism. Report of a patient with a tail-like lipoma and review of 200 cases in the literature. *Arch Dermatol* 1978; **114**: 573–7.

65 Torrelo A, Zambrano A, Happle R. Cutis marmorata telangiectatica congenita and extensive mongolian spots: type 5 phacomatosis pigmentovascularis. *Br J Dermatol* 2003; **148**: 342–5.

66 Turner JT, Cohen MM Jr, Biesecker LG. Reassessment of the Proteus syndrome literature: application of diagnostic criteria to published cases. *Am J Med Genet A* 2004; **130**: 111–22.
67 Ville D, Enjolras O, Chiron C, Dulac O. Prophylactic antiepileptic treatment in Sturge–Weber disease. *Seizure* 2002; **11**: 145–50.
68 Waner M. Recent developments in lasers and the treatment of birthmarks. *Arch Dis Child* 2003; **88**: 372–4.
69 Wiedemann HR, Burgio GR, Aldenhoff P, Kunze J, Kaufmann HJ, Schirg E. The proteus syndrome. Partial gigantism of the hands and/or feet, nevi, hemihypertrophy, subcutaneous tumors, macrocephaly or other skull anomalies and possible accelerated growth and visceral affections. *Eur J Pediatr* 1983; **140**: 5–12.
70 Wilcox WR, Banikazemi M, Guffon N, Waldek S, Lee P, Linthorst GE et al. Long-term safety and efficacy of enzyme replacement therapy for Fabry disease. *Am J Hum Genet* 2004; **75**: 65–74.

CHAPTER III.B

Venous Malformations (VM)

III.B.1 Common Venous Malformations

Introduction and Clinical Patterns

Venous malformations (VM) are hemodynamically inactive, slow-flow vascular malformations involving the collecting side of the vascular network. They are the most common vascular malformation seen in clinics for vascular anomalies. This localized defect in vascular morphogenesis is characterized by enlarged and distorted venous channels, with irregular lack of smooth muscle cells around the flat continuous layer of endothelial cells in their walls (5).

Most VMs occur sporadically. Rare familial cases exist: these account for about 1% of all VMs (3). A VM is usually visible at birth, as a minor bluish patch or plaque, or as a network of dilated veins. It slowly worsens over the life of the patient to varying degrees. The overload of distorted venous channels within the dermal layers give the skin or mucous membranes the characteristic blue hue. The blue color becomes particularly significant when the dilated venous-like channels invade the superficial dermis. This blue color is obvious on skin as well as on the mucous membranes of the mouth, conjunctiva and genitalia. A VM never regresses, unlike hemangioma and various vascular tumors present at birth or developing in infancy. It affects males and females equally.

VMs are localized or extensive, minor or distorting, flat or spongy, single or multiple. They involve skin, mucous membranes, soft tissues and particularly muscles, joints and bones, and even viscera. Depending on the size and site of their lesion, patients complain of swelling and pain sensation. Stiffness and pain upon awakening are common symptoms in patients with extremity VM. VMs swell with physical exertion and when the region is dependent, in fact in every situation when blood pressure increases. Deformation of anatomical structures happens slowly over the years. With a VM in the cheek, facial features are altered by the soft-tissue filling and bony deformity results from a mass-compressing effect. Skin temperature is usually normal or mildly increased. There is no thrill, no bruit like in AVM. Head-and-neck VM and trunk-and-limbs VM have different clinical consequences due to the unique environment they occur in (20, 21, 31).

Worsening over the years is due to the progressive "opening" of the distorted, poorly defined and interconnecting anomalous venous network that dissects the normal tissues.

Pathology

Whatever their location, the pathological features of VM are similar (40). Macroscopic evaluation of surgical specimens may be deceptive, as the blood content of the lesion is lost during surgery. The lesion may be elusive or appear as soft sponge-like fibrous tissue, unless modified by thrombosis or embolization or containing spherical phleboliths. Histologically, VMs are badly delimited, made of interconnecting slit-like or open lumen, dissecting the host tissues and surrounding some normal elements (arteries, nerves, muscle bundles, etc.). The frequent intralesional thrombosis may be organized as concentric laminated collagen deposits that are prone to calcification (phleboliths), or as thin fibrous papillary fronds (Masson intravascular papillary hyperplasia).

In rare cases the vascular channels are more grouped together, packed against each other without intervening normal constituents of the host tissue, forming fairly delineated nodules. This type of nodular VM, often called "cavernoma" when localized in the central nervous system, is rarely diagnosed preoperatively as a VM in the skin and soft tissues and may be operated on as a cyst or a tumor.

Investigations

First of all, one should stress the point that the best imaging tool for VM is MRI.

Ultrasonography and color doppler give information on the angioarchitecture, vessel density, peak flow velocities, and resistive indexes (32). It easily distinguishes between hemangioma and vascular malformations, and between VM and fast-flow anomalies. Heterogeneous echogenicity and ill-defined hypoechoic lacunar or tubular pattern are noted. Arterial structures are not identified. Calcifications are detected.

CT SCANS with iodinated contrast detect soft-tissues and skeletal alterations, but the images are not specific for a VM.

MRI with spin–echo T1-weighted images allowing anatomical evaluation, and fat saturation T2-weighted sequences characteristic of slow-flow lesions, visualizes the VM in axial, sagittal, and coronal sections. In a majority of patients MRI is the only indispensable radiological investigation to ensure the diagnosis and delineate the VM. On T1-sequences the VM gives an intermediate signal, hypo- or isointense to muscles. On T2-sequences with fat saturation, a VM is composed of well-delineated venous pouches with high signal intensity (17). Round areas of absent signal (black dots) correspond to phleboliths (round calcification secondary to thrombi). Thrombus and hemosiderin deposits modify the signal. MRI demonstrates the involved structures and the extent of the vascular anomaly. Muscle involvement by the VM may be localized or diffusely distributed to a muscle or a group of muscles, and the abnormal venous network creates either large pouches or multiple small hyperintense areas outlined by fibrous septa. Gadolinium contrast infusion enhances the VM lesions in T1-weighted sequences, a finding that distinguishes between VM and lymphatic malformations (LM), or in the craniofacial area between VM and various cystic lesions (thyroglosal duct, cysts of pharyngeal arch, etc.).

DIGITAL COMPUTED ARTERIOGRAM is not recommended as it usually poorly fills a VM; in large spongy VM the late venous phase of the femoral arteriogram shows the contrast collecting or pudding in the anomalous network (9).

PHLEBOGRAPHY reveals the abnormal veins of VMs located in the extremities, but it does not precisely demonstrate their anatomical location and the size of the lesion, and therefore has limited usefulness in comparison to Doppler plus MRI evaluation. "Direct percutaneous puncture of the malformation with contrast injection" gives a phlebogram that best shows the VM and its drainage prior to sclerotherapy (10, 17, 34).

VM can be associated with "modifications of the blood coagulation profile," e.g. an activation of coagulation in the distorted and enlarged stagnant venous channels, with consumption of coagulation factors (29). This localized intravascular coagulation (LIC) due to local conditions has to be distinguished from disseminated intravascular coagulation (DIC) linked with general conditions such as septicemia, and from KMP (Table 15). The slow flow and increased blood volume within the VM are responsible for blood stagnation and activation of the intravascular coagulation. Consequences are: local thrombotic episodes with pain, activation of coagulation factors and consumption of inhibitors, and consumption of coagulation factors potentiating blood loss from the VM (29).

Table 15 Differences between the Kasabach–Merritt syndrome (KMS) or phenomenon (KMP) and the VM/LM-associated localized chronic intravascular coagulopathy (LIC).

	KMP	*VM/LM LIC*
Age of occurrence	Infancy	Flares from birth to old age
Pathologic subset	A tumor: tufted angioma or kaposiform hemangioendothelioma	A vascular malformation: VM or LM, usually an extensive one in the limbs or trunk
Platelet counts	Very low (5000–10000/mm^3)	Moderately low (usually around 80000–100000/mm^3
Other coagulopathic anomalies	High D-dimers, low fibrinogen	Very high D-dimers, very low fibrinogen
Pathogenesis	Platelet trapping inside the tumor	Abnormal channel wall function
Clinical patterns and risks	The tumor (usually congenital) becomes suddenly raised, shiny, bruising, and occasionally inflammatory purpura Visceral bleeding	Intralesional bruise, local pain, phlebolith formation secondary to thrombosis may progress to DIC with hemorrhages, in case of trauma, surgical treatment, embolization/ sclerotherapy
Therapeutic management	Tumor resection when feasible Pharmacological treatment (GS, IFN, VCR, etc.)	LMWH Pharmacological treatments totally ineffective
Course	Residual tumor (usually minor) after cure of the KMP	VM and LM persist lifelong
Remark	This phenomenon matches the original description by Kasabach and Merritt in 1940	This phenomenon should not be called KMP/KMS, as is often done in the literature: this brings a risk of therapeutic mismanagement

VM= venous malformation; LM= lymphatic malformation; DIC= disseminated intravascular coagulopathy; GS =glucocorticosteroids; IFN= interferon alpha 2a or 2b; VCR= vincristine; LMWH= low-molecular-weight heparin.

D-dimers increase and fibrinogen level is low, while platelet count is variably lowered. Improving these parameters counteracts the clinical problems: patients are moderately anticoagulated with low-molecular-weight heparin in a preventive dosage (for example enoxaparine 100 units/kg once a day, and we monitor anti Xa activity to reach a target value of 0.5 u/ml) (29). This LIC is common in extensive limb and trunk VMs, and, for unknown reasons, seems unusual in cephalic ones.

Treatment

Treatment depends on the location and likely consequences of the lesion. It relies on sclerotherapy and surgery. Selective catheterization of slow-flow lesions is difficult, and, therefore, arterial embolization is now very seldom used. The best strategy for treatment is intralesional treatment after direct puncture of the lesions (1, 18, 39, 41). Various sclerosant injections have been used, mainly Ethibloc® (a mixture of the corn protein zein, ethanol, contrast medium, and additives (19, 35)) and absolute ethanol.

Acrylic polymers are not suitable for VM sclerotherapy; however, just before resection of some VMs they are sometimes preferred, as they help limit bleeding and better delineate the lesion, they also cause less immediate post-treatment inflammation and edema than Ethibloc or ethanol (10). The adjunctive technique consists of introducing platinum coils in very large VM before injecting the sclerosant, and sometimes inflating a balloon in a large collecting vein, during the intralesional injection of ethanol, to reduce the washout of the sclerosant (28). Ethanol is the best sclerosant but it carries a serious risk of side-effects, locally (swelling, necrosis and scarring, nerve injury) and systemically (pulmonary vasospasm, pulmonary embolism, myocardial toxicity, CNS depression, etc.) (10). In the literature the currently admitted "safe" limit dose was 1 ml/kg of body-weight of ethanol for sclerotherapy (27, 28). This dose is in fact probably unsafe and should be redefined. Rare lethal complications have happened with lower dosages (15). The dose of 1 ml/kg also results in an alcohol-intoxicated state, which can pose risks during and after the procedure (28). Procedures are performed under fluoroscopic control with real-time digital subtraction. For safety, a procedure with ethanol requires the use of an adjuvant to visualize this X-ray-undetectable sclerosant (37). The treatment is given under general anesthesia with careful monitoring. Some small lesions are treated utilizing "detergent sclerosants" that are milder than ethanol (12, 36) – either sodium tetradecyl sulfate (Sotradecol or Trombovar®) or polidocanol (Lauromacrogol or Aetoxisclerol®) – also aiming at destroying the endothelium. These sclerosants are given every 2 or 3 weeks, with either local (contact) anesthesia and/or neuroleptanalgesia, or without anesthesia, and they are effective enough for bluish cutaneous VM, with the advantage of carrying a more minor risk of necrosis of the skin than Ethibloc or ethanol. Microfoam prepared with polidocanol seems to have few local side-effects, as this mixture allows reduction of the amount of injected sclerosant (13, 14). US-guided sclerotherapy avoids misdirected injections and provides the best results.

For cephalic VMs, treatment begins as soon as deformity or functional problems (mainly misalignment of teeth) develop. Multiple sessions are required, combining sclerotherapy and surgical procedures, with varying timing. In addition, open-bite deformity requires orthodontic management and sometimes orthognathic surgery is also performed after the secondary teeth erupt.

The final aim of this long-lasting treatment is to maintain or restore facial symmetry and improve the patient's quality of life, reducing the painful episodes of swelling of the VM. Good resolution of small and medium-sized VMs in the trunk or limbs, involving skin and/or muscles, may be obtained with percutaneous sclerotherapy (41). However, large VMs in the extremities or trunk, affecting skin, muscles, and joints, cannot be eradicated without functional risk and marked scarring; in this case treatments are palliative, sclerotherapy limiting areas of pain, or excision of some bulges improving shape. Sclerotherapy and resection help alleviate volume and symptoms in some parts of the lesion, but can never suppress it. Elastic stockings are indispensable: they provide comfort by reducing the venous pressure, and they may reduce the risk of intralesional thrombosis and ensuing pain.

III.B.2 Syndromic Venous Malformations, Nosology

A number of syndromes have long been associated or confused with common VM. Some are familial, others are sporadic.

III.B.2.1 BEAN SYNDROME OR BLUE RUBBER BLEB NAEVUS SYNDROME

Blue rubber bleb naevus (BRBN) syndrome consists principally of multiple circumscribed venous lesions disseminating on skin, of three types: dark blue often keratotic spots, blebs of normal skin color, and large venous or venous and lymphatic masses resembling common VM. The second important aspect is bleeding from lesions of the gastrointestinal tract. Many other sites of involvement have been reported but they are all uncommon. BRBN has long been described in the literature as familial, probably because of a confusion with VMCM. In the literature several cases reported as BRBN are probably different diseases (mainly VMCM, glomuvenous malformation or Maffucci syndrome (see pages 174–6). Bean syndrome occurs sporadically in our experience with a large number of patients. Both sexes are equally affected. Vascular skin abnormalities are usually visible from birth, and they rapidly increase in number. This proliferation may continue lifelong. Among the gastrointestinal (GI) lesions, the small bowel ones are the most frequent (22, 23), but GI distribution may display a widespread involvement in many patients. Easy bleeding causes anemia and severe iron deficiency (melena, rectal bleeding, gastric blood vomiting). Other reported visceral locations include: the brain, bladder, liver, spleen, lung, heart, etc. All these lesions are often reported as "hemangiomas," which is misleading: they encompass venous channels and they are VMs. Imaging is characteristic of a VM: in addition to the small blue "nipples" and "buttons" (26) the lesions may also create a large soft bluish mass and affect the muscles. MRI clearly shows them as well-circumscribed, septated, strongly hyperintense masses on T2. Gastrointestinal lesions are evaluated using endoscopy, and capsular videoendoscopy, barium studies, nuclear imaging, CT, MRI, or selective mesenteric artery angiograms (26). Intestinal lesions are treated when anemia is severe. Bleeding requires blood transfusions when conservative treatment (iron supplementation) is insufficient. Other complications include intussusception, infarction, and volvulus. Endoscopic sclerotherapy and laser photocoagulation or intestinal resection are applied, but new lesions often develop with time (16). A chronic intravascular coagulopathy, identical to what happens with large VM in an extremity, often manifests early in childhood (and even at birth) with high D-dimers, very low fibrinogen levels and a moderate thrombocytopenia; it enhances intestinal bleeding and can be improved using low-molecular-weight heparin treatment.

III.B.2.2 FAMILIAL CUTANEOUS AND MUCOUS VENOUS MALFORMATIONS

In familial cutaneous and mucous venous malformations (VMCM) patients display multiple skin, mucosa, and muscle venous malformations, in an apparently haphazard distribution. They do not usually have a visceral location. Histologically, the lesions are identical to common sporadic VMs. Vikkula et al. (38) identified a single aminoacid change in the endothelial-specific angiopoietin receptor TIE2/TEK, leading to a gain-of-function genomic mutation. The mutated gene, located on 9p21, is the cause of this rare familial autosomal dominant vascular malformation (OMIM 600195), the occurrence being about 1% of all VM (3).

III.B.2.3 GLOMUVENOUS MALFORMATIONS (GVM)

A venous malformation (VM) is composed of malformed venous channels lined by a media which is focally deficient in smooth muscle cells. In contrast, glomuvenous malformations (GVM) have a variable increased number of layers of rounded or cuboidal cells in their walls, long known as glomus cells. These are alpha-actin positive smooth muscle cells. In the past, these lesions were called glomus tumors or glomangiomas. They have now been renamed glomuvenous malformations (GVMs) to stress the fact that they are malformations and not tumors as suggested by the suffix "-oma" (3, 5).

GVM (OMIM 138000) is familial in 64% of cases (3). This autosomal dominant disorder has a high penetrance in affected families. Brouillard et al. (5) localized the VMGLOM locus on chromosome 1p21–22, and identified the mutated gene as the glomulin gene; they first published the pedigrees of 20 affected families, indicating the affected patients and unaffected carriers, based on screening for mutations in the *glomulin* performed on genomic DNA and cDNA. A second publication based on 43 families (6) stresses the fact that four common *glomulin* mutations cover two-thirds of GVM familial cases. In addition, a second-hit mutation was demonstrated in the lesion of a patient. Therefore, it is suggested that if the somatic mutation (the second hit) occurs early in the development of the embryo this would explain the large segmental GVM, if it occurs late it would result in small scattered GVM, and the paradominant mode of inheritance would also explain the existence of unaffected carriers in some families. The disease is due to loss-of-function mutations of the *glomulin gene* (7). The skin is the main location for GVM, but the oral mucosa may be affected. Muscles are rarely and only superficially permeated, contrary to what occurs with common VM. On MRI, lesions of GVM give and intermediate signal on T1 and hypersignal on T2. the T1-sequence after gadolinium injection shows homogeneous hypersignal. No clinical and histological difference exists between the sporadic and hereditary cases. Management relies on resection, as sclerotherapy is rarely beneficial.

III.B.2.4 MAFFUCCI SYNDROME

The disease is rare and sporadic, chronic, usually benign but disabling, affecting both sexes equally. The first signs appear in childhood. The skin displays soft or firm blue nodules, which are shown to be true VM by investigation: the presence of phleboliths on plain radiography, hypersignal on T2-sequences with MRI, small capillary tufts at the late venous phase of the angiogram. From the pathological point of view skin lesions exhibit two different anomalies. There are areas where large irregular venous-type vessels (a VM) dissect the dermis and subcutis. In other areas nodules or strips of dense spindle cells correspond to the spindle cell hemangioendothelioma (SCH), sometimes developing inside a large venous channel (33). We currently do not know if SCH is a constant pathologic feature in Maffucci syndrome or if it occurs (or complicates?) only in some patients. The second most important clinical feature is enchondroma distorting the bones. Enchondroma is the incapability of cartilage to build normal bone. Radiographically there are translucent metaphyseal and diaphyseal masses. The hands and feet are affected in nearly 90% of patients, while one third of them have long-bone involvement creating distortion and dwarfism. Neurological complications may occur with cranial involvement. Enchondrosarcoma occurs; however, this malignant change may have been overestimated (30% of cases) in the literature.

Figures

VENOUS MALFORMATIONS
Pathology of Common VM

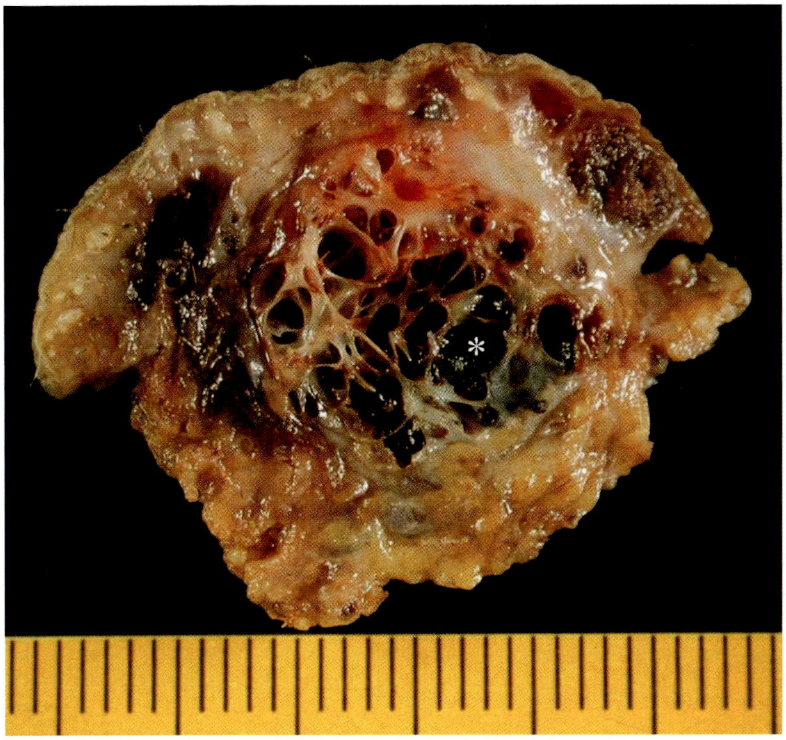

Gross specimen of a venous malformation in the dermis. Venous malformations usually collapse when operated on. In this specimen the vascular lumen remained opened, probably due to fibrosis, and the spongy architecture of the lesion is apparent. The cavities are communicating, are separated by thin or thick septa and contain some recent thrombus (*).

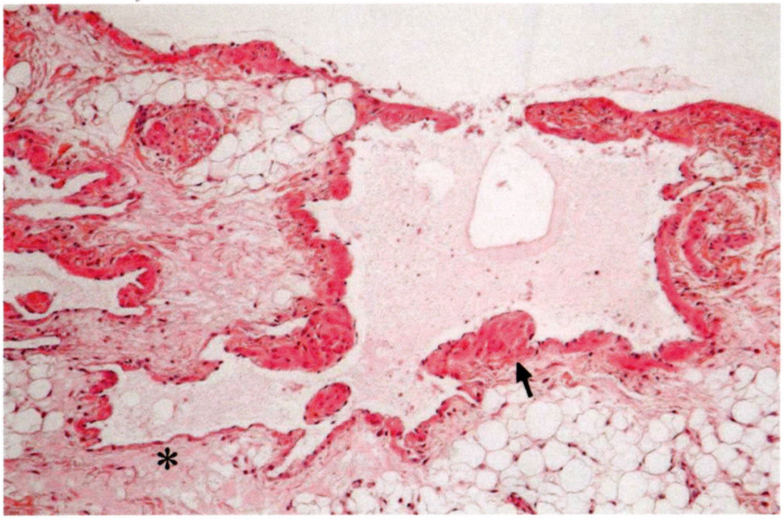

The lumens of the malformed vessels are irregular, their walls are thin and present areas with a muscular media (arrow) alternating with areas devoid of smooth-muscle cells (*).

Pathology of Common VM

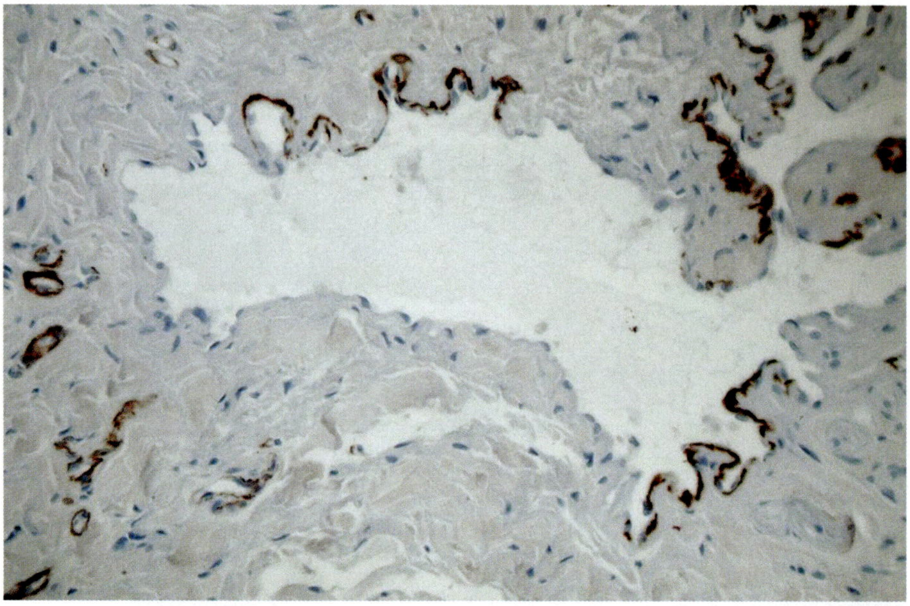

Immunohistochemistry with an anti-alpha smooth-muscle cell actin antibody (decorating the smooth-muscle cells in brown) highlights the defective character of the media, with large areas devoid of smooth-muscle cells.

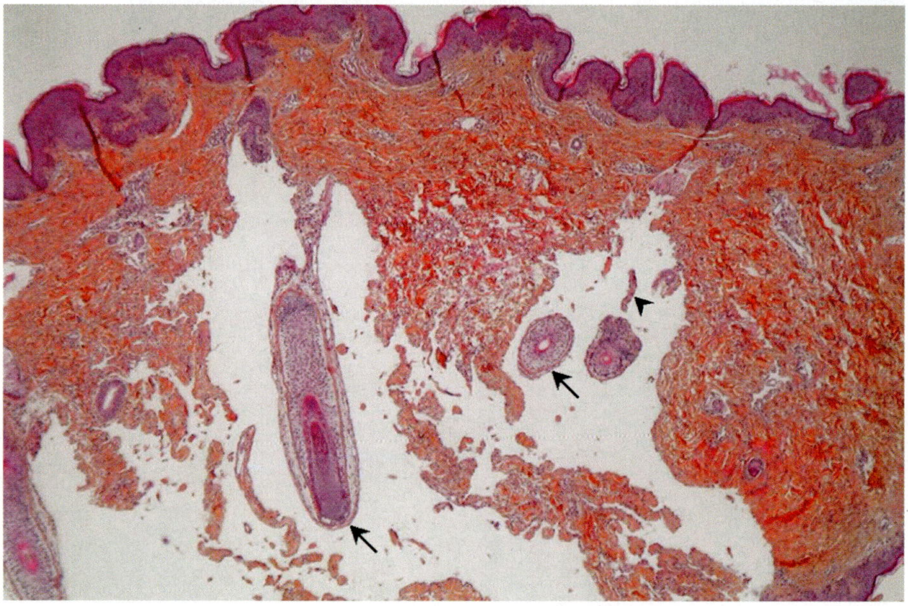

Venous malformation of the skin. The lesion seems to replace the dermis collagen. Hair follicles (arrows) and a small nerve (arrowhead) are floating in the cavities.

Pathology of Common VM

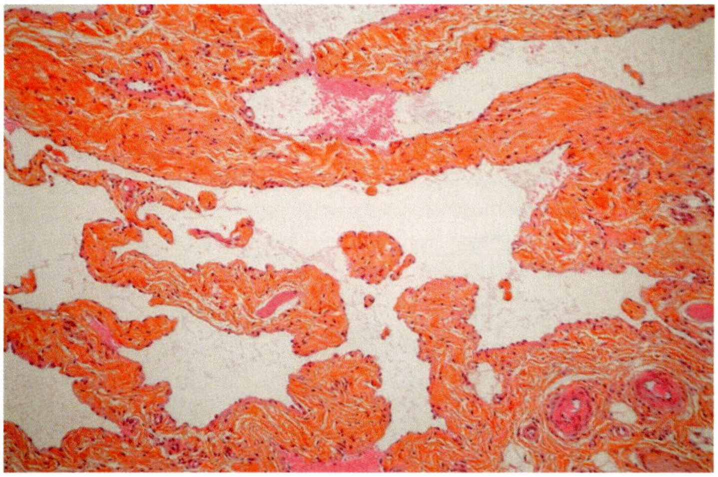

Venous malformation of the lip. The anastomosing vascular channels dissect the dermis. Their walls are nearly devoid of smooth-muscle cells.

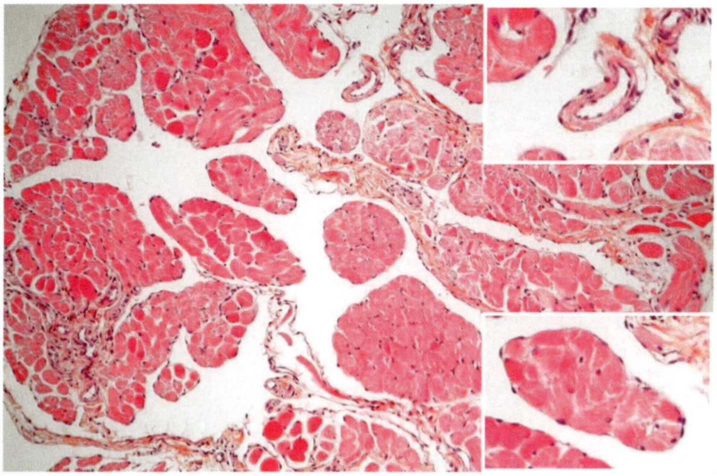

Venous malformation of the tongue. The thin-walled vascular channels separate the fascicles of the tongue muscle. Some fascicles (lower inset) and some arterioles (upper inset) are passing through the lesion, completely surrounded by the cavities.

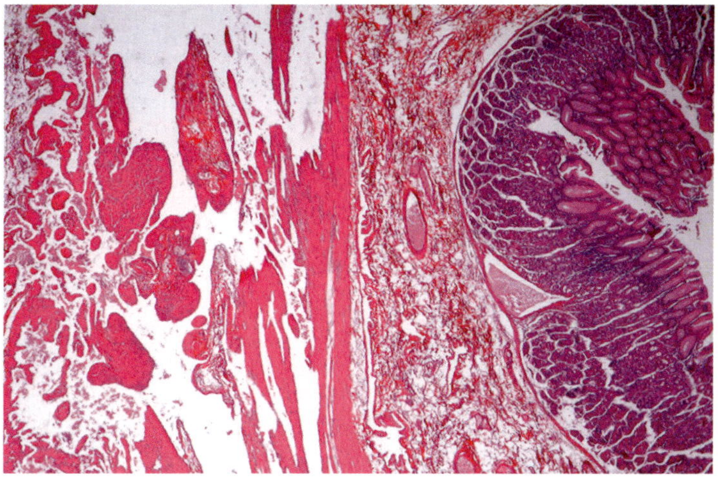

Nearly all organs or tissues may be affected by venous malformation. This is an example of venous malformation of the stomach, dissecting the muscularis proper.

Pathology of Common VM

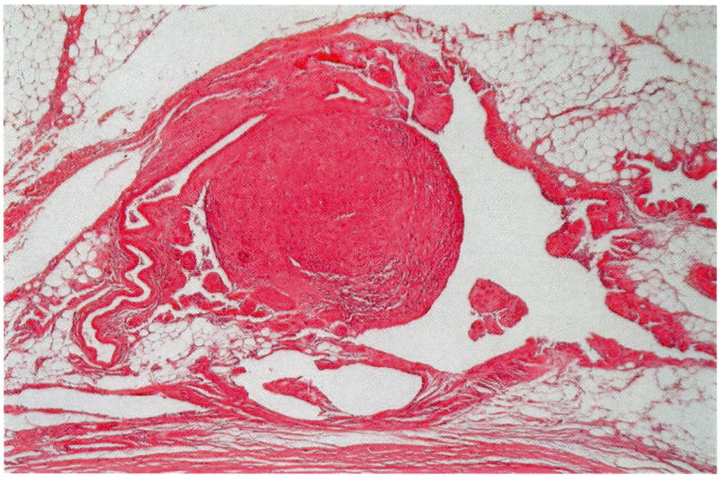

Organizing thrombus in a venous malformation. The thrombus is spherical but is not yet collagenized nor calcified.

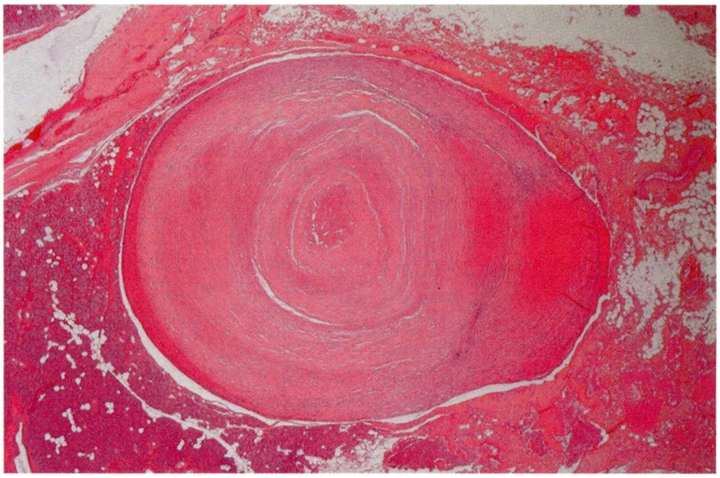

This organized thrombus in a parotid venous malformation is made of concentric laminated collagen deposits with calcification (phlebolith).

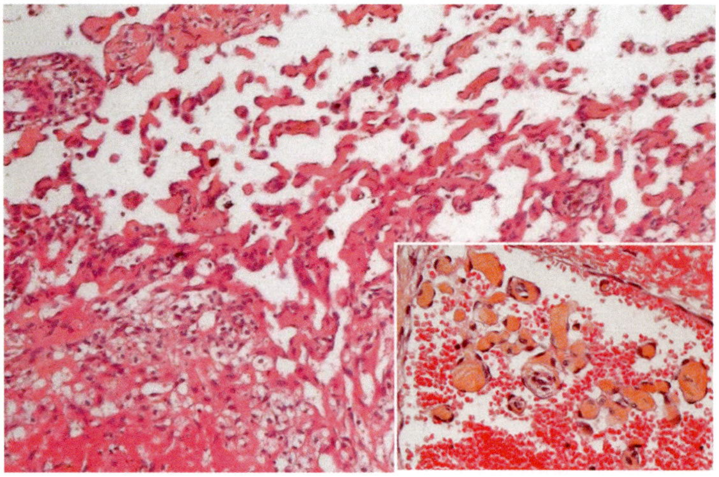

In some cases, the thrombus organizes forming fibrous papillary fronds named Masson's intravascular papillary hyperplasia, which may simulate an angiosarcoma. The inset shows the fibrous core of the papillae covered by a thin monolayered endothelium.

Clinical Patterns, Investigations, and Treatment

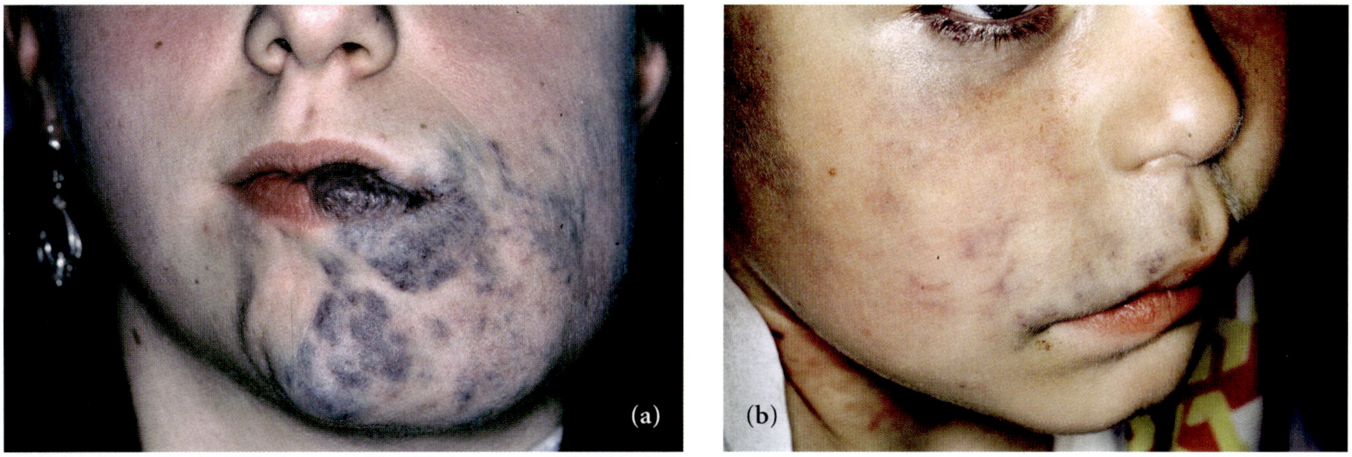

In the cephalic area VMs are usually unilateral, but some are bilateral, and may also be associated with another trunk or limb location of VM. The blue color of a facial VM is easily observed in skin. The full lesion may appear blue (a). In patient (b) there is some swelling of the cheek, which is fully involved by VM, but the blue hue mainly affects the lower lid and upper lip, a very common presentation.

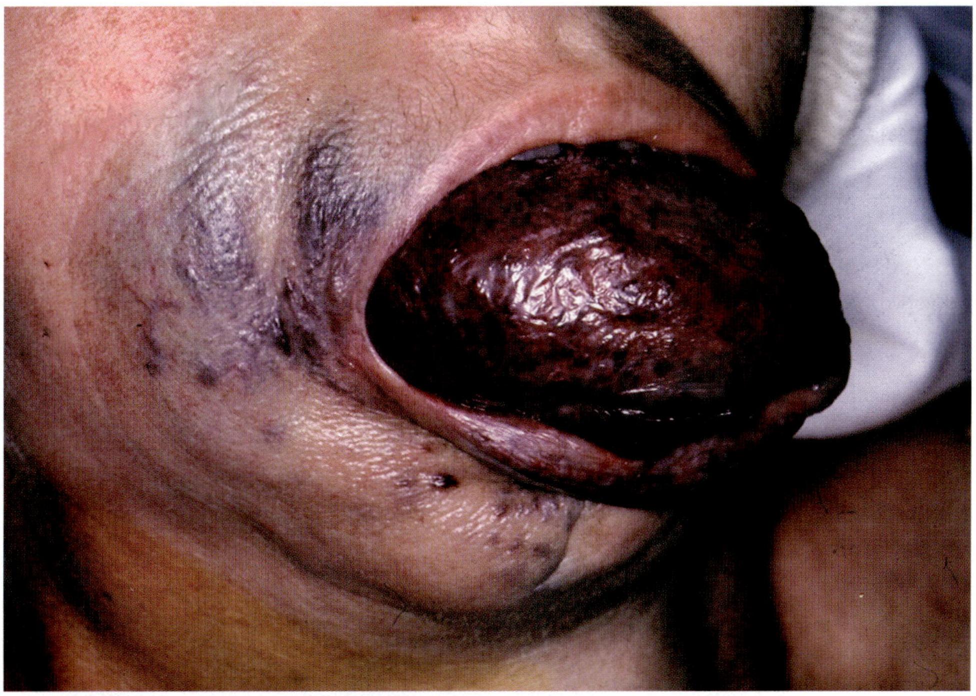

The blue hue is also clearly seen on the affected mucosa: in the mouth area the surface of the tongue is of a deep blue.

Clinical Patterns, Investigations, and Treatment

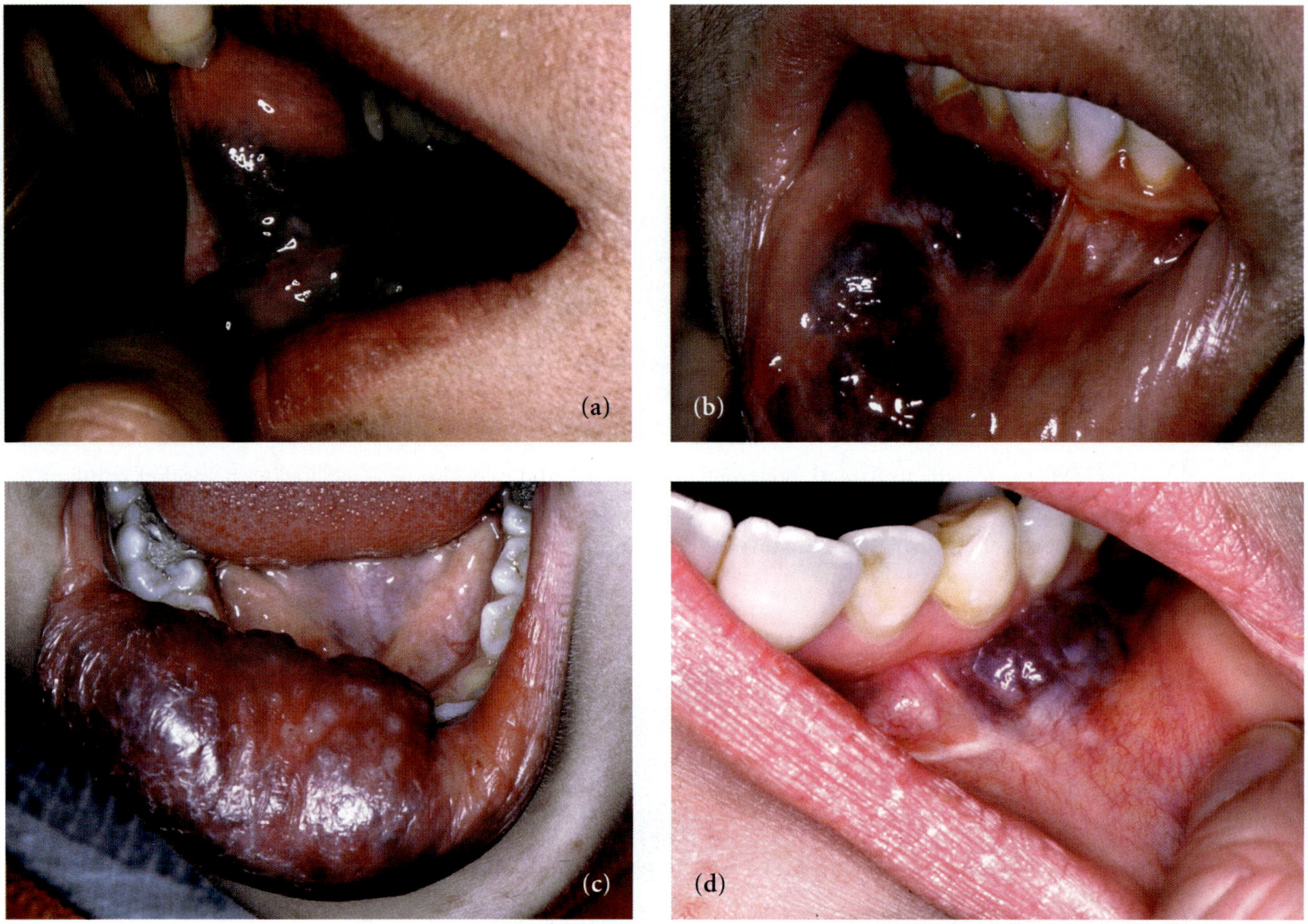

VMs of the mucosal aspect of the cheek (a), lip (b, c), and gums (d) also have a more or less blue hue.

Palate lesions, as well as pharyngeal and parapharyngeal involvement, create a risk of sleep apnea syndrome. This patient was diagnosed as having a severe sleep apnea syndrome which required direct sclerotherapy of the VM, under the protection of tracheostomy; this was not fully effective in this patient who still needs to wear facial equipment for ventilation with positive pressure at night.

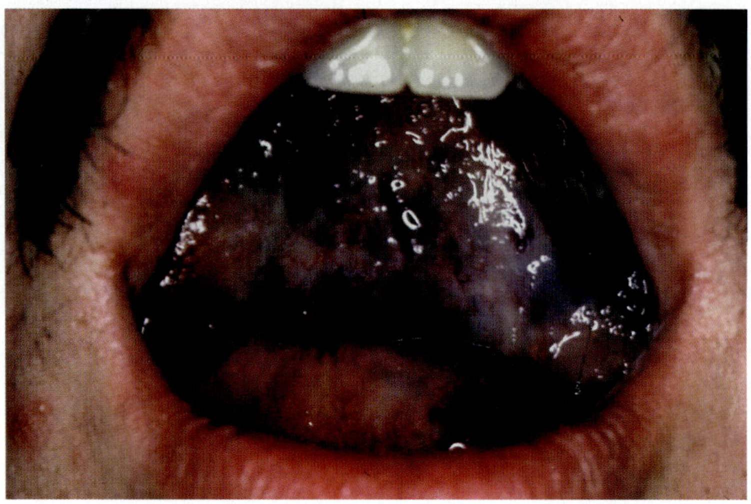

Clinical Patterns, Investigations, and Treatment

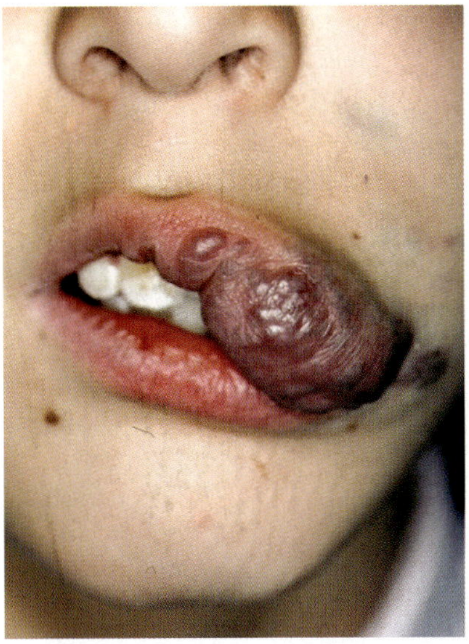

Half of the upper lip is involved, unilaterally, creating a venous macrocheily, softness, and swelling.

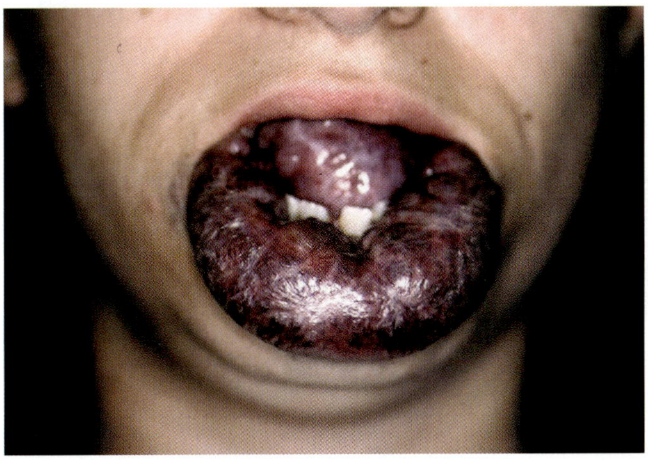

Distortion, expansion, and swelling of the lip, incompetence and severe open bite deformity with class III malocclusion were the consequences of a lower lip and tongue VM.

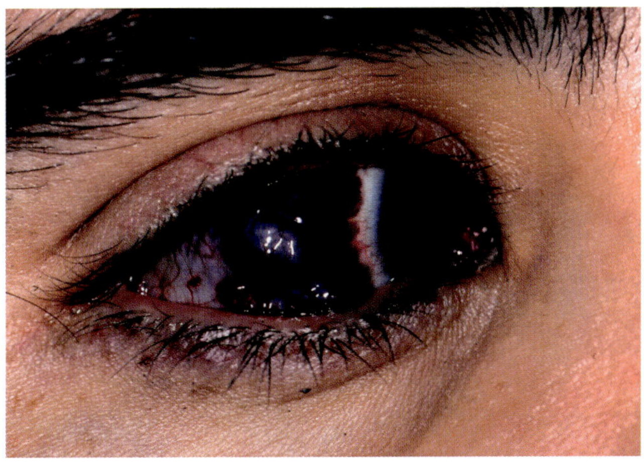

VM is sometimes visible on the conjunctiva, and this is cosmetically disabling and difficult to treat.

Clinical Patterns, Investigations, and Treatment

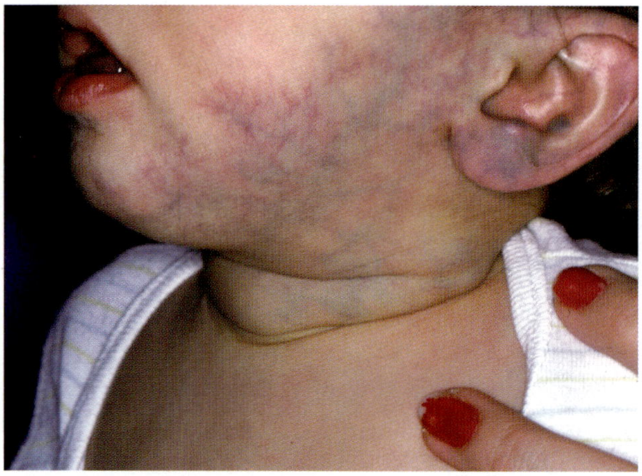

VM in the neck often appears as a faint stain in infancy, creating a subtle network of arborescent capillaries and veins; with time it will generate larger blue lesions permeating the skin.

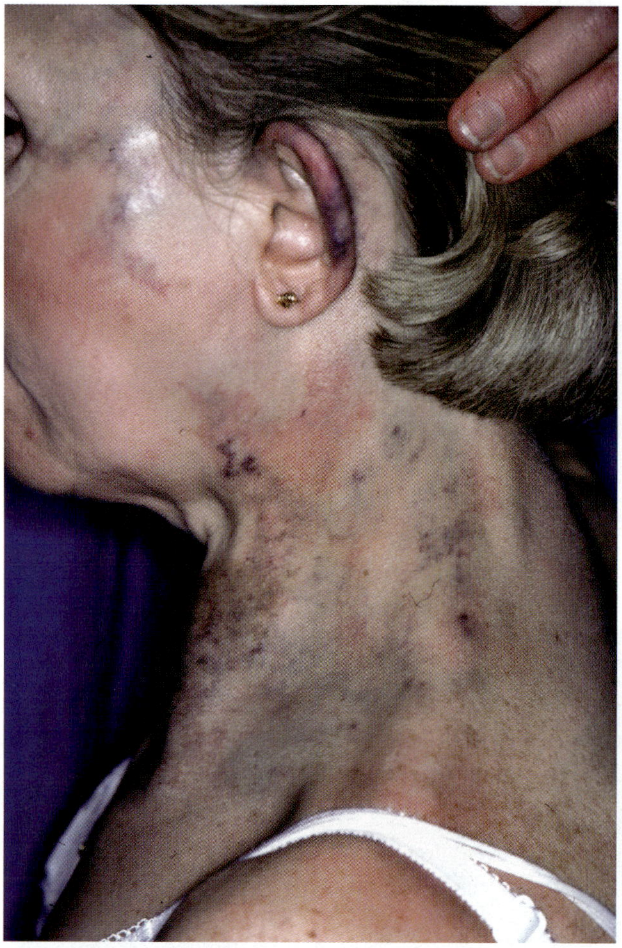

In adults a VM in the neck is usually thick, filling muscles, invading the parapharyngeal areas and encircling the respiratory tract.

Clinical Patterns, Investigations, and Treatment

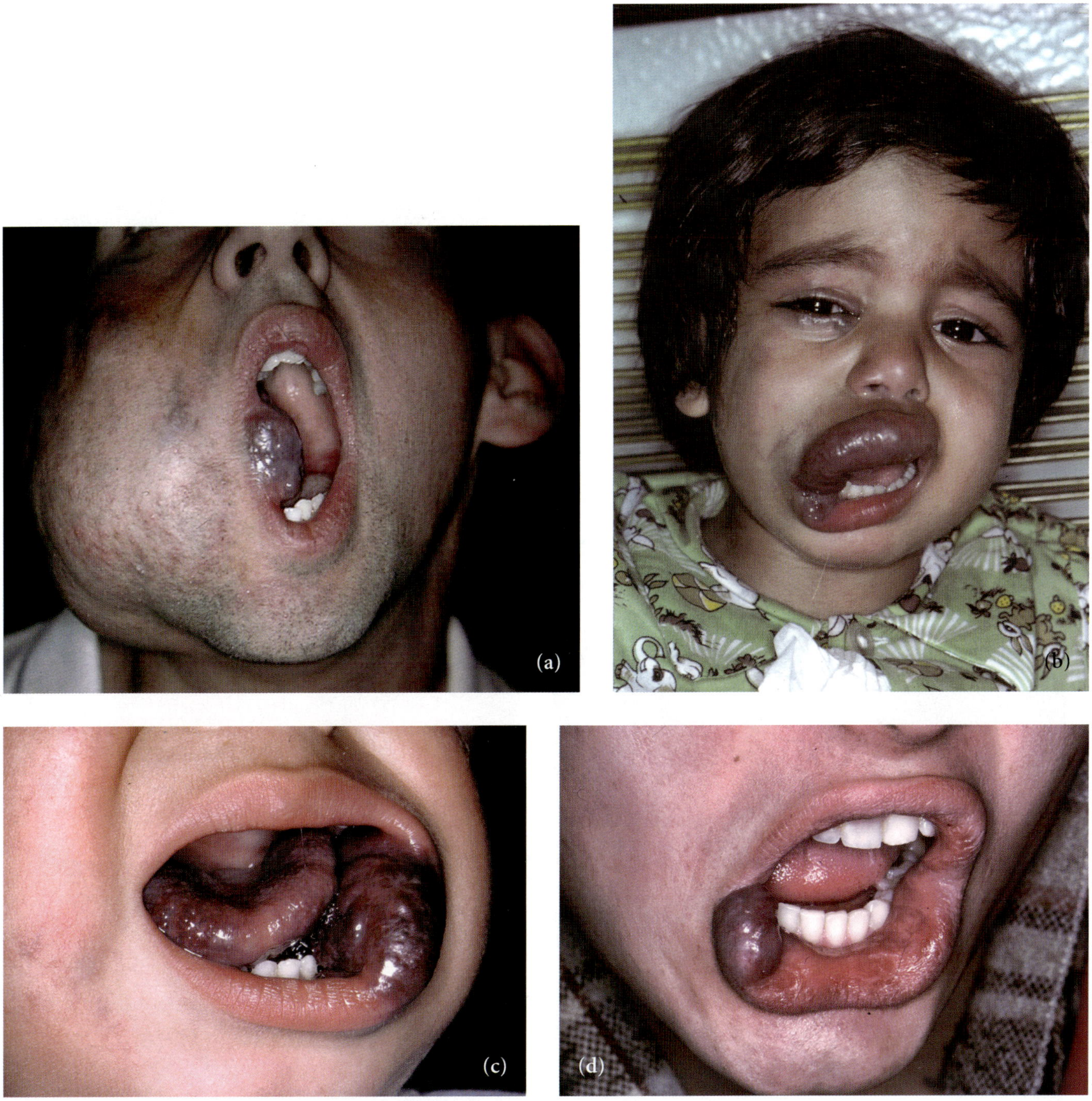

VMs swell with physical effort, giving a sensation of fullness and pain, this may occur when the patient puts his head back (a), when a child cries (b, c), and even when speaking (d). All this progressively creates permanent deformities.

Clinical Patterns, Investigations, and Treatment

Due to a mass effect on the developing jaws, malocclusion with open bite deformity commonly complicates extensive VM in the cheek and tongue. The open bite deformity will need years of specific management, when the secondary teeth have all erupted, while treating in parallel the soft-tissues lesions (VM of lip and cheek). Treatment combines orthodontics and orthognathic surgery.

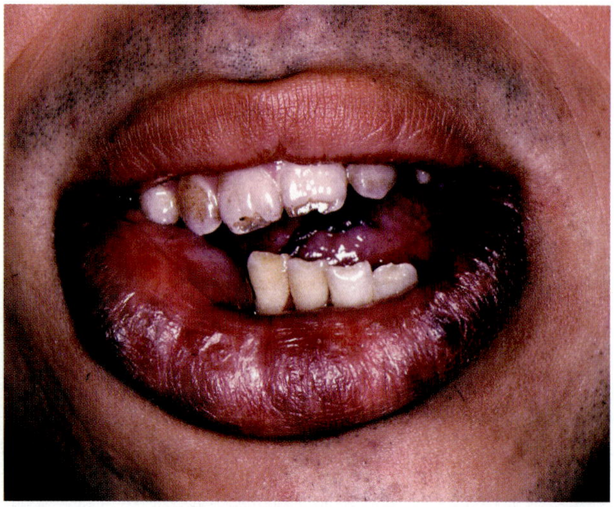

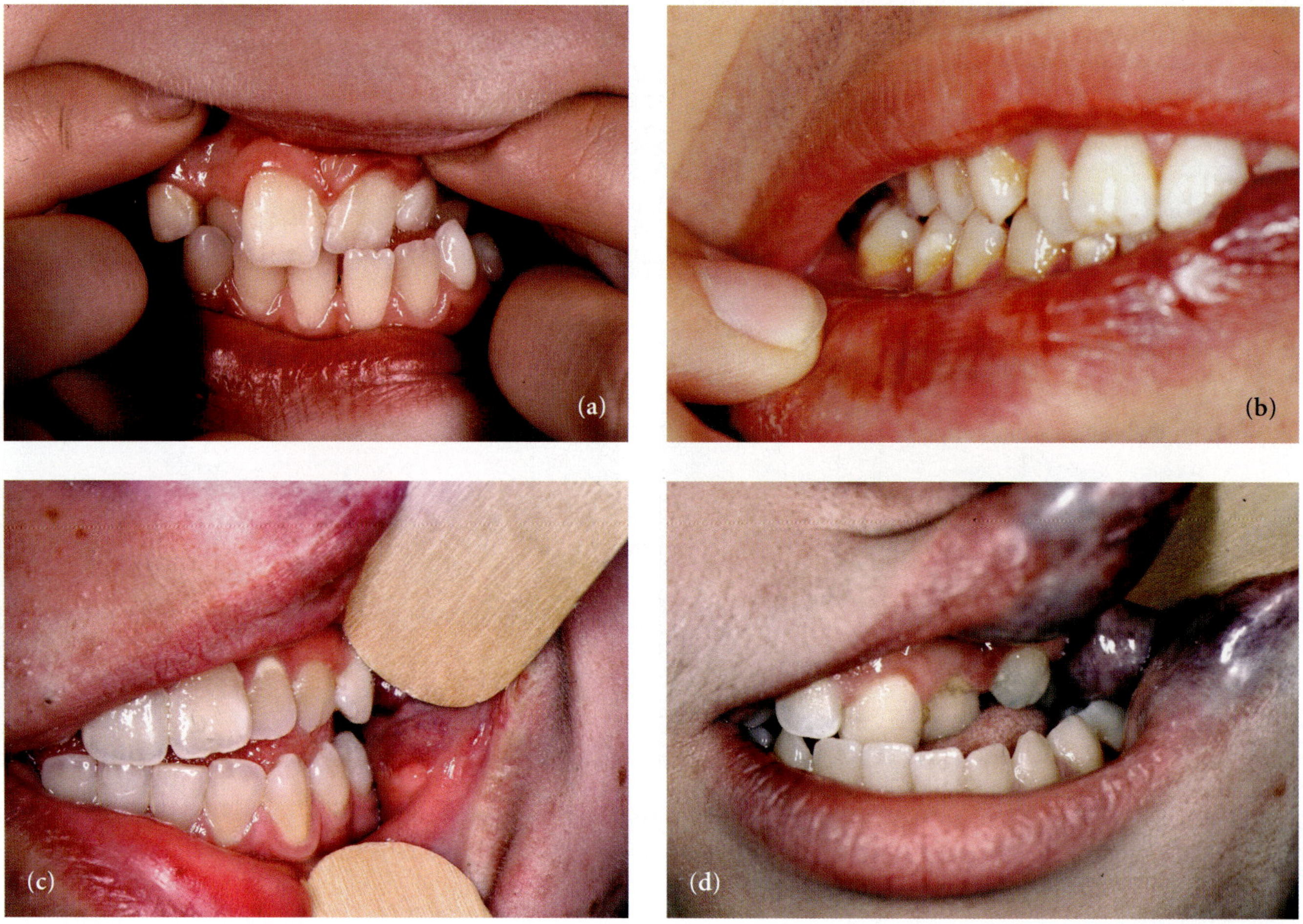

Dental misalignment, and a shift in the dental midline are the first signs of the mass effect of a facial VM on facial bones, then malocclusion develops, usually a lateral open bite. This montage shows various consequences of the mass effect created by VM in the cheek and tongue.

Clinical Patterns, Investigations, and Treatment

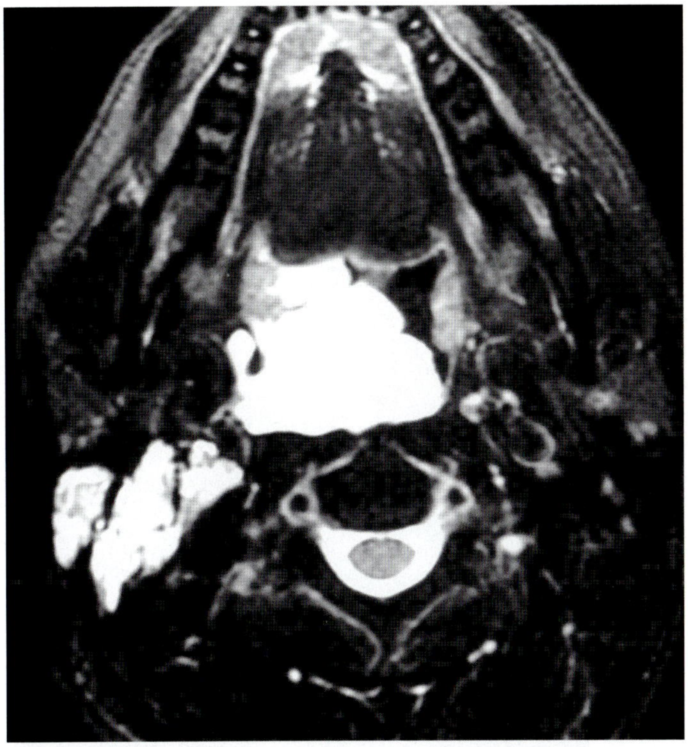

A large VM in the mouth area and neck may extend to the velum, the palate, and the posterior area, affecting the pharynx and parapharynx, as shown on this MRI scan, SE-T2-weighted image (white areas). The patient can have a normal appearing neck but severe breathing problems at night, with snoring and sleep apnea, and the need for several pillows, to raise the head, neck, and back.

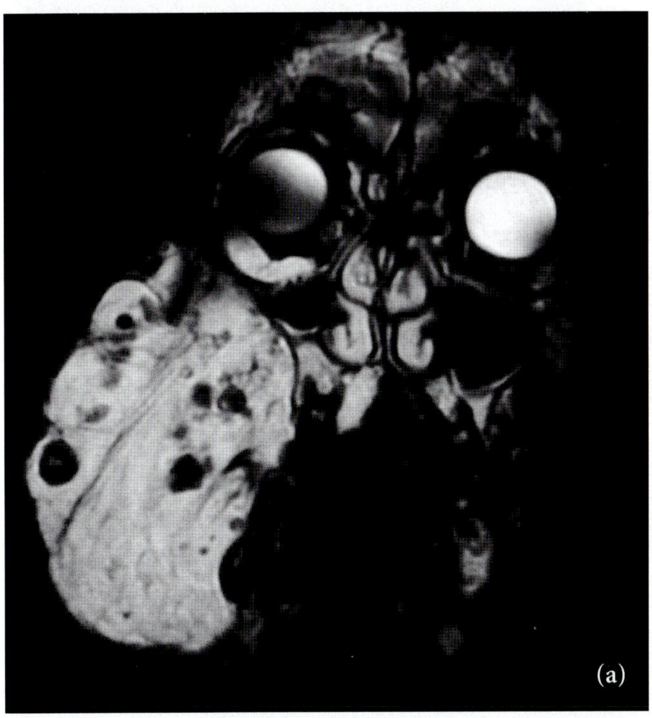

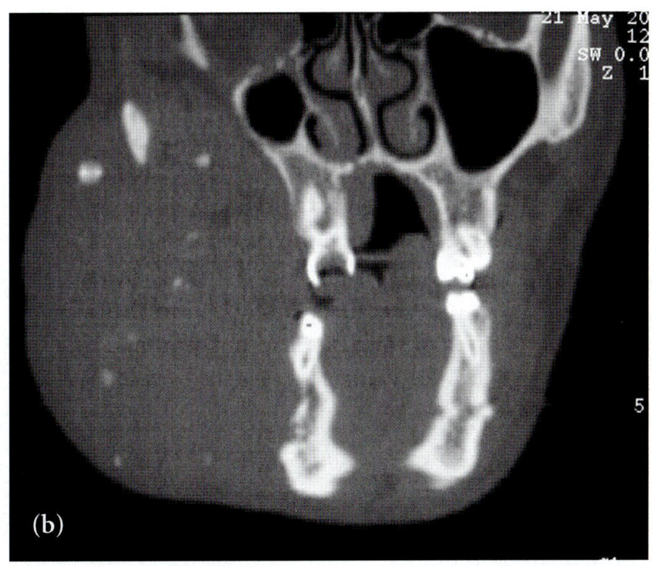

MRI is the best imaging tool: the venous pouches appear hyperintense (white) on spin–echo T2-weighted sequences, while black dots correspond to phleboliths (round calcifications) (a). Phleboliths are also seen on the CT scan (b), as well as distortion of the right facial bones due to a mass effect.

Clinical Patterns, Investigations, and Treatment

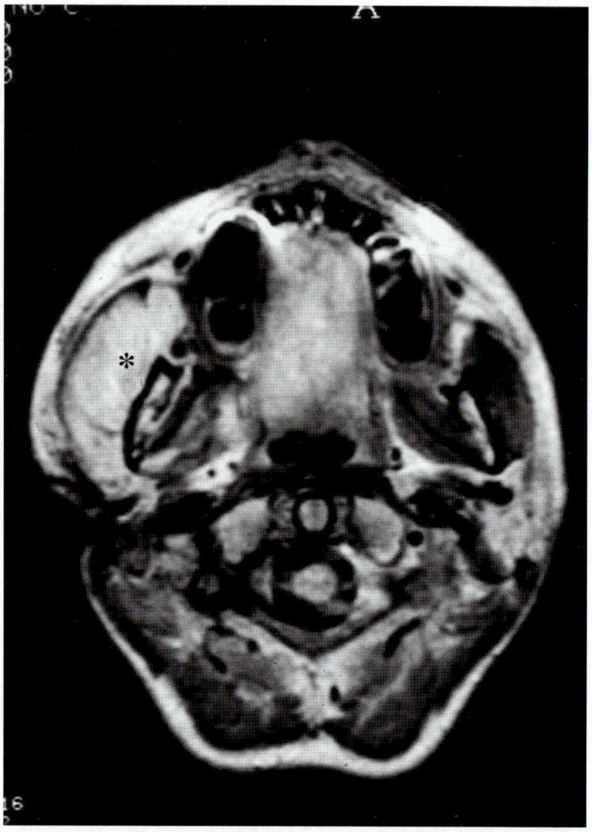

In this patient complaining of intermittent swelling and pain in the cheek; MRI, T2-weighted sequence, showed a VM restricted to the masseter (∗).

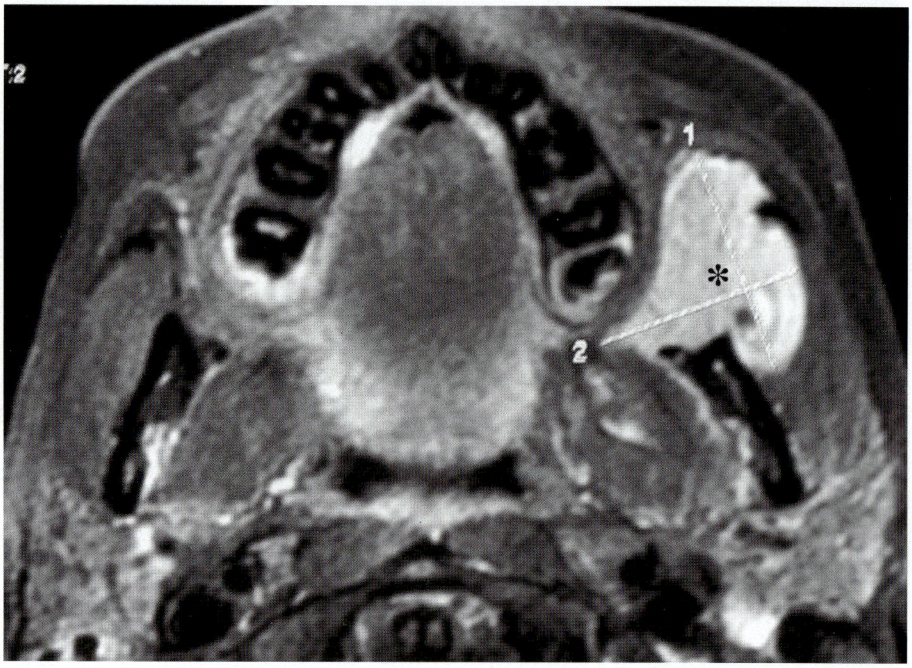

MRI, T2-weighted sequence with fat suppression, shows in this patient a VM involving the left fat pad in the cheek (∗). This may allow an interesting therapeutic approach: the surgical removal of the fat pad, including the VM, performed through a small mucosal incision allowing extirpation of the fat pad (with no visible external scar and no risk to the facial nerve), gives good remodeling of the cheek.

Clinical Patterns, Investigations, and Treatment

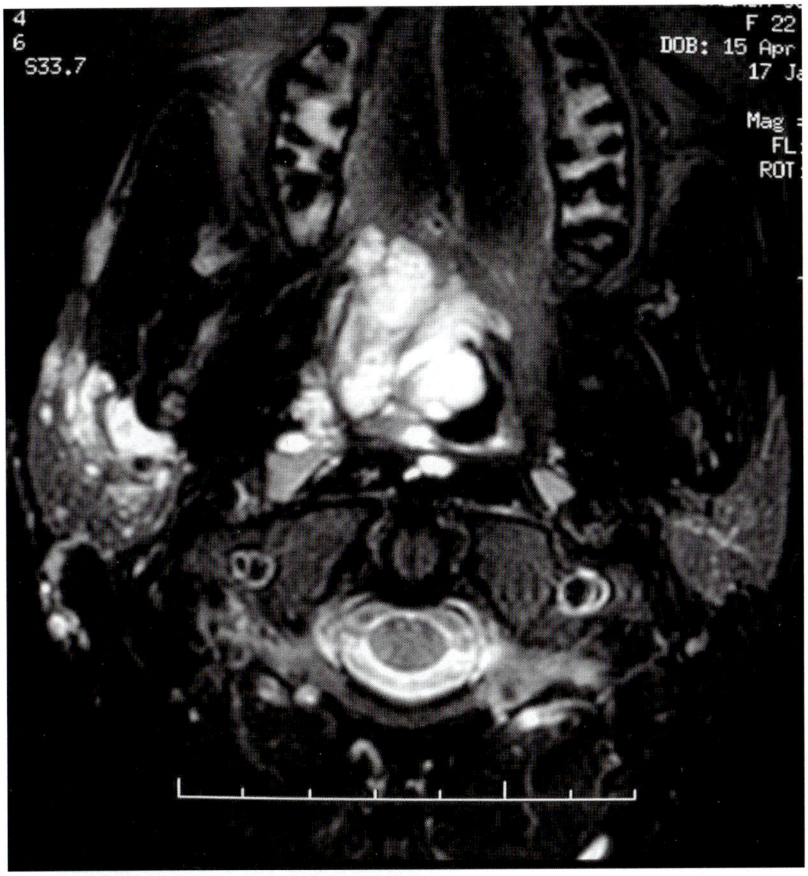

MRI in this patient with VM in the entire neck revealed not only deep lesions around the respiratory tract, but also VM close to the parotid gland, a finding suggesting a high risk of facial palsy if ethanol sclerosing treatment of this part of the VM is planned.

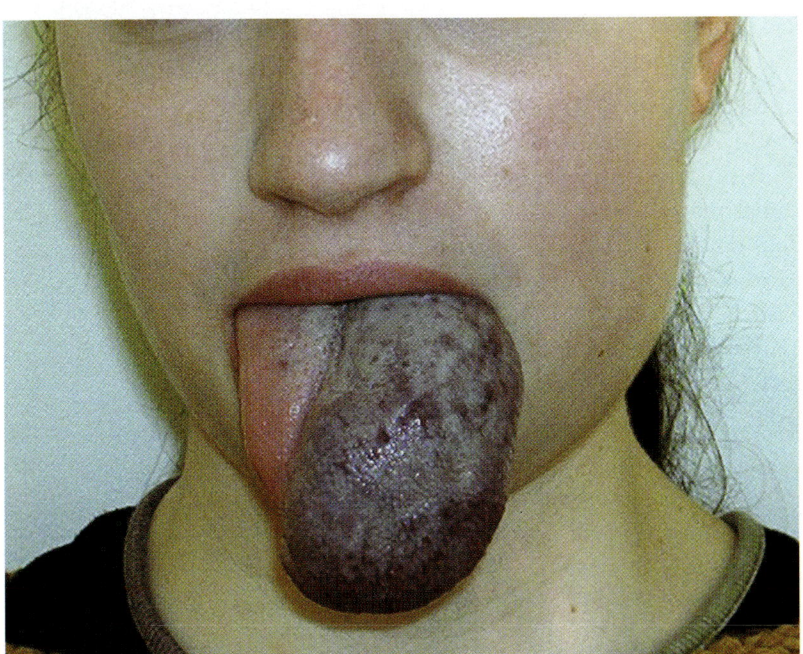

VM on the mobile part of the tongue creates dental malposition and malocclusion due to the mass effect and pressure, but it rarely impairs speech, while VM of the base of the tongue and pharynx can cause difficulties in swallowing, airway compromise, and sleep apnea syndrome.

Clinical Patterns, Investigations, and Treatment

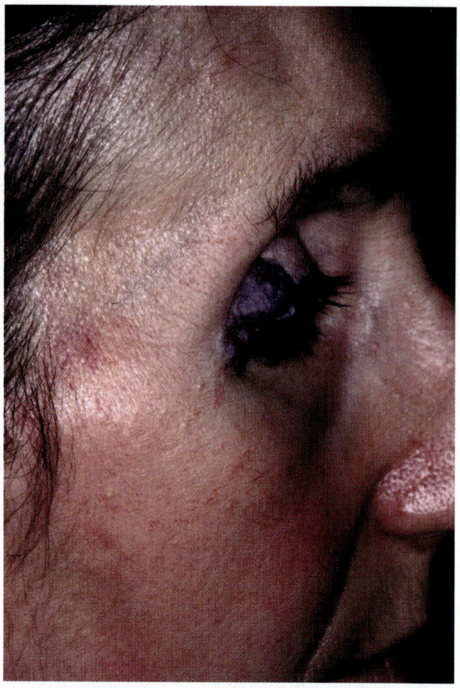

Intraorbital VMs vary in size depending on head position, and this progressively expands and enlarges the orbit, resulting in enophthalmia when the patients are standing, and exophthalmos when they rest or lie back. Pain is often significant but vision is usually not impaired. Optic nerve compression very rarely results from an intraorbital VM encompassing the optic nerve.

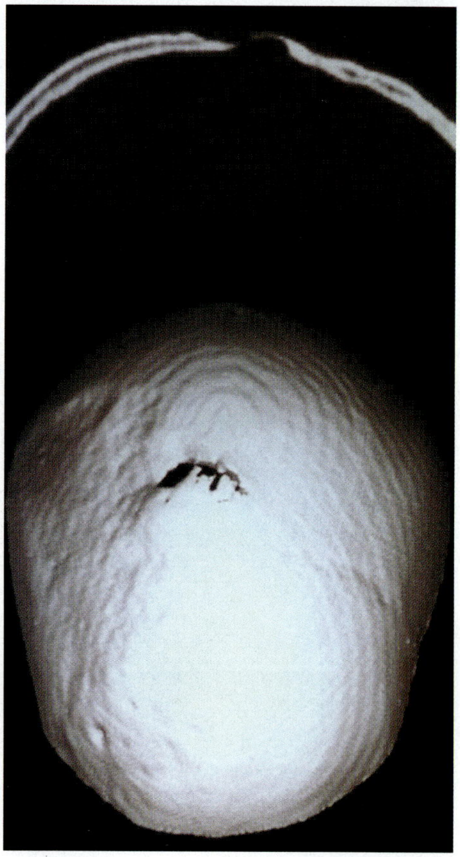

Bony defects are present in about 20% of VMs involving the scalp or forehead (4). In this case the sinus pericranii underlying the VM was detected by CT bone windows and 3-D reconstruction delineated it. A sinus pericranii creates a communication between extracranial and intracranial venous systems (11). VM located within the diploe creates a soft mass that rapidly fluctuates depending on head position. With MRI the intraosseous venous lakes give an intradiploic hypersignal on T2, sometimes in association with an underlying intracranial dural increased T2 signal (2). Endovascular treatment of sinus pericranii is only effective in patients with focal defect, while those with diffuse bony VM had recurrence or failure of treatment (8).

Clinical Patterns, Investigations, and Treatment

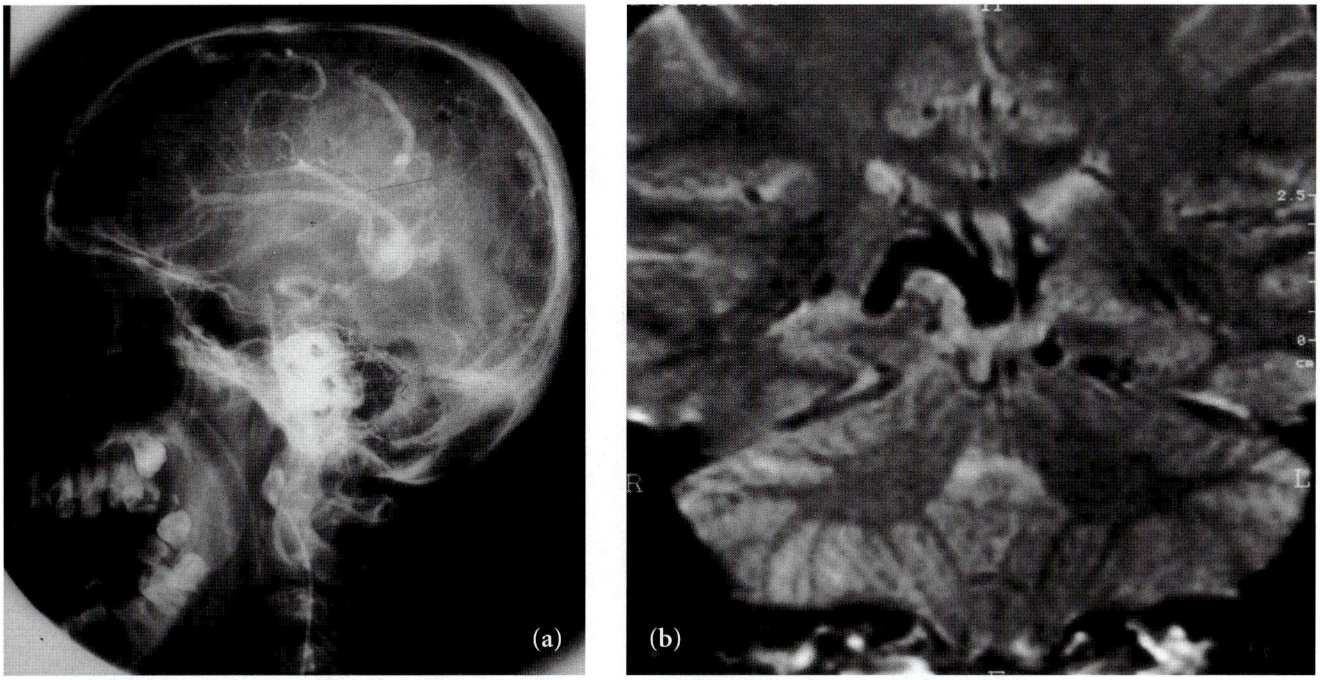

Cerebral developmental venous anomaly (DVA) consists of dilated intramedullary veins converging into a large draining vein. This uncommon trajectory of the brain venous drainage occurs in less than 0.5% of the general population, while in our experience it is observed in 20% patients with head and neck VMs. In patients with cephalic VMs, DVAs usually consist of ectatic and dilated veins converging into the drainage system of the deep brain (4). In contrast to cerebral "cavernoma" (previously known as "angiographically occult" vascular malformation), opacification of DVA appears in the angiographic venous phase, as do normal veins. DVA is imaged using CT and MRI with MRA. Patients with DVA usually complain of headaches, but they are not at risk of cerebral hemorrhage, seizures or neurological deficit.

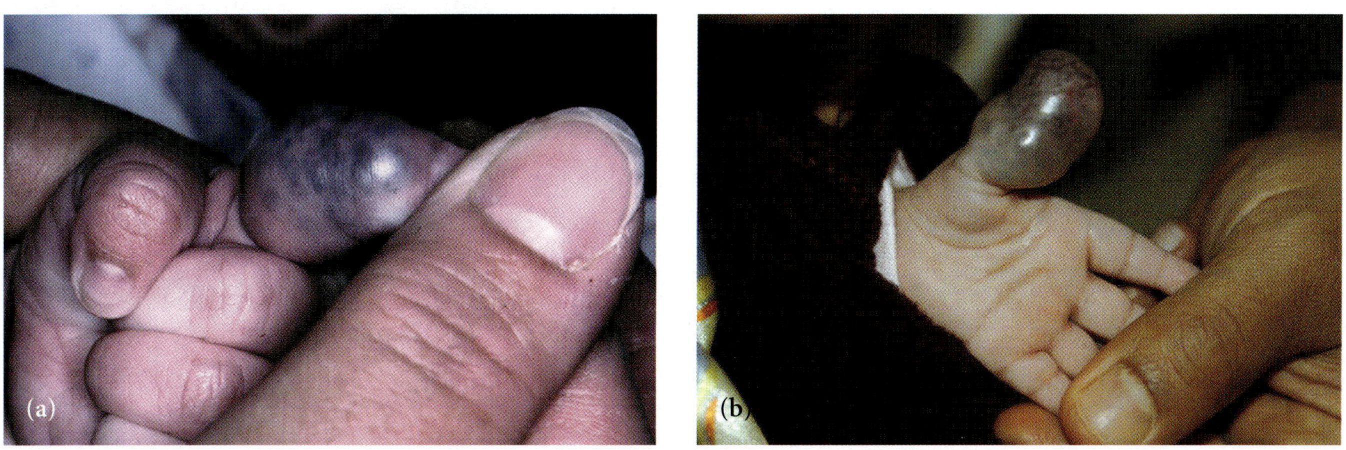

These very limited VMs in a finger were both present at birth; the blue color is distinctive: it indicates that the malformed venous channels permeate the skin reaching the very superficial dermis. Treatment of such a lesion in a child is nearly impossible.

Clinical Patterns, Investigations, and Treatment

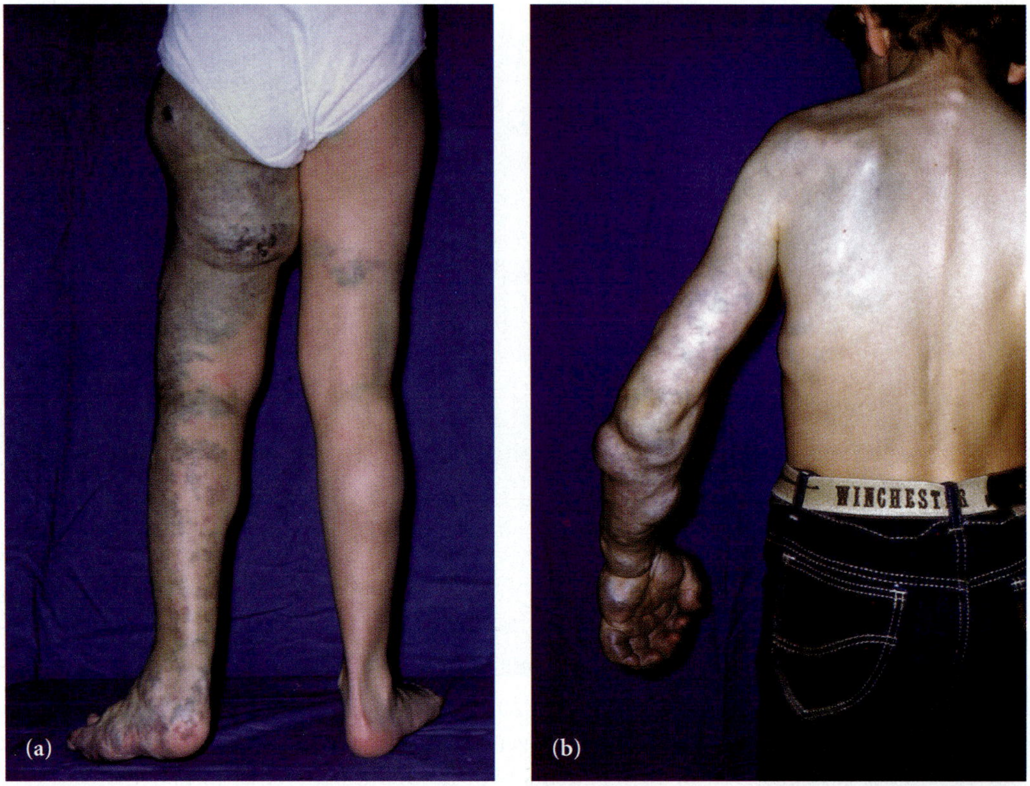

(a) (b)

VM can affect an entire upper or lower extremity and the adjacent trunk. It brings about swelling of the soft tissues, deformity, some increase in limb girth, but no limb length discrepancy. In time function is affected, with pain; symptoms are increased after exercising and upon waking in the morning and tend to abate with rest. Elastic garments for both the hand and the arm, or leg and foot, are absolutely indispensable, as they bring comfort, limit swelling and pain, and reduce the consequence of the localized intravascular coagulopathy (LIC).

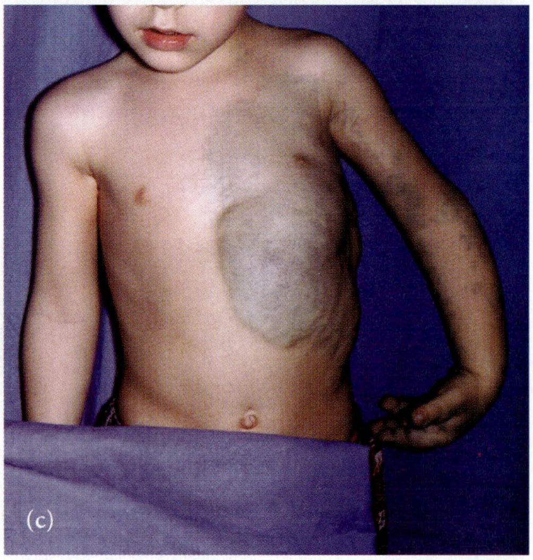

(c)

Clinical Patterns, Investigations, and Treatment

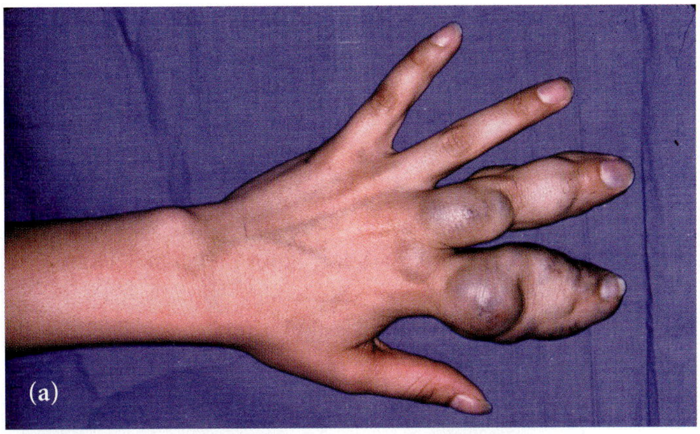

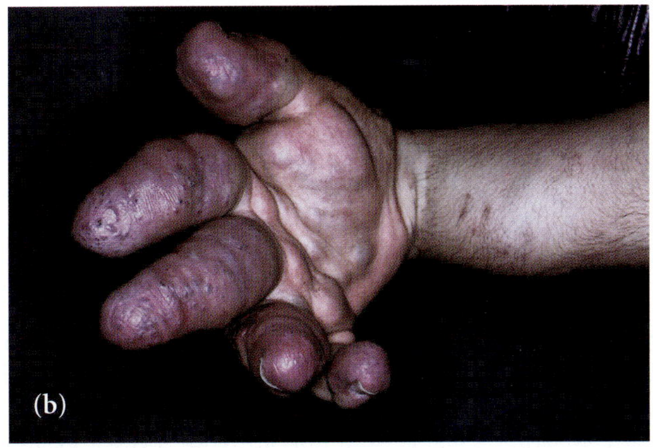

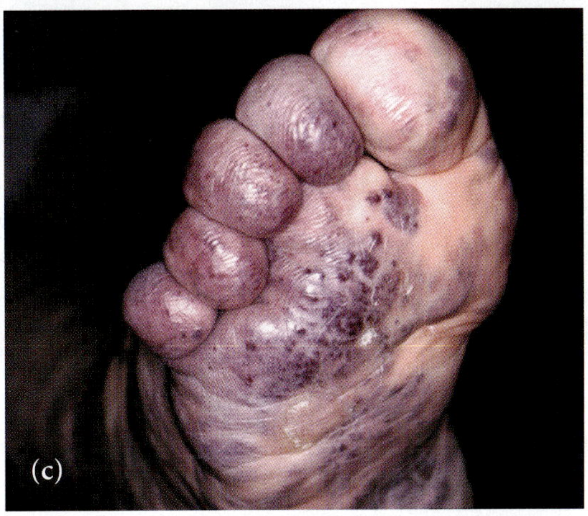

Upper limb VM, when distal, causes enlarged blue fingers with sagging skin, in a segmental pattern (a, b). At the foot and toe level VM also distends the soft tissues and gives the skin a deep blue color (c).

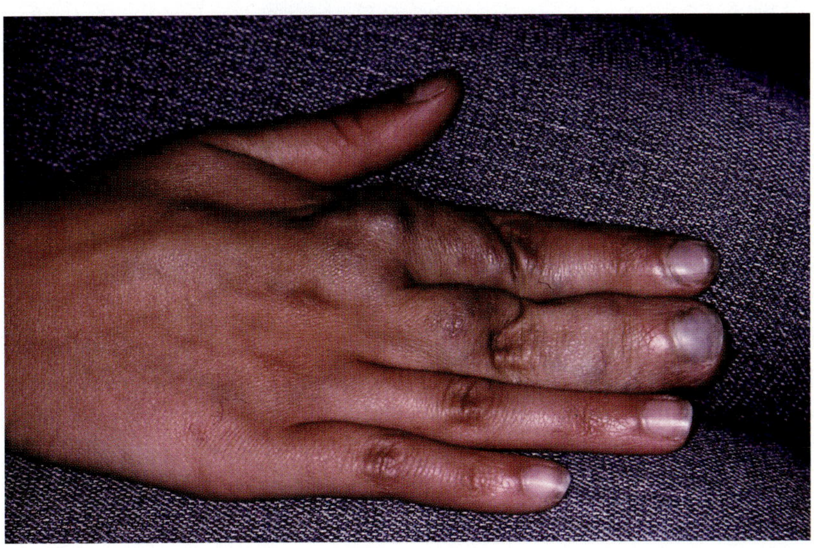

Blue nail is observed when the VM extends to the tip of the finger: this is sometimes mistaken for cyanosis when all fingers are affected.

Clinical Patterns, Investigations, and Treatment

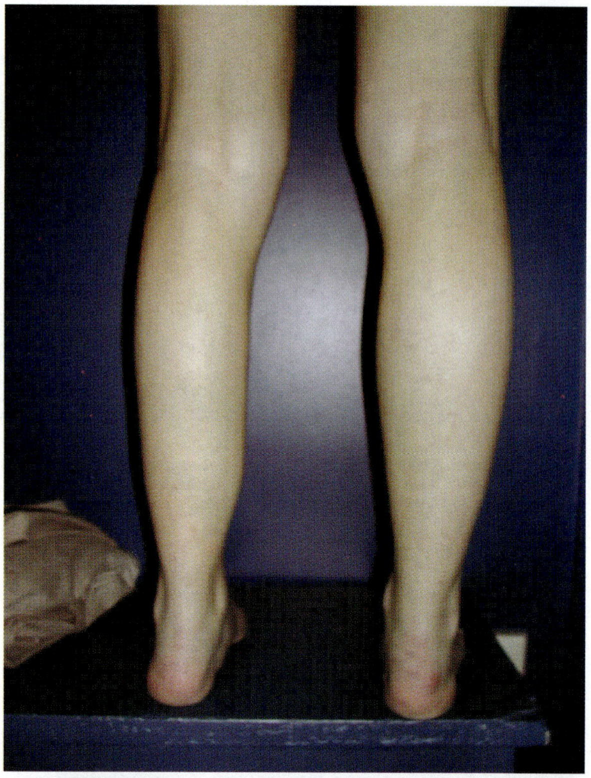

Amyotrophy is a common and early finding in a child with intramuscular extremity VM, particularly in lower limb locations: surprisingly it can occur not only with extensive skin and muscles VMs affecting a whole limb but also with a small localized intramuscular VM under normal skin, as was the case in this child.

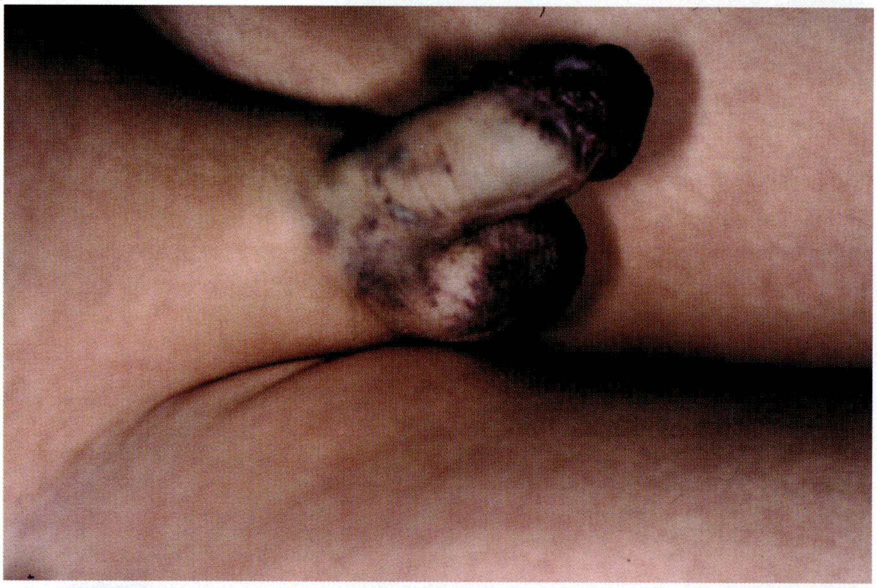

VMs in the male genitalia create cosmetic problems. They also have psychological consequences and in some patients cause erectile difficulties in adolescence and adulthood, with effects on their sex life.

Clinical Patterns, Investigations, and Treatment

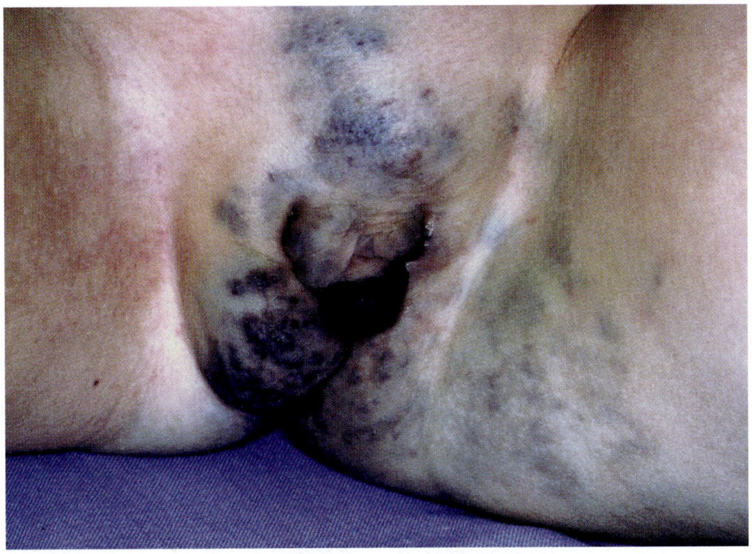

VM in the vulva is usually associated with VM of the lower extremity and/or gluteal area. The blue color and the swelling increase during adolescence and with pregnancy. However, in a majority of women the lesions are strictly located to the vulva and vaginal delivery is possible (after MRI control, during the third trimester to check if there is no involvement of uterus, cervix, or vagina).

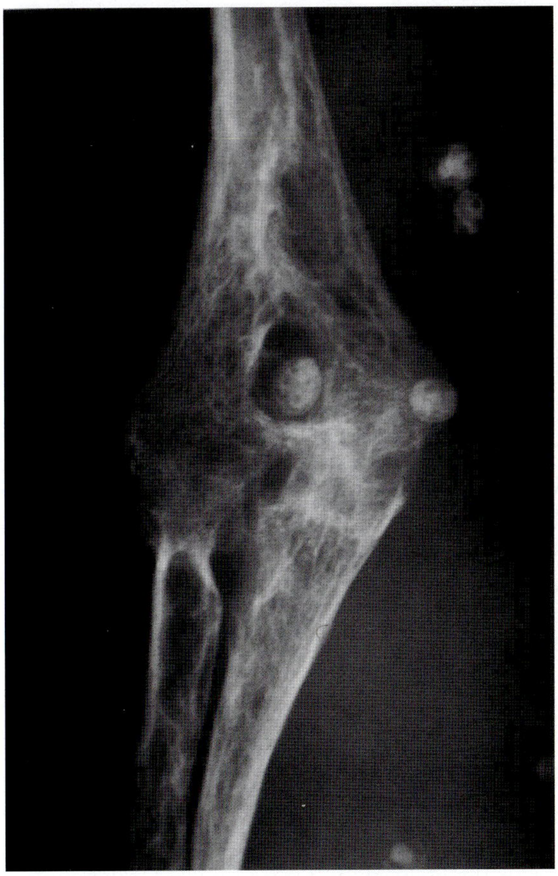

This plain radiograph of an extensive VM of the arm of a young man shows not only phleboliths but also osteolytic lesions and weakening of the bony shaft; in this situation a pathological fracture can occur with minor trauma (20). However, according to Hein (25) after studying a group of 176 patients with VM of skeletal muscles, skeletal problems such as fracture or deformation are rare. Plain radiographs sometimes also show a periosteal reaction in adolescents and adults with diffuse limb VMs. These reactive changes sometimes mimic osteoid osteoma.

Clinical Patterns, Investigations, and Treatment

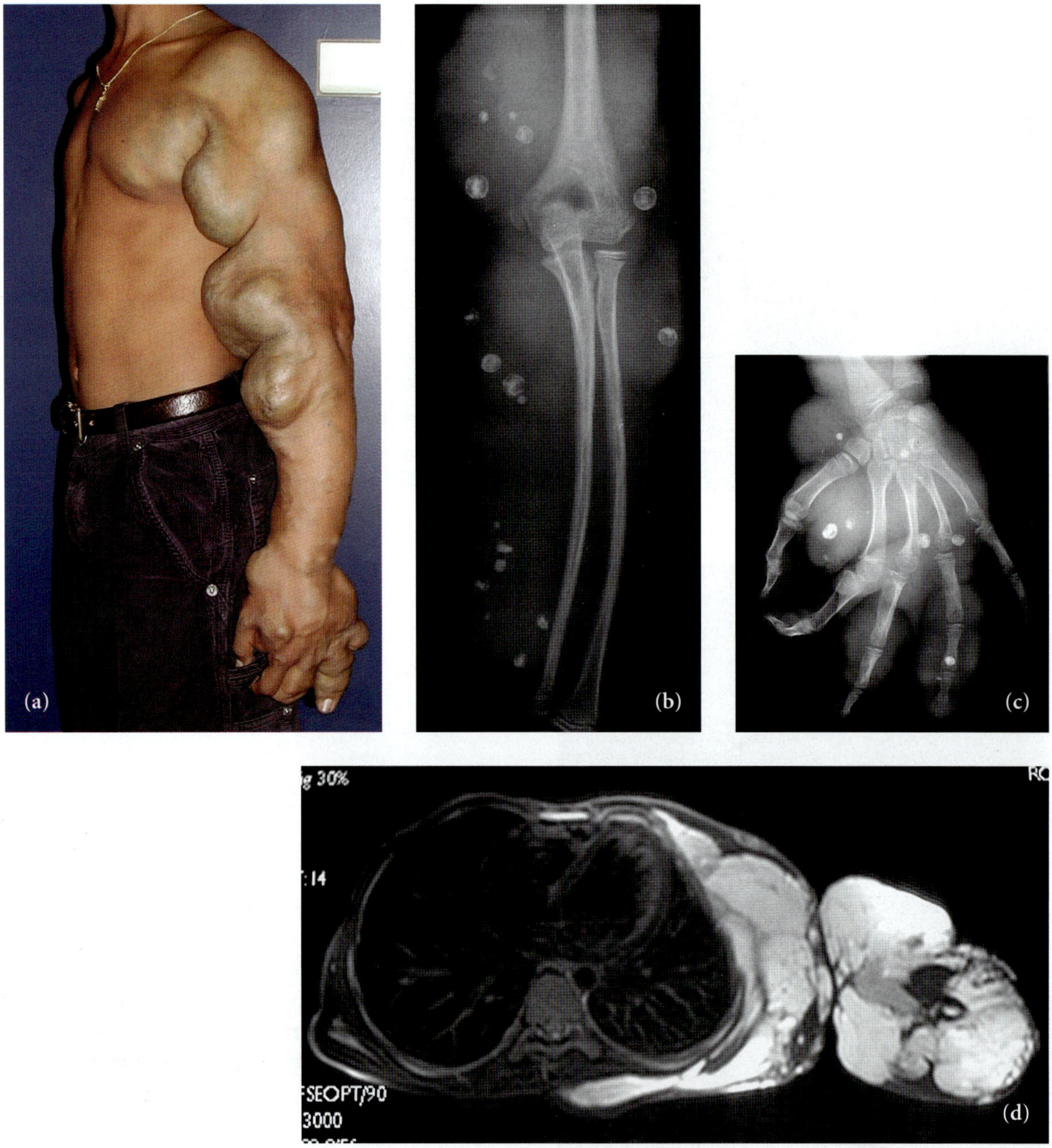

Such a diffuse involvement of the arm and trunk in this young man (a) precludes surgical treatment: muscles are all extensively filled and excision will be too disabling. The extent of the VM also does not allow us to offer efficient percutaneous sclerotherapy: this challenging treatment will end in fairly deceptive results, and there is also a high risk of adverse effects, particularly migration of the embolic material with possible nerve damage or pulmonary embolism. In this case, elastic garments are indispensable, as well as medical treatment (low-molecular-weight heparin injections) because of flares of the associated localized intravascular coagulopathy (LIC): the heparin treatment minimizes pain, a common complaint linked to episodes of venous thrombosis. In most cases thrombosis affects superficial veins, but occasionally deep vein thrombosis happens, carrying, rarely, a risk of pulmonary embolism. Thrombosis precedes phlebolith formation (b, c). T2-sequence of MRI (d) shows the VM filling the muscles.

Clinical Patterns, Investigations, and Treatment

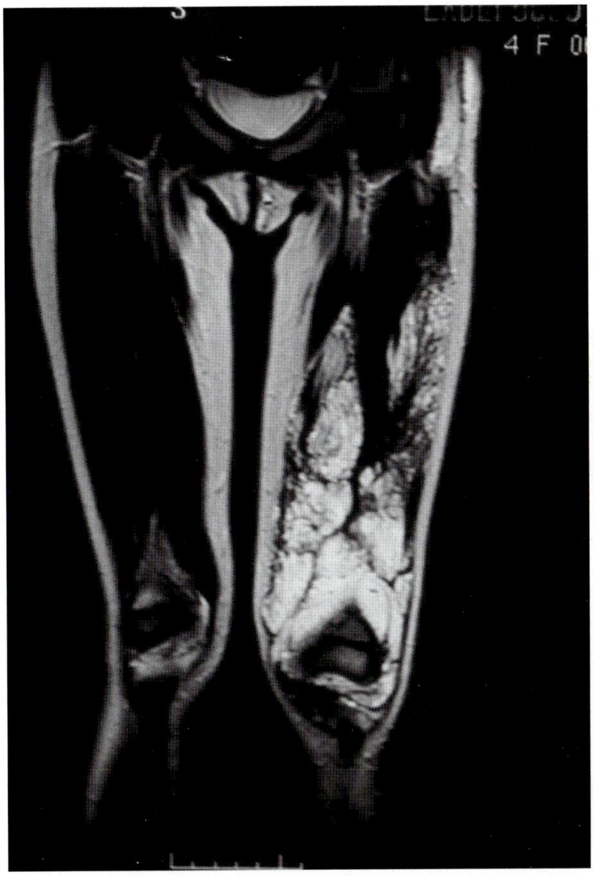

MRI is mandatory to clearly delineate a VM in an extremity or trunk; there is no longer a need for angiography. The VM involving the muscles in the thigh and the knee joint appears as well-delineated white pouches with the hypersignal on SE-T2-weighted sequences with fat suppression.

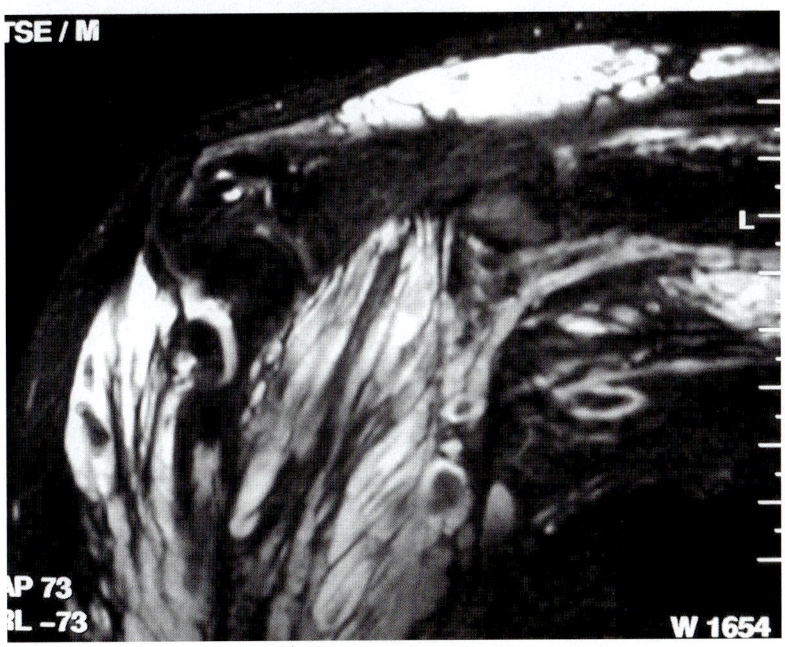

This VM in the shoulder permeates all muscular structures with channels being somewhat linear, with multiple intervening fibrous septa.

Clinical Patterns, Investigations, and Treatment

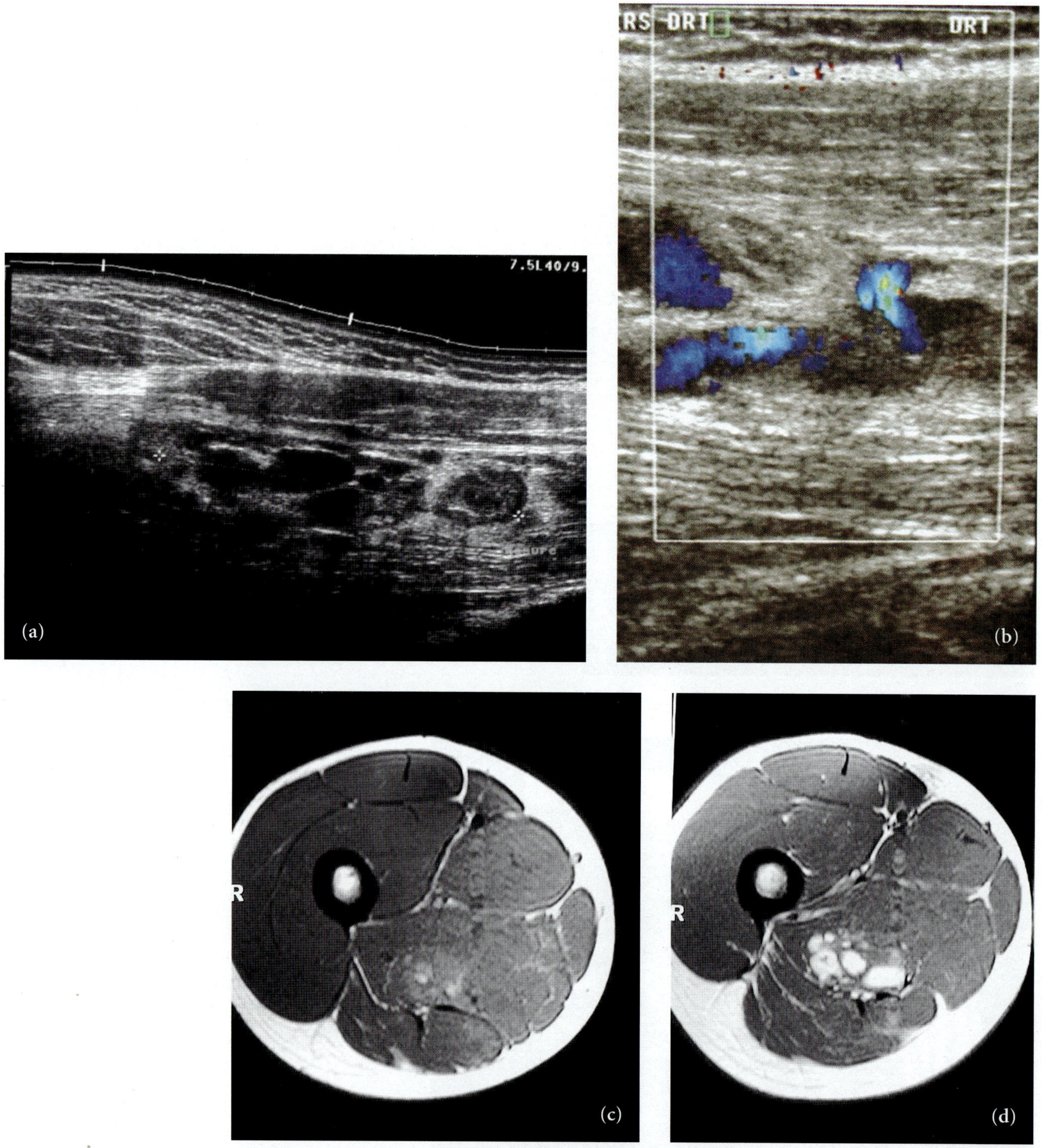

This is an example of the full work-up required for a VM located in the thigh; the lesion is detected by US (a) and Doppler (b), a venous flow is barely visible on the MRI T1 sequence (c), but clearly shown on the SE T1-sequence after gadolinium injection (d). *Figure continues at top of page 201.*

Clinical Patterns, Investigations, and Treatment

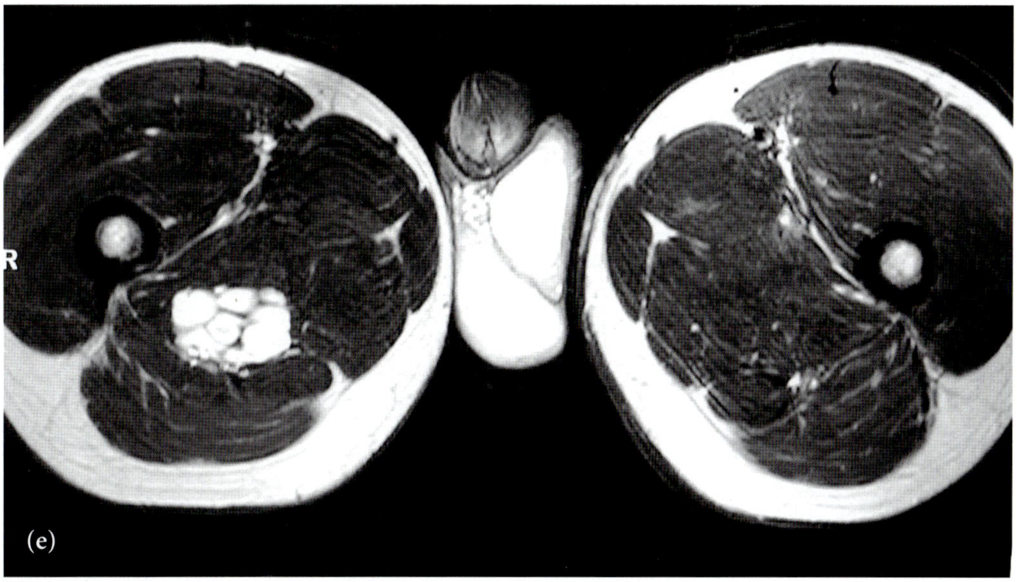

(e)

Continued from page 200: on the SE T2-sequence the VM is hyperintense to surrounding muscles (e)

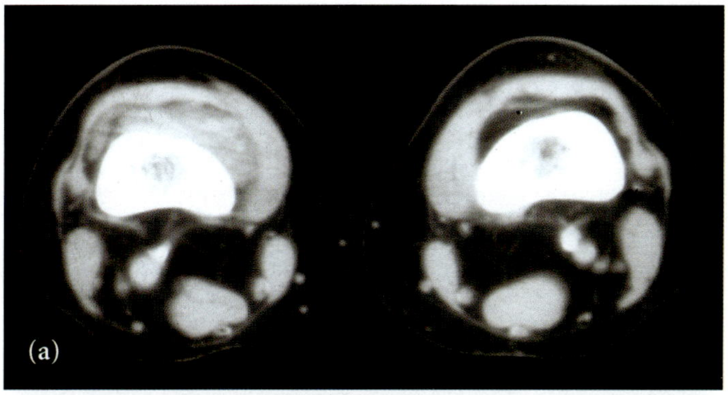

(a)

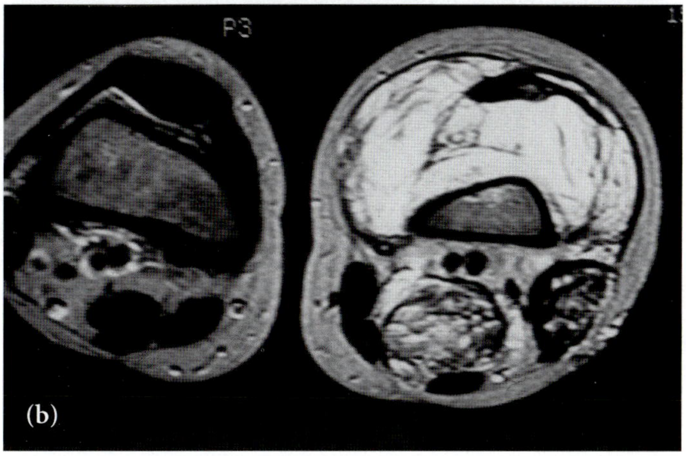

(b)

This knee joint VM is shown by both CT scans and MRI. Knee joint VM is usually first suspected in children around 6 to 10 years of age: they report intermittent swelling and pain of the joint; in addition, recurrent episodes linked to joint effusions and hemarthrosis result in stiffness, instability and progressive ankylosis. However, without effective treatment, this ends in tender flexion and ankylosis of the joint, and terminates in permanent flexion contracture in the worst cases. These symptoms first resolve with bed rest in a day and are more severe with intrasynovial VM involvement.

Clinical Patterns, Investigations, and Treatment

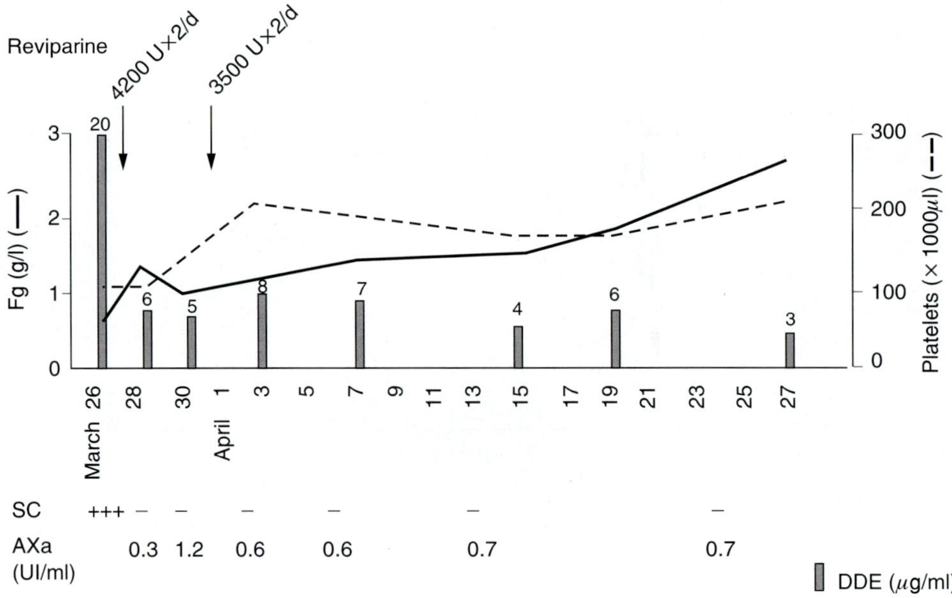

Hemarthrosis is severe in patients with joint VM and VM-associated chronic localized intravascular coagulopathy (LIC). Treatment of episodes of LIC is best carried out using low-molecular-weight heparin as indicated in this scheme: clinical improvement followed the normalization of D-dimers and fibrinogen only when a low molecular weight heparin (reviparine) was introduced (courtesy of Dr. E. Mazoyer, Hôpital Avicenne, APHP Paris, France).

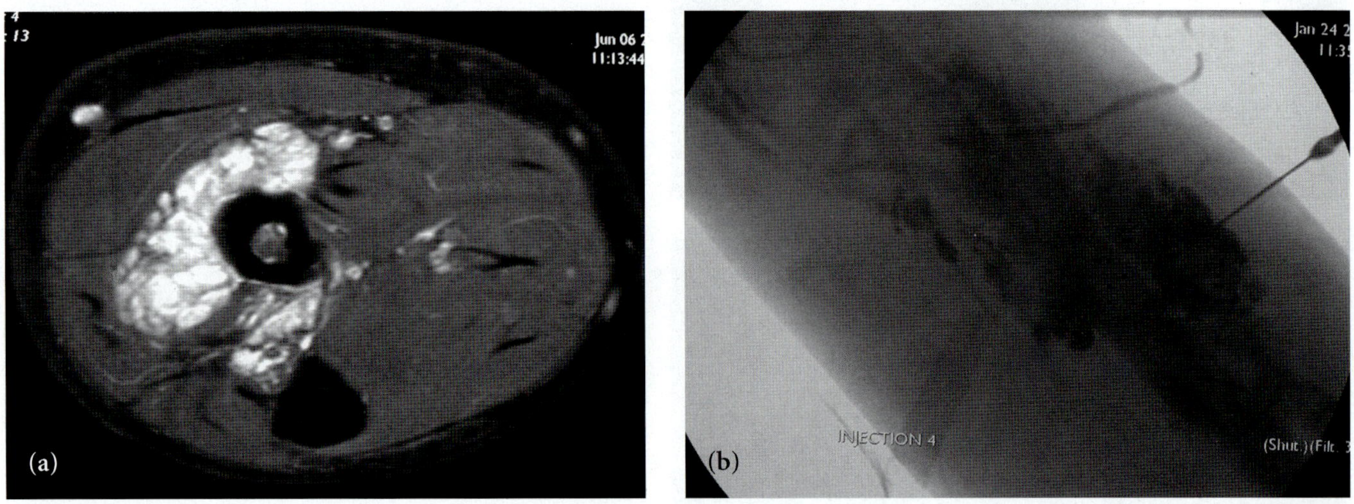

For intramuscular VM in an extremity, direct injection of ethanol, under fluoroscopic control, may be considered. Using compression and a tourniquet prevents the rapid dispersal of ethanol. According to Puig et al. (34), when there is no direct communication with the adjacent venous system as visualized by direct contrast injection (type-I VM) we can expect complication-free sclerotherapy. When there is rapid drainage of the VM into regular veins (type-2 VM) there is a risk of dangerous migration of the sclerosant, which can be controlled technically during the procedure. When the VM drains into dilated veins (type-3 VM) sclerotherapy should not be used because the risk of diffusion is significant, with a risk of local nerve palsy, and pulmonary embolism.

Clinical Patterns, Investigations, and Treatment

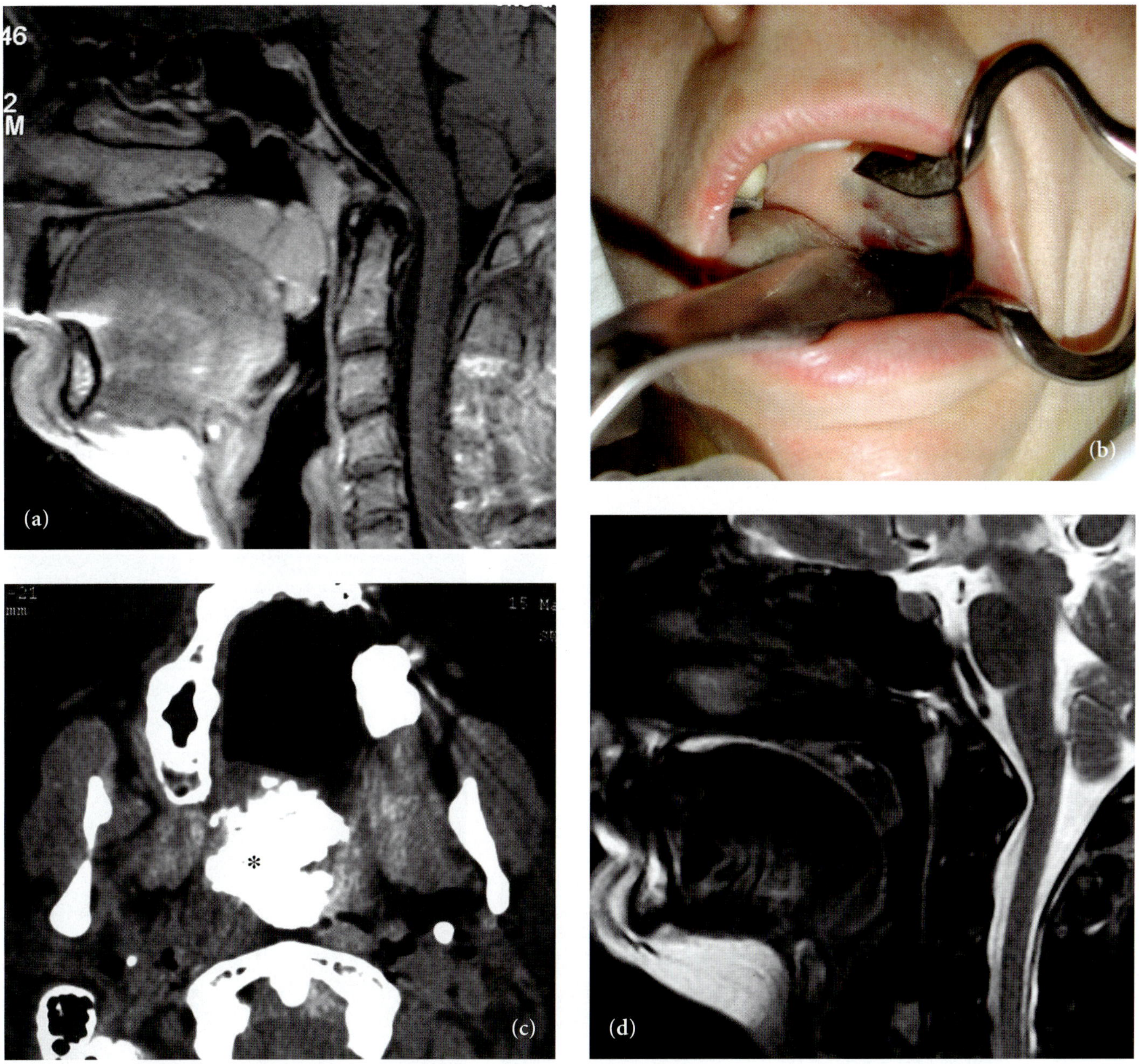

A soft-palate VM, shown on MRI scan (a), induced severe dyspnea. As surgical removal of the VM-enlarged soft palate could cause important functional impairment, it was contraindicated, and thus direct sclerotherapy was decided on. The soft palate was accessed by direct puncture (b) and a mixture of ethanol, Ethibloc® and lipiodol was injected, after a tracheostomy because of the expected serious inflammatory reaction with risk of breathing impairment. Tracheostomy is also recommended when there is bulking of the posterior tongue and pharyngeal VM, creating a risk of local wound and hemorrhage during intubation for general anesthesia. CT immediately after sclerosis showed filling of the VM with the sclerosing (∗) agent (c). Nearly complete resolution of the VM was shown on MRI scan in (d) 3 months later, while the functional symptoms had disappeared.

Clinical Patterns, Investigations, and Treatment

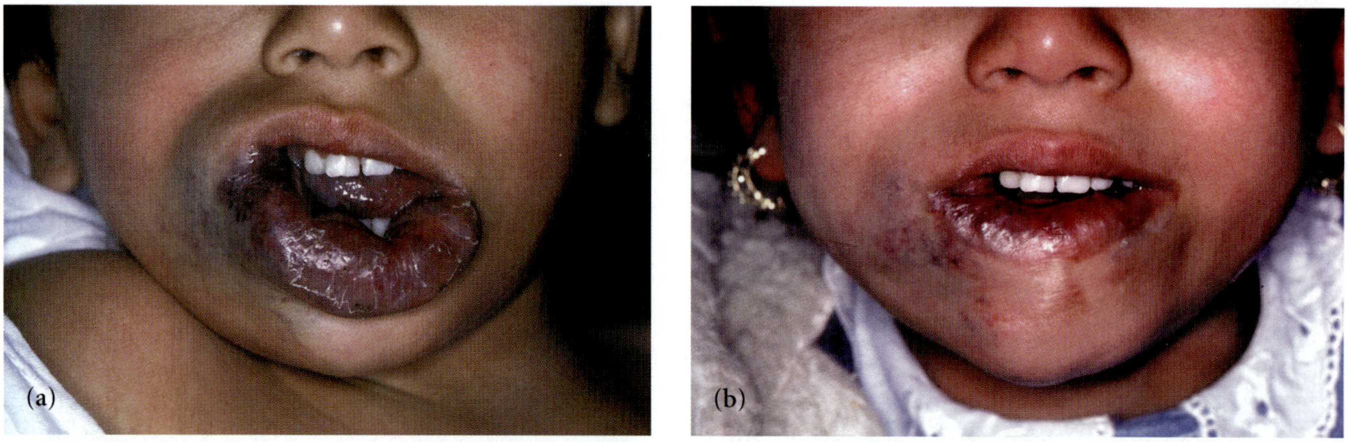

This girl waited 3 months after pre-operative sclerotherapy with Ethibloc® and ethanol, to create some fibrosis and minimize intraoperative bleeding. Then, repair of the shape of the lip was carried out. However, as the VM was filling her whole lower lip, it was impossible to completely resect the lesion. Thus, some residual VM in the lip is prone to swell again, requiring further sclerosing treatments in the future.

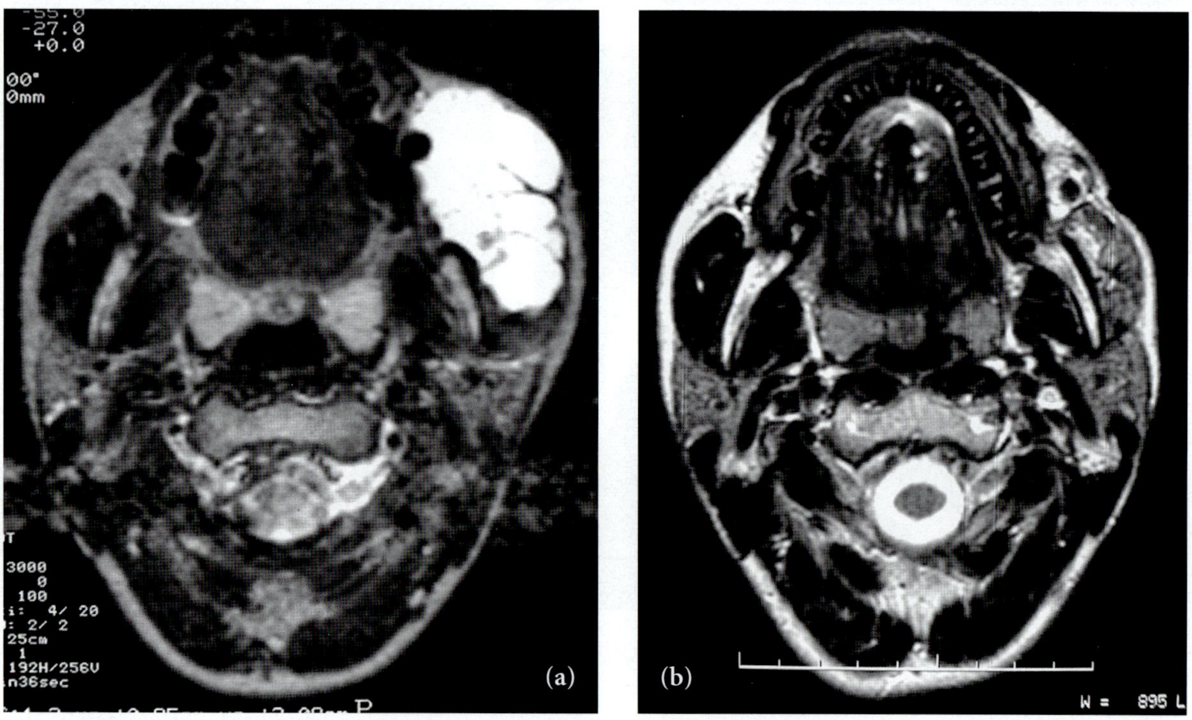

This intramasseter VM was treated with percutaneous sclerotherapy. The sclerosing agent is a mixture of 80% ethanol, and 10% lipiodol to allow visualization during injection, and 10% Ethibloc® to stabilize the mixture. Swelling of the VM is usual after sclerosis and is due to an intense inflammatory reaction. The duration of swelling is variable, from a few days to several weeks, depending on the amount of injected sclerosing agent and on individual susceptibility. Complete destruction of the VM may be achieved, as in this patient. This allowed this young woman to recover a symmetrical face. The procedure had some adverse effects: pain for 2 weeks and a temporary block of the temporomandibular joint with trismus.

Clinical Patterns, Investigations, and Treatment

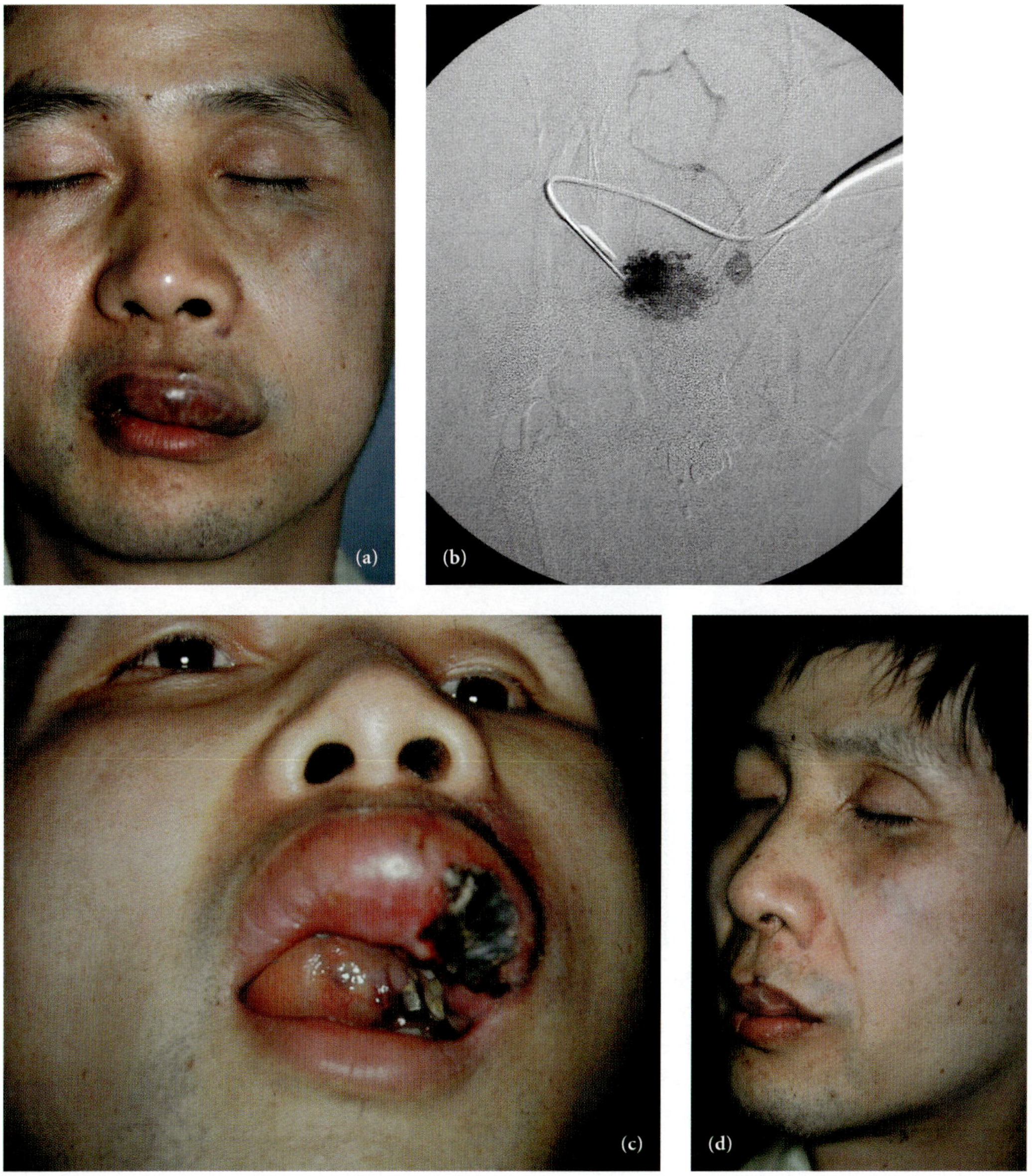

This lip VM (a) was treated using ethanol sclerotherapy (b). The complication of two necrotic ulcers (of the lip and palate) occurred (c). After spontaneous healing the lip was correctly reshaped with no need for complementary resection (d). Direct injection of pure ethanol into a VM is effective but potentially dangerous (1). In addition to possible local complications, severe systemic complications such as renal, neurological or pulmonary toxicity, rhabdomyolysis, myocardial depression, atrial arrhytmias, ventricular tachycardia and cardiac arrest, and even death have been reported. Therefore close monitoring is indispensable during and after the sclerosing procedure. Some, but not all, of these general complications seem related to high doses of ethanol, above 0.5 ml/kg.

Clinical Patterns, Investigations, and Treatment

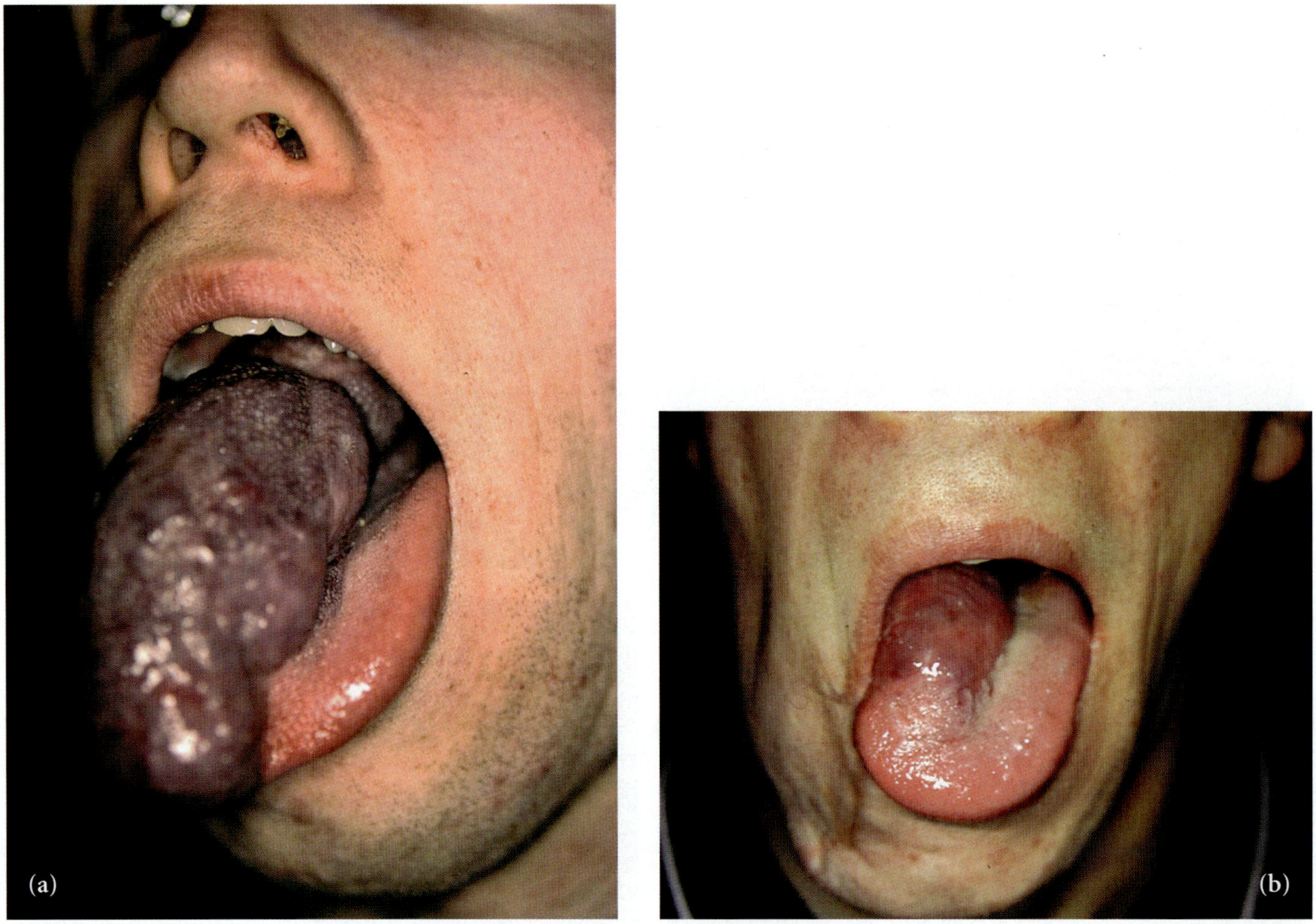

Ethanol sclerotherapy is usually effective. Ethanol destroys the endothelium causing cell death, thrombosis, inflammation, parietal necrosis, and subsequent vascular occlusion (28). The procedure is very painful and thus it is performed under general anesthesia. Careful monitoring is mandatory during the procedure and in the recovery room because serious systemic alcohol contamination occurs during the procedure (24). In this case (a) the sclerosing treatment prepared for resection of the tongue VM (b). When the base of the tongue and upper respiratory tract is significantly compromised by the VM, control of the airway during and after the therapeutic injections is necessary. In some patients a tracheostomy is performed prior to the interventional treatment and is maintained as long as necessary.

Clinical Patterns, Investigations, and Treatment

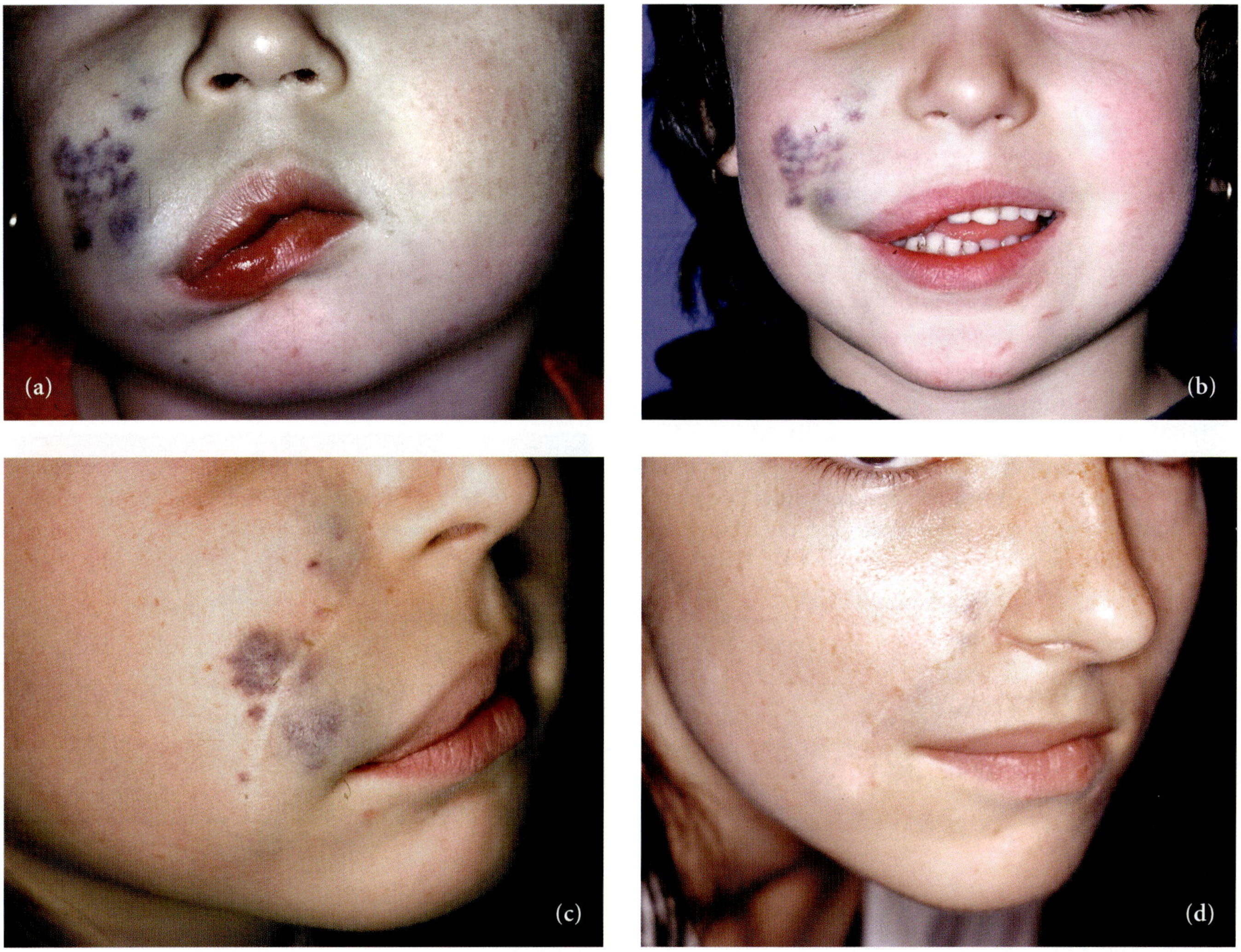

Results of 15 years of therapeutic management including multiple use of direct puncture sclerotherapy with Ethibloc®, various surgical procedures, with progressive excision of areas of VM bumping in the mouth, and blue skin locations on the cheek. In addition orthodontic management was followed by bi-maxillary surgical treatment. With the use of Ethibloc®, inflammation, swelling, and bruising are immediate and last from weeks to a few months. Usually surgery takes place a few weeks later. Local complications of this sclerosing agent occur in about 10% of procedures and they include skin necrosis, aseptic chronic drainage, and finally some degree of scarring. Peripheral nerve damage is extremely rare with Ethibloc®, by contrast with absolute ethanol sclerotherapy. Fever commonly occurs after the procedure, but no severe systemic complications have been reported with Ethibloc®.

Clinical Patterns, Investigations and Treatment

VM in the knee synovia is responsible for effusion and hemarthrosis, and pain. Episodes of stiffness and restriction of joint motion are observed in active children as early as 6–10 years of age. In the long term degenerative joint disease and destructive bone changes will impair function of the involved joint. To prevent this, partial synovectomy and excision of the VM embedded in the synovia (a) is carried out. Removal requires careful dissection from the femoral bone and muscles; (b) when involved periostum is excised. After 3 months of intense physical therapy, the child often recovers painless joint mobility (courtesy of Dr. Claude Laurian, Hôpital Saint Joseph, Paris, France).

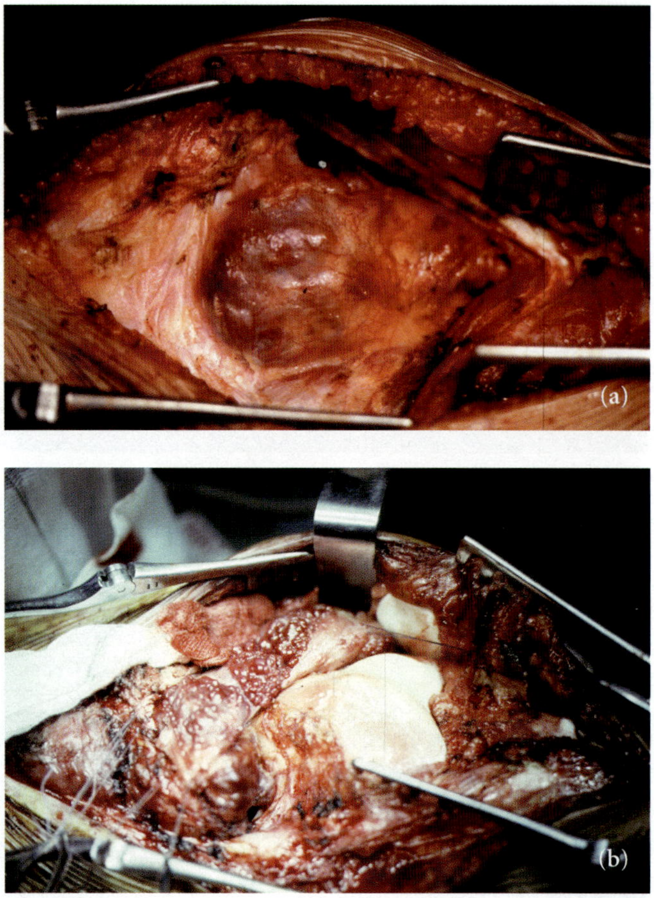

This woman has a VM occupying the mid-face (the nose and upper lip), the right cheek and right periocular region. She first had a single-stage treatment (sclerotherapy with Ethibloc® and ethanol) (operator: Dr. Annouk Bisdorff, Hôpital Lariboisière, APHP Paris, France) followed by excision of her large upper lip VM, with excellent remodeling of the mouth (operator: Dr. Dominique Deffrennes, Hôpital Lariboisière, APHP Paris, France). She also had an injection of polidocanol foam in the upper lid and cheek VM, with clear reduction of their size. Full nose involvement is quite uncommon: usually facial VMs do not affect the midline of the nose; in this case MRI showed a nasal meningo-encephalocele, in addition to the superficial VM, a finding that makes treatment of the nose VM perilous.

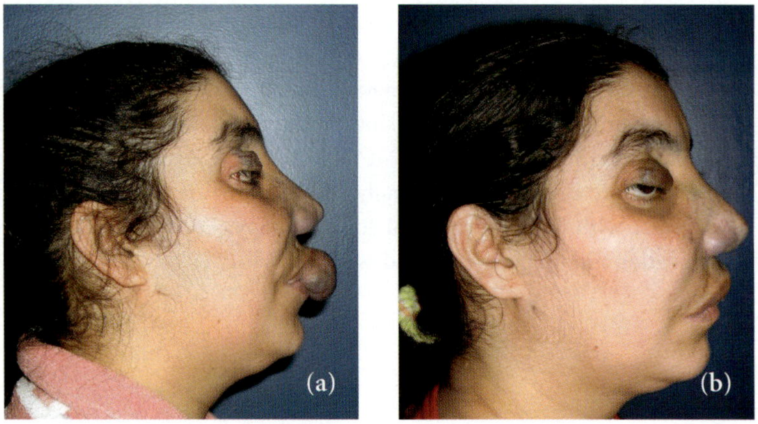

Clinical Patterns, Investigations, and Treatment

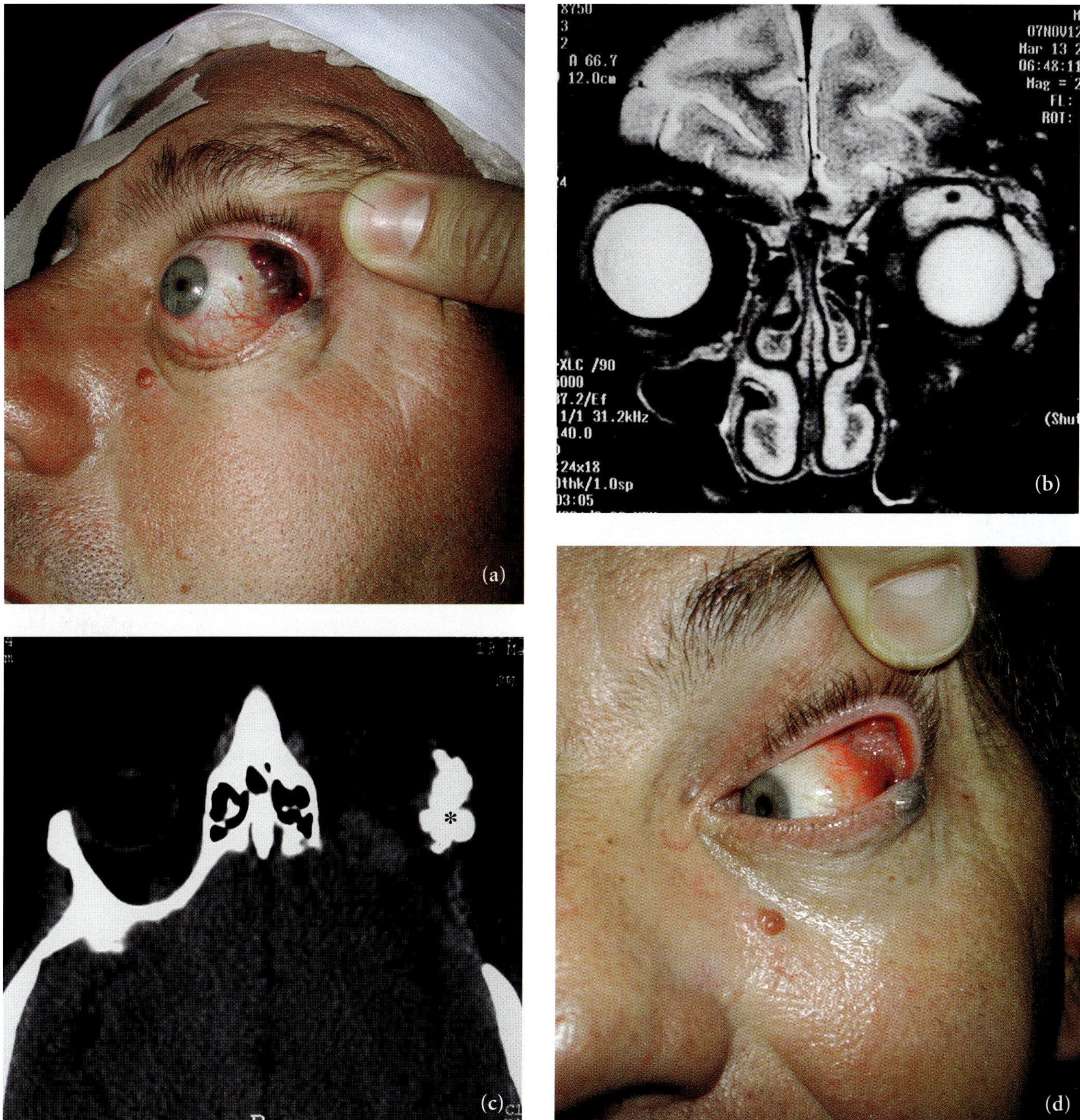

Orbital VM inducing severe headaches and exophthalmos (a, b). Sclerosis was used, taking extreme care to avoid diffusion of the sclerosing agent, which was ethanol. Injection of ethanol can only be used if the ophthalmic vein is not directly connected to the VM. CT shows the compartment treated ∗ (c). Complete waning of this compartment and of exophthalmos was achieved 2 months later (d).

Clinical Patterns, Investigations, and Treatment

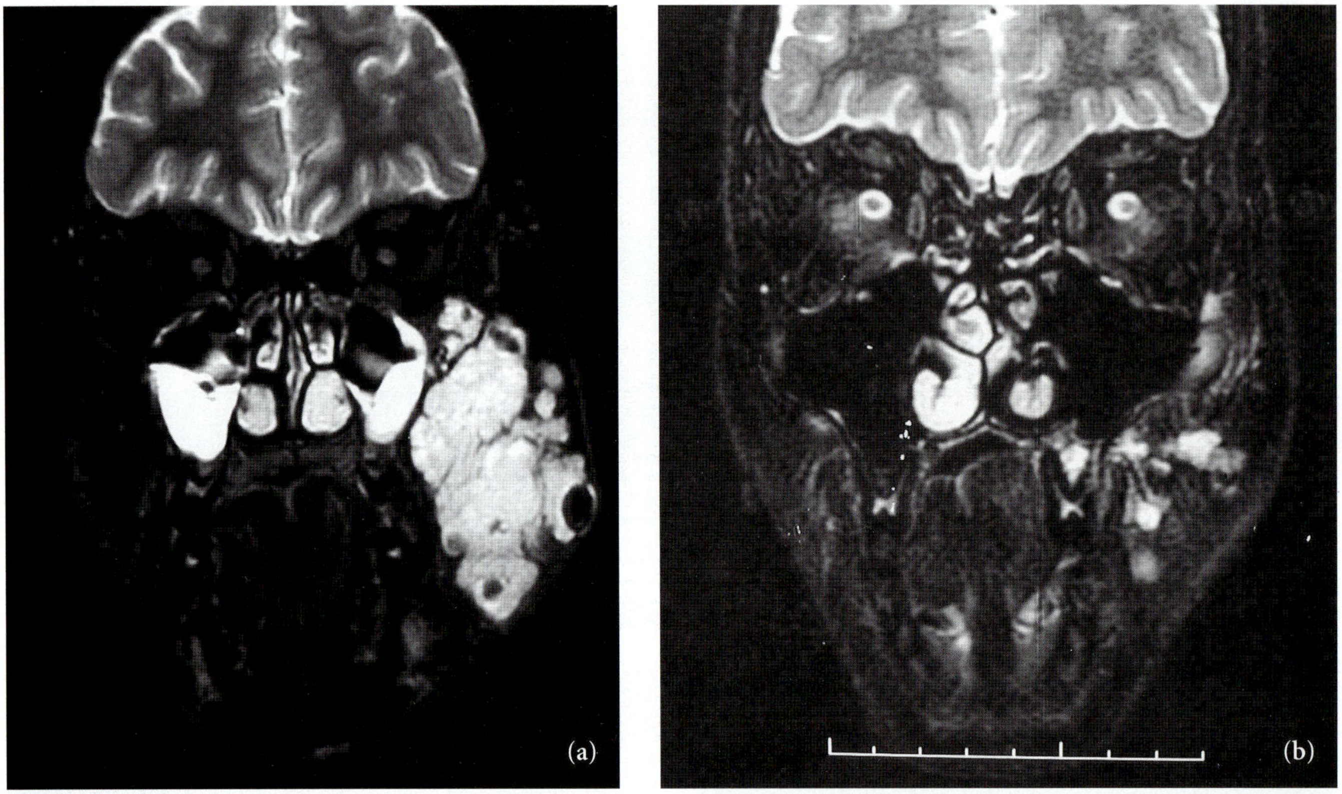

VM of the cheek inducing dental malocclusion. The sclerosing agent is injected progressively under fluoroscopy, filling the VM until the normal surrounding veins are opacified. This requires temporarily stopping the infusion of the sclerosing agent, which may be continued after a short delay in order to fill other compartments of the VM. Important regression of the VM may be obtained, as confirmed on MRI with regression of the hyperintense signal on T2-sequences.

Pathology of Bean Syndrome

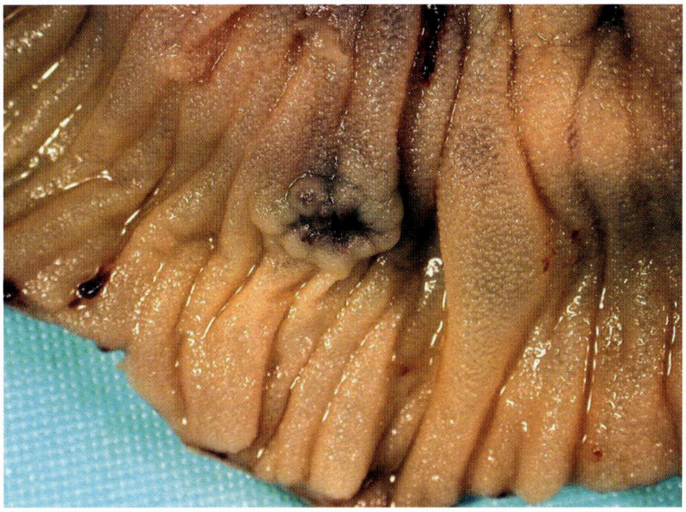

Small bowel specimen in BRBN syndrome, showing one of numerous bowel VMs.

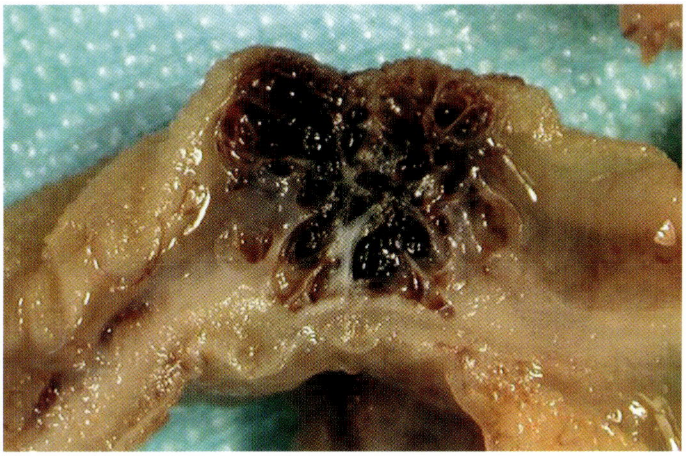

Macroscopic transection of the same lesion. The VM in Bean syndrome is better delineated than in common VM and affects the submucosa and muscularis proper. Some cavities contain thrombus.

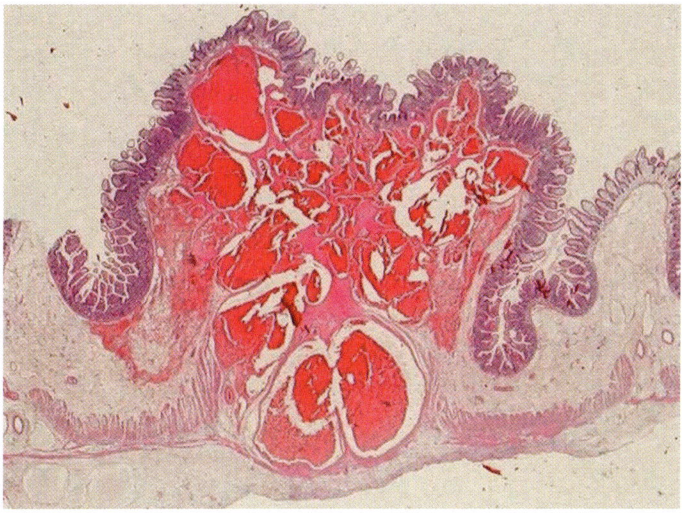

Low-power histological view of another small bowel lesion in the same patient. The thin-walled dilated venous cavities occupy the submucosa and musularis proper. The involvement of the mucosa is not apparent at this magnification.

Pathology of Bean Syndrome

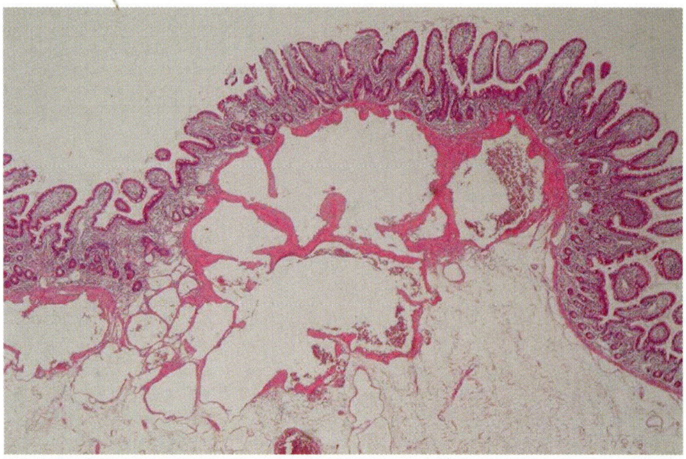

Small bowel lesion situated in the submucosa. The smooth-muscle cells of walls of the venous lakes merge with those of the muscularis mucosae. Some discontinuities of the venous wall/muscularis mucosae are seen, through which the lesion extends to the mucosa.

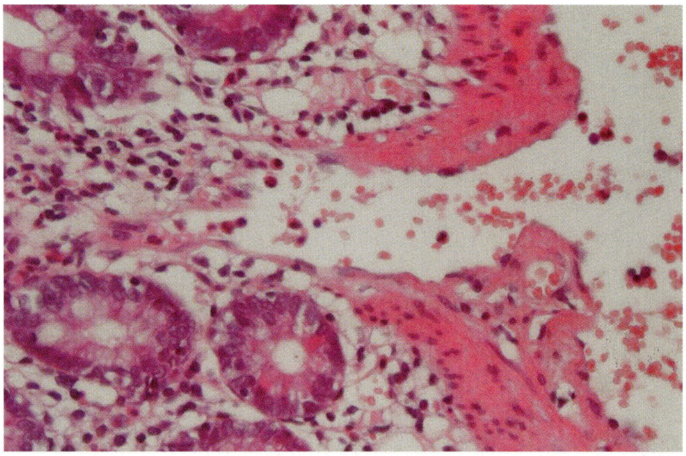

Direct communication between a dilated capillary of the mucosa and the cavities of a small bowel VM (at the right). This may explain the propensity of these lesions to bleed.

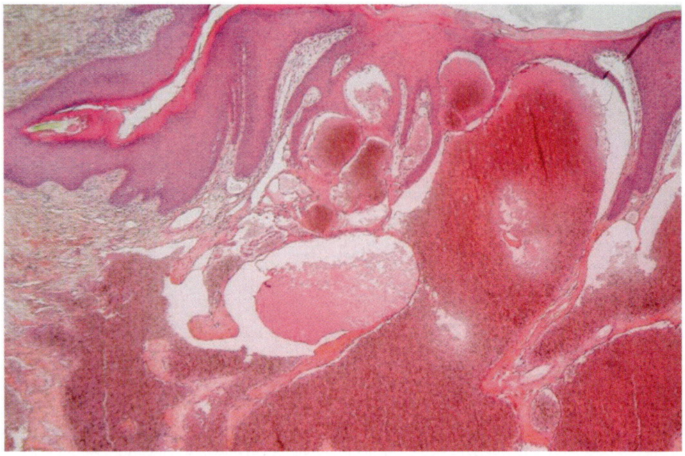

Superficial cutaneous lesion in Bean syndrome. While the deep venous lesions are similar to common VM, the superficial ones are more delineated, made up of closely packed thin-walled dilated vessels, occupying the papillary dermis, raising up a hyperkeratotic epidermis.

Clinical Aspects of Bean Syndrome

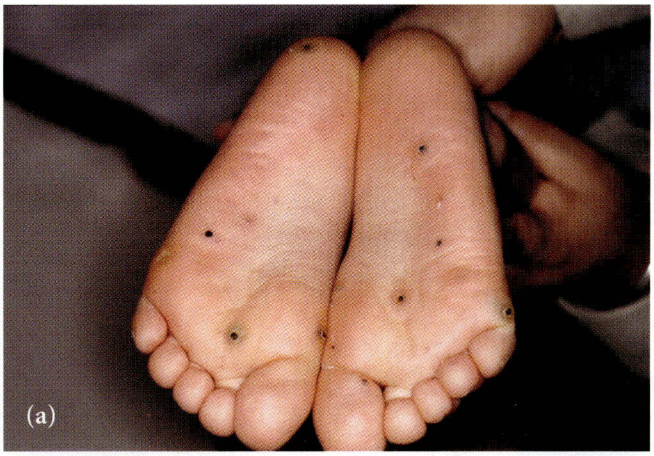
(a)

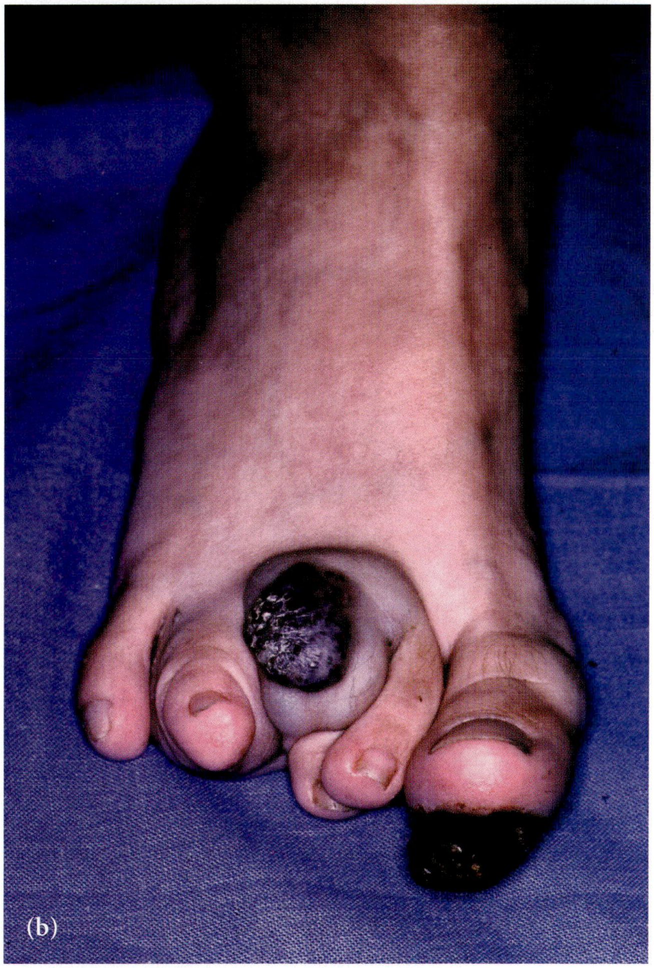
(b)

Dark-blue spots disseminate on the skin in Bean syndrome. They rapidly increase in number over the years, and first appear soon after birth. Some skin lesions have a rubber-like nipple aspect (rubber blebs). The dark-blue venous spots arise everywhere on the skin, including the face and scalp, and early in life the palms and soles. The blue papules and nodules often have a keratotic surface, and exhibit a transepidermal elimination of a dark-blue crust, then the blue spot re-emerges.

Clinical Aspects of Bean Syndrome

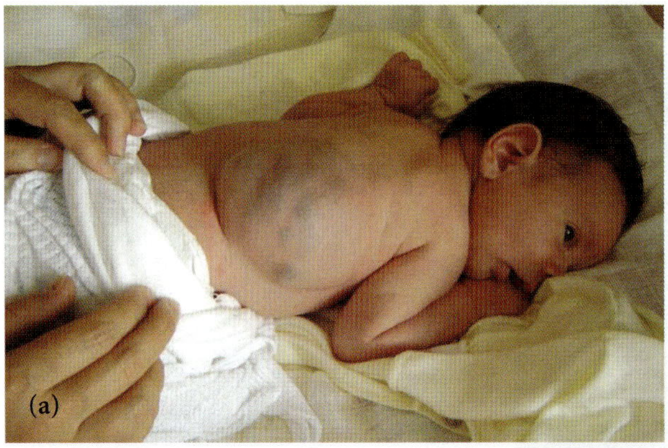

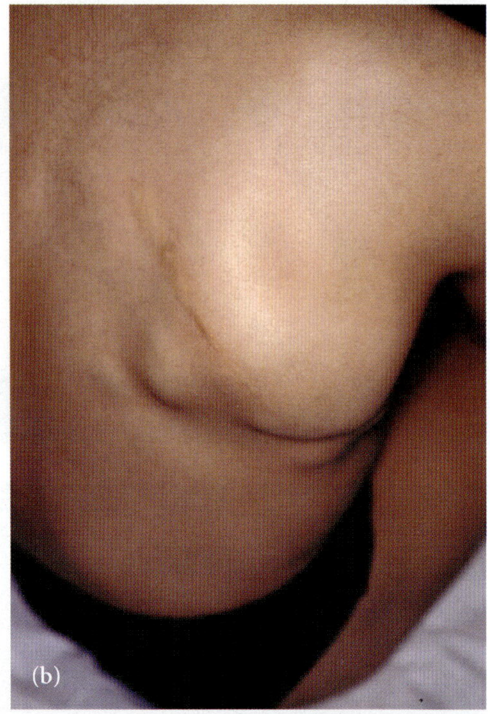

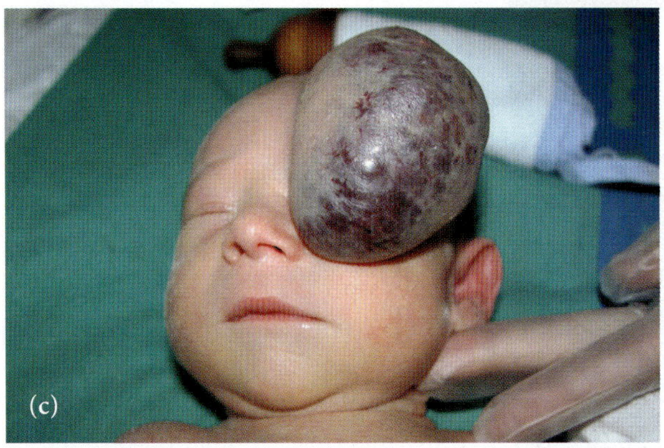

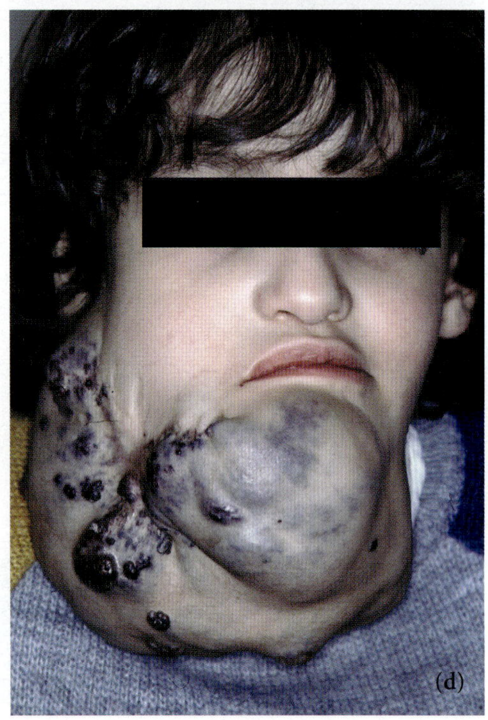

A patient with Bean syndrome may have a large venous mass, present from birth, in association with the blue spots. The mass may be located under apparently normal skin (a, b) (courtesy of Dr. L. Kitanovski, Slovenia), or may be of a deep blue hue (c) (courtesy of Dr. E. Baselga, Hospital de la Santa Creu I Sant Pau, Barcelona, Spain). Resection, when incomplete is followed by some re-swelling of the venous mass. Sometimes blue spots are superimposed on a large mass of VM (d).

Pathology of Glomuvenous Malformation

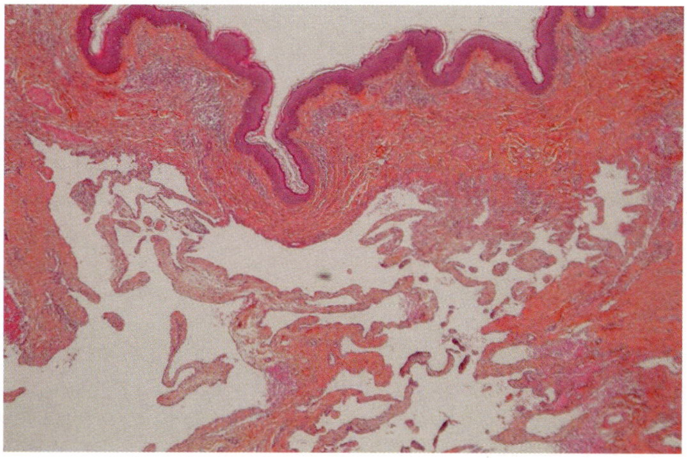

Microscopic view of a GVM. At this low magnification, GVM is made of large thin-walled interconnecting vascular channels, indistinguishable from common VM.

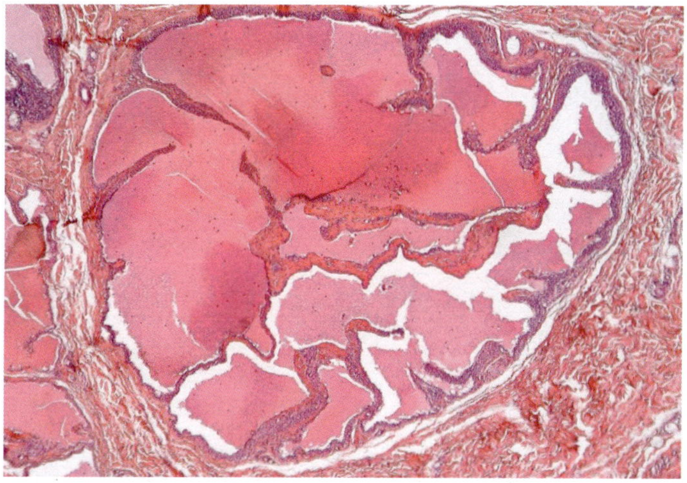

In some areas, GVM may present a more nodular distribution. The wall of the cavities appears thick and cellular, especially at the right of the figure.

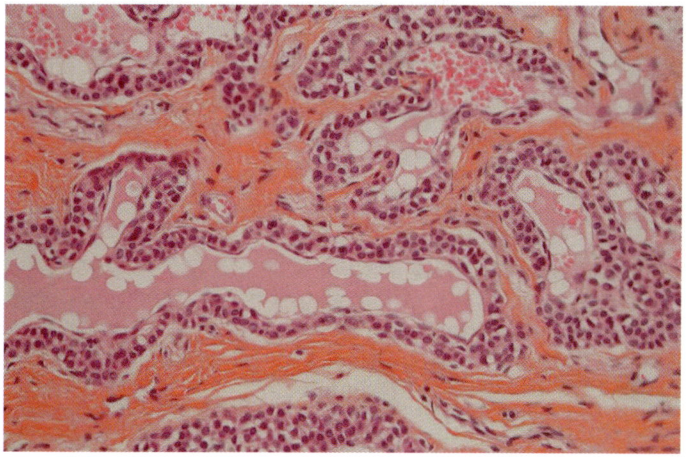

The walls of GVM are covered by endothelial cells, characteristically lined by media made of one or several rows of cuboidal glomus cells, with round nuclei and pale eosinophilic cytoplasm.

Pathology of Glomuvenous Malformation

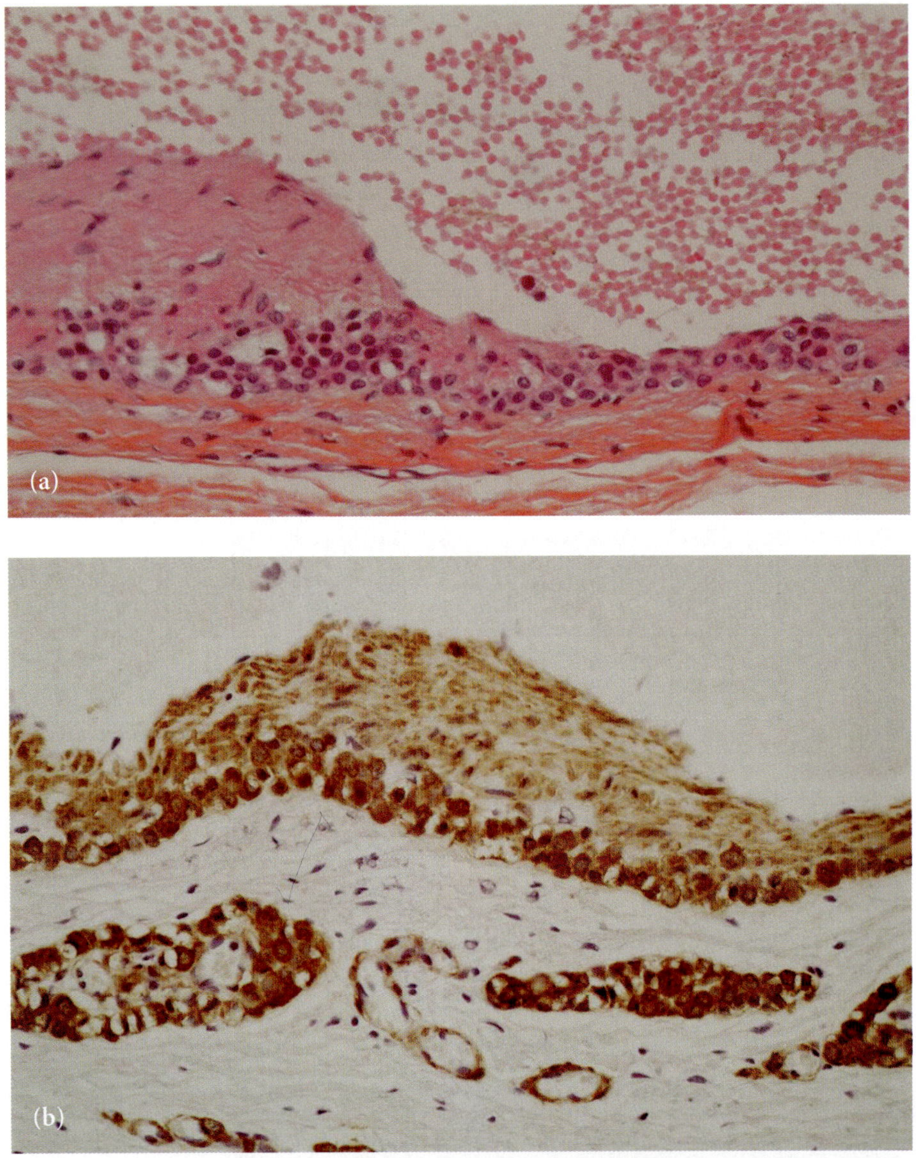

In places, the cuboidal glomus cells continue with more-common media made of spindled smooth muscle cells (a). Both types of cells contain smooth-mucscle cell actine (immunohistochemistry using anti smooth-muscle cell antibody is on (b).

Pathology of Glomuvenous Malformation

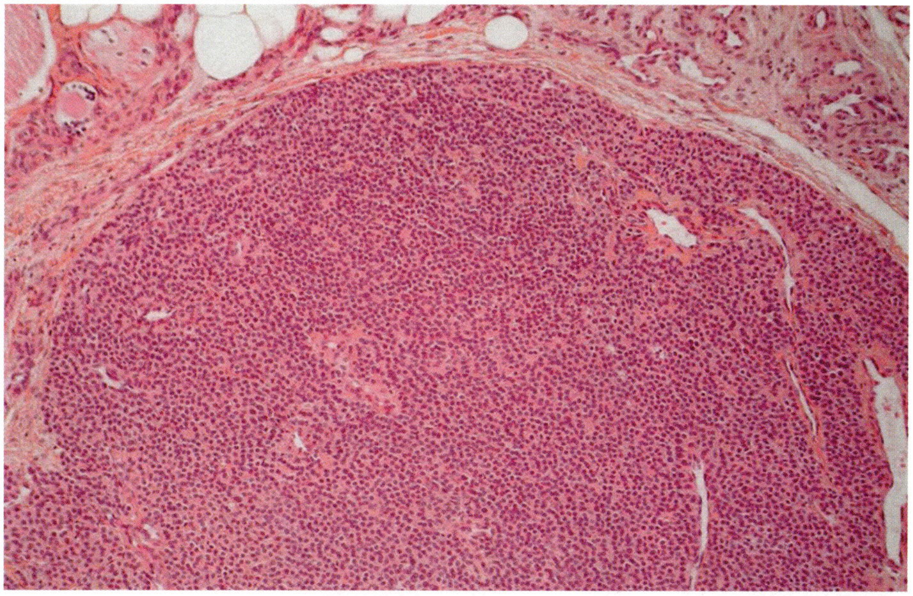

Some GVM are made of solid sheets of glomus cells, with few veins.

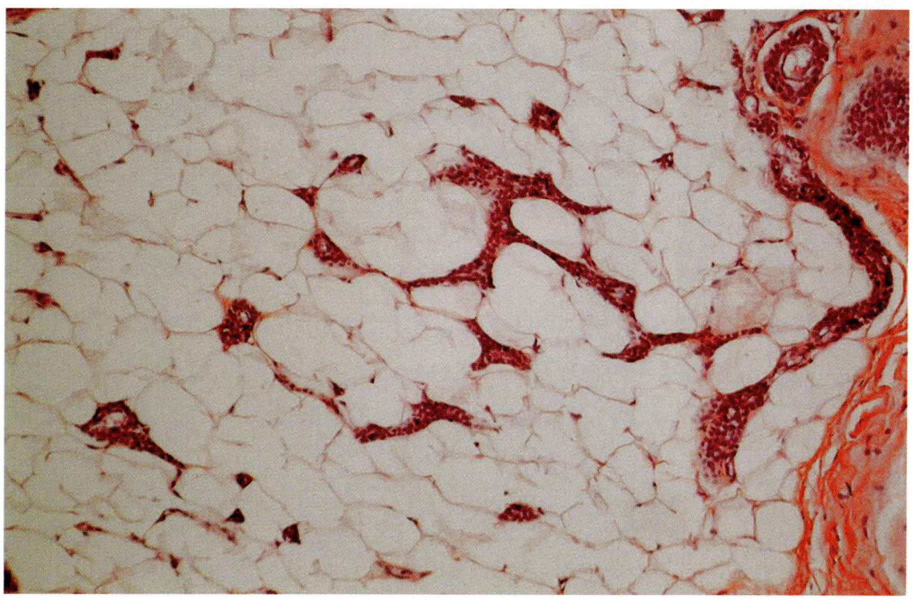

The glomus cells can be found not only in the media of vein-like vessels, but also in the wall of arteries or of capillary-size vessels, as in this case.

Clinical Aspects of Glomuvenous Malformation

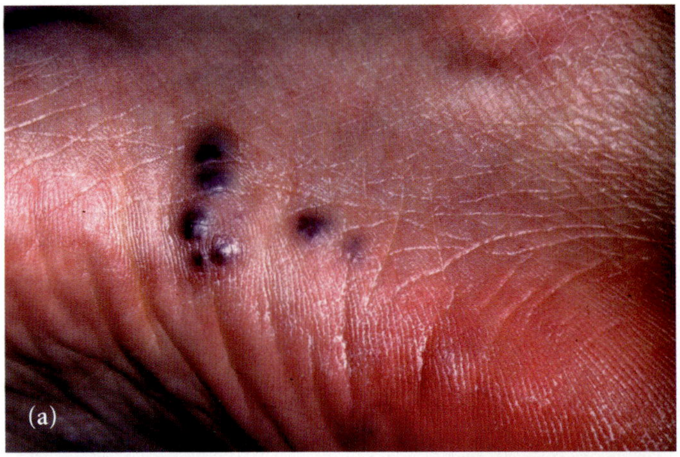

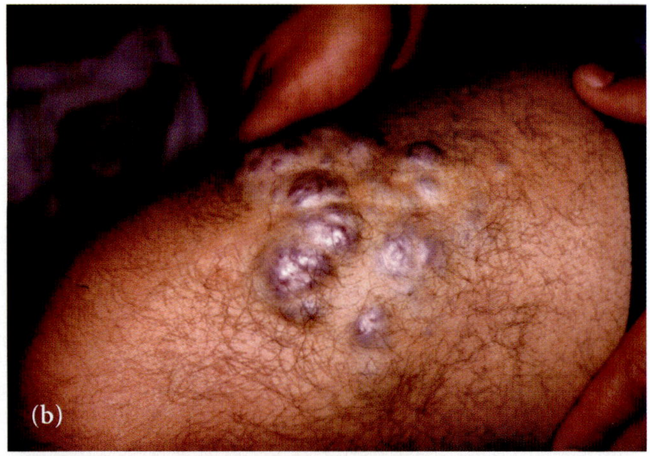

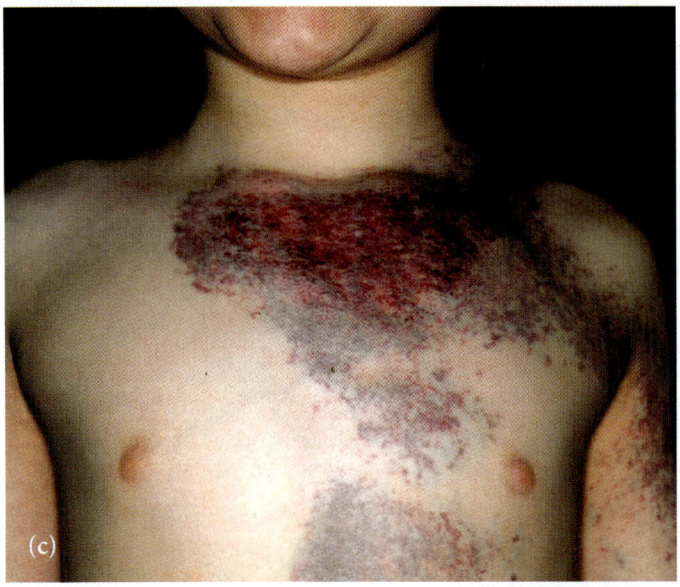

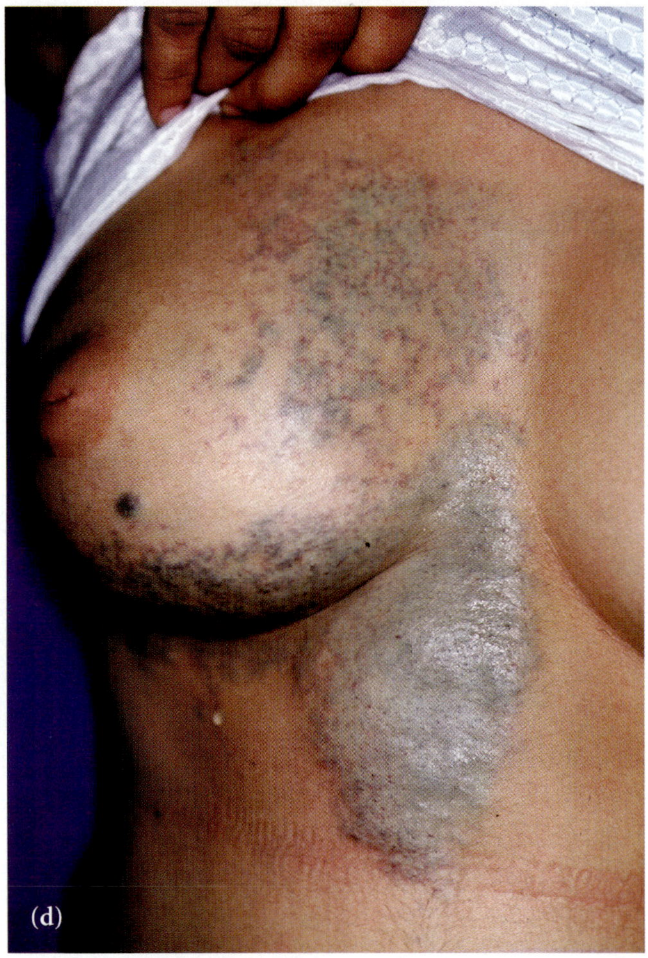

This montage illustrates various patterns of GVM. Some GVM patients display small blue papules or nodules reminiscent of Bean syndrome but without the hyperkeratosis and transepidermal elimination (a, b). Others have deep blue to purple nodules scattered over the skin (sometimes a single lesion). And some have large, segmental or not, plaque-like lesions (c,d). No specific location exists and the large plaque-like lesions observed in a segmental distribution may occur over the face, trunk, or limbs (30).

Clinical Aspects of Glomuvenous Malformation

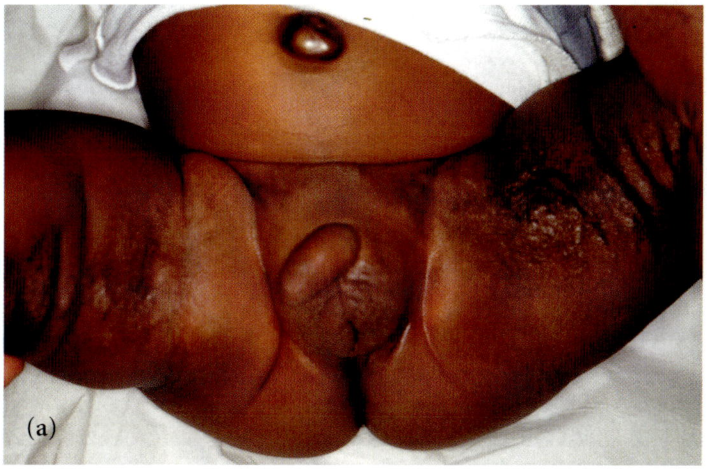

(a)

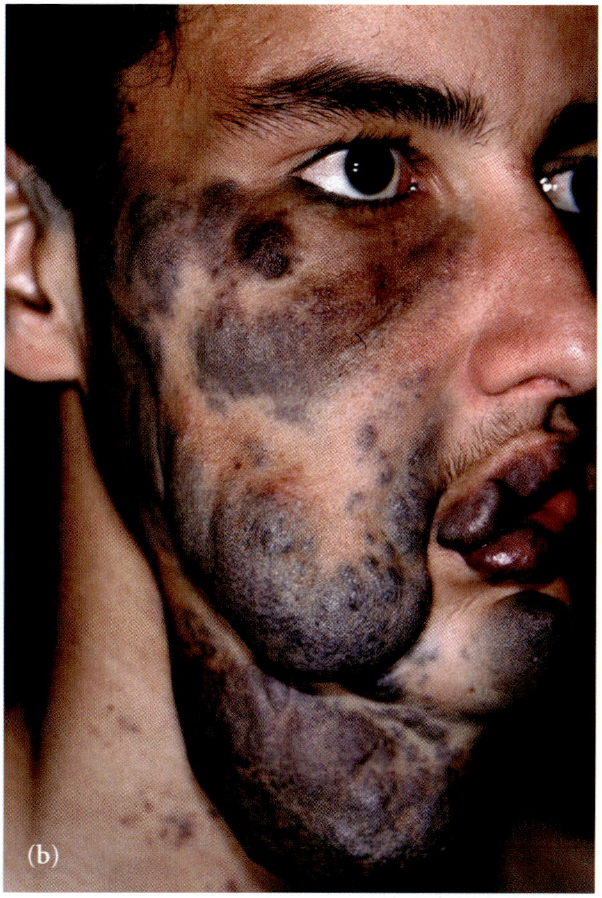

(b)

Diagnosis of GVM may be clinically difficult in patients with dark skin, like in this infant with internal aspects of both legs and perineum affected (a). When huge sagging lesions expand as in this young man the diagnosis is also tricky (b). Compared to VM, GVM is less compressible and not easily emptied by compression, it shows less discoloration during manipulation, and it does not swell when dependent. Tenderness on palpation or sudden contact is the main symptom differentiating it from VM skin lesions.

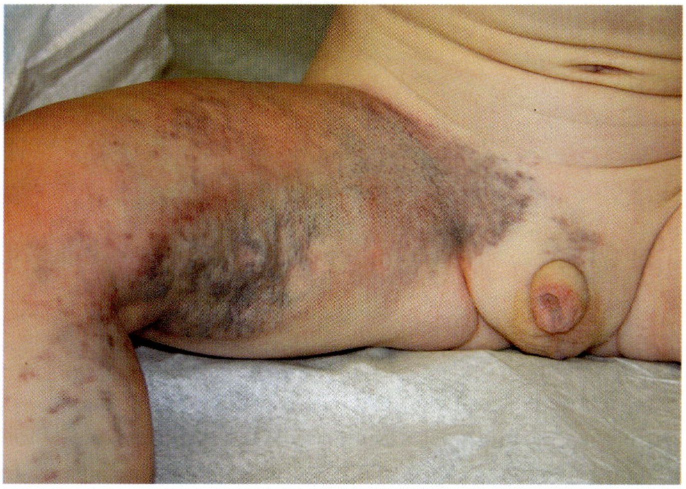

In infancy GVM are minor and diagnosis is difficult. Even the large plaque-like thick GVM are often inconspicuous at birth: large pink macules or subtle azure plaques. Later their appearance is distinctive with the blue hue increasing and the infiltration of the skin becoming prominent (courtesy of Dr. S. Mallory, St Louis, USA).

Clinical Aspects of Glomuvenous Malformation

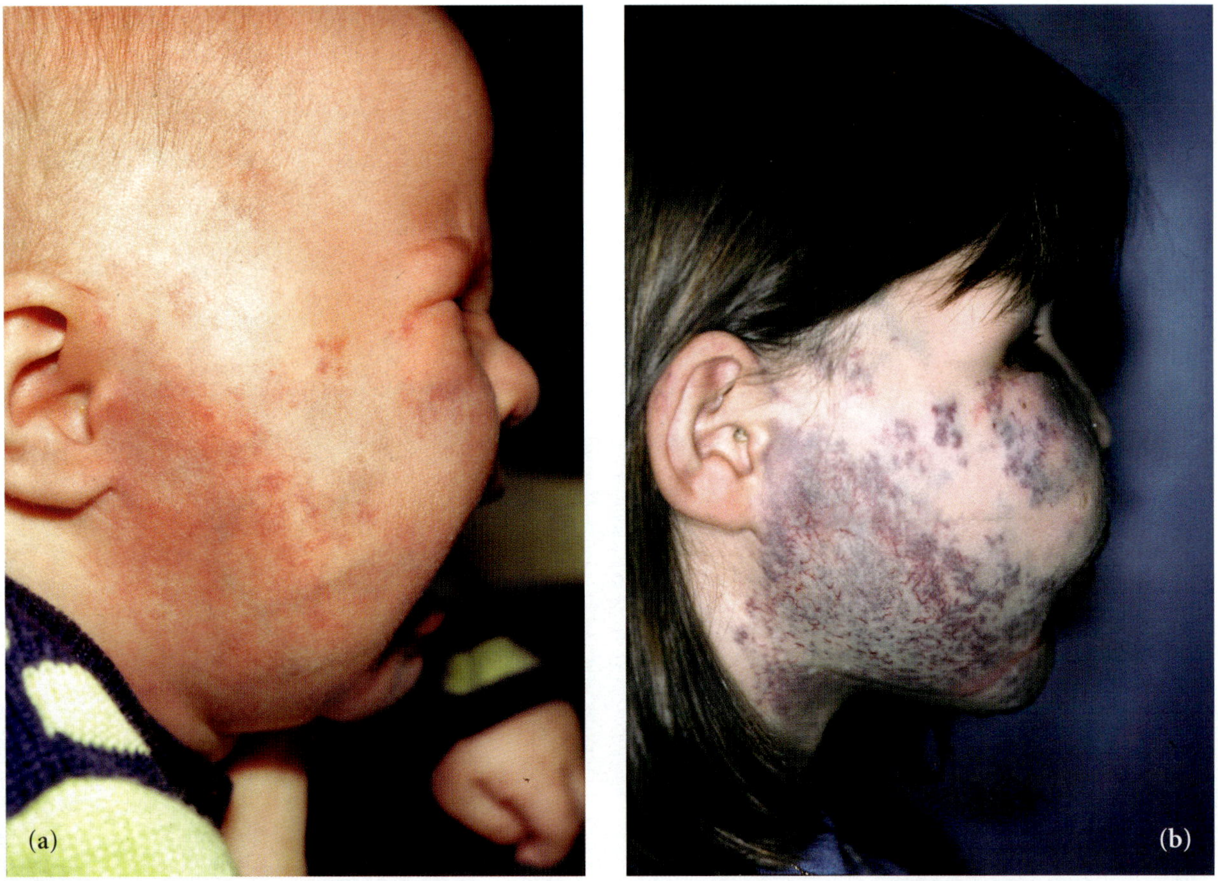

GVM develops and thickens from infancy into childhood and into adulthood, becoming raised with a cobblestone appearance; the color turns from pink or purple to deep blue: (a) and (b) show the thickening of this inconspicuous facial lesion at birth, first misdiagnosed as CM or a precursor of infantile hemangioma, and its appearance at 7 years of age after a first resection, with a thick blue lesion in the cheek.

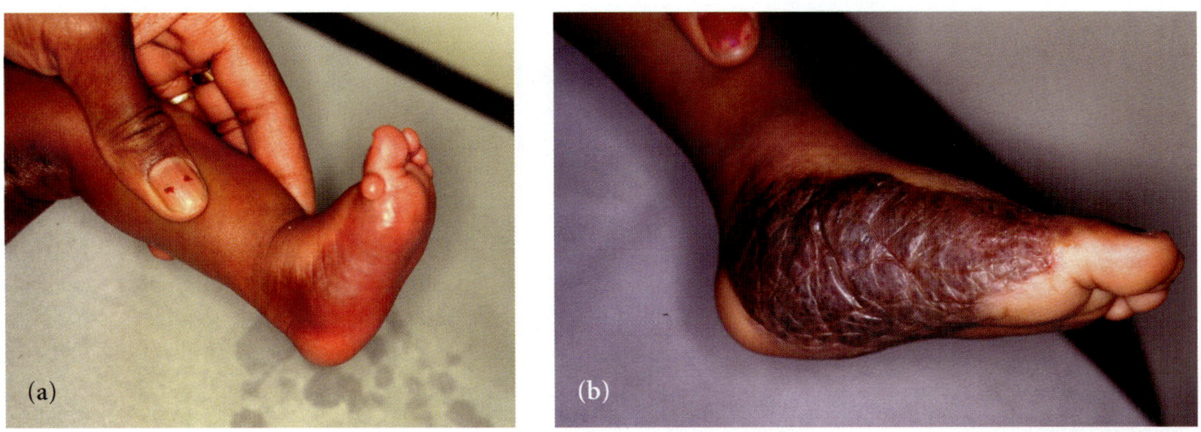

GVM in this African boy involved symmetrically the internal aspects both two legs and feet, as well as the perineum (see also figure (a) p. 217, same boy). At birth, (a) shows the shiny plaque-like lesion on one of the foot and a sixth toe (which was excised); one year later (b) the diagnosis of GVM became evident with the blue color and the aggregating papules.

MAFFUCCI SYNDROME
Pathology

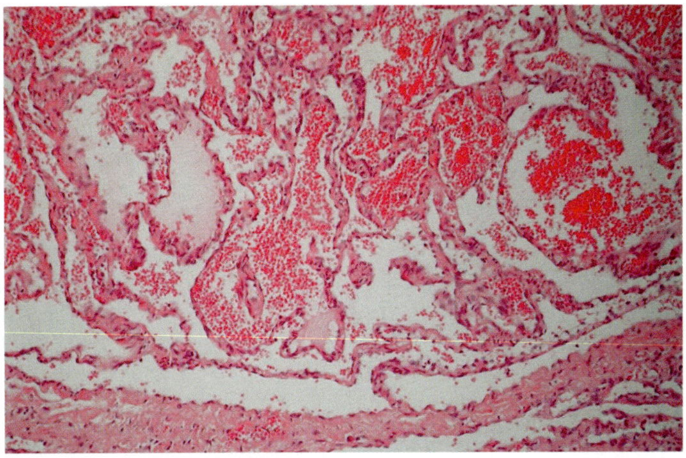

Spindle cell hemangioma (SCH) in a patient with Maffucci syndrome. The lesion is nodular and made of open thin-walled vessels containing red blood cells and separated by thin fibrous septa.

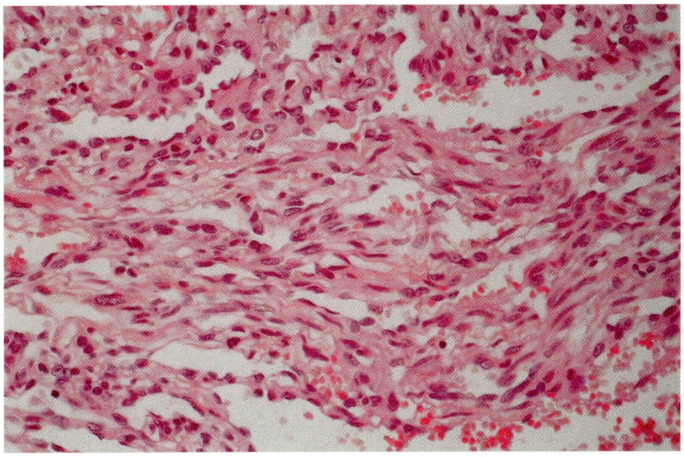

In some areas, rarely representing most of the lesion, the septa are thick and contain elongated spindle cells, separated by slit-like vascular lumen.

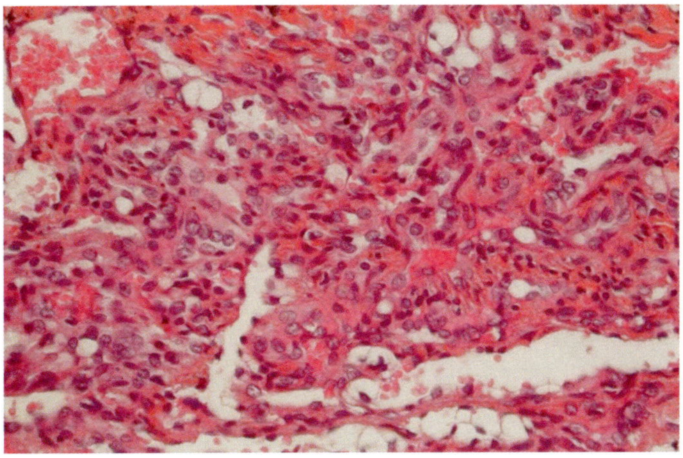

Some epithelioid endothelial cells are sometimes present, with a large eosinophilic or amphophilic cytoplasm and occasional intracytoplasmic clear vacuoles.

Pathology

SCH often extend into the lumen of malformed or normal-appearing veins.

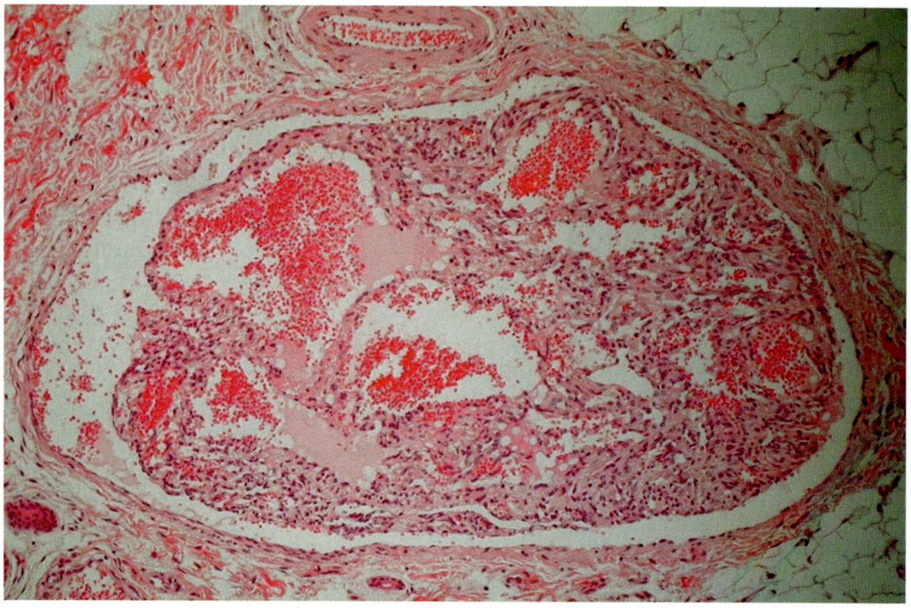

SCH, like VM, may contain phleboliths.

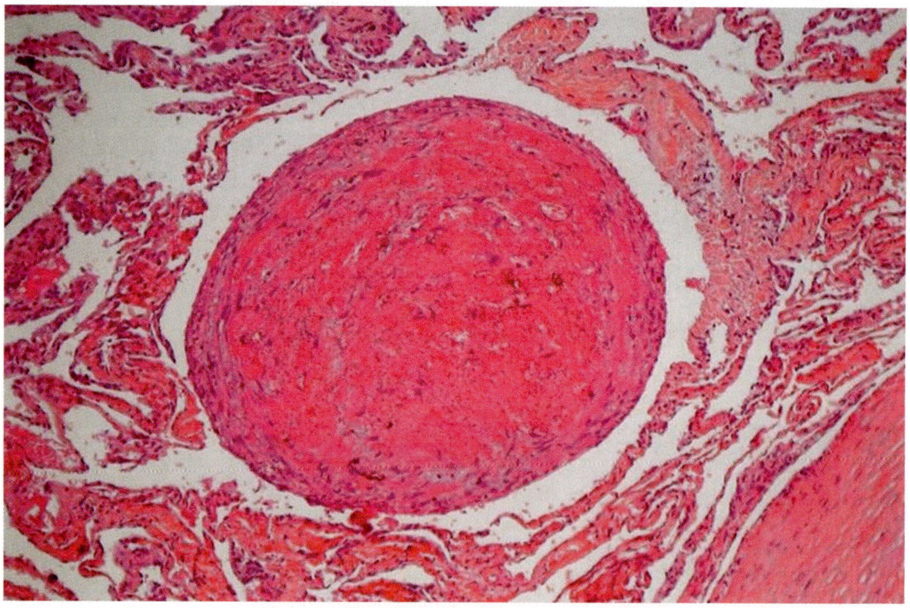

Clinical aspects

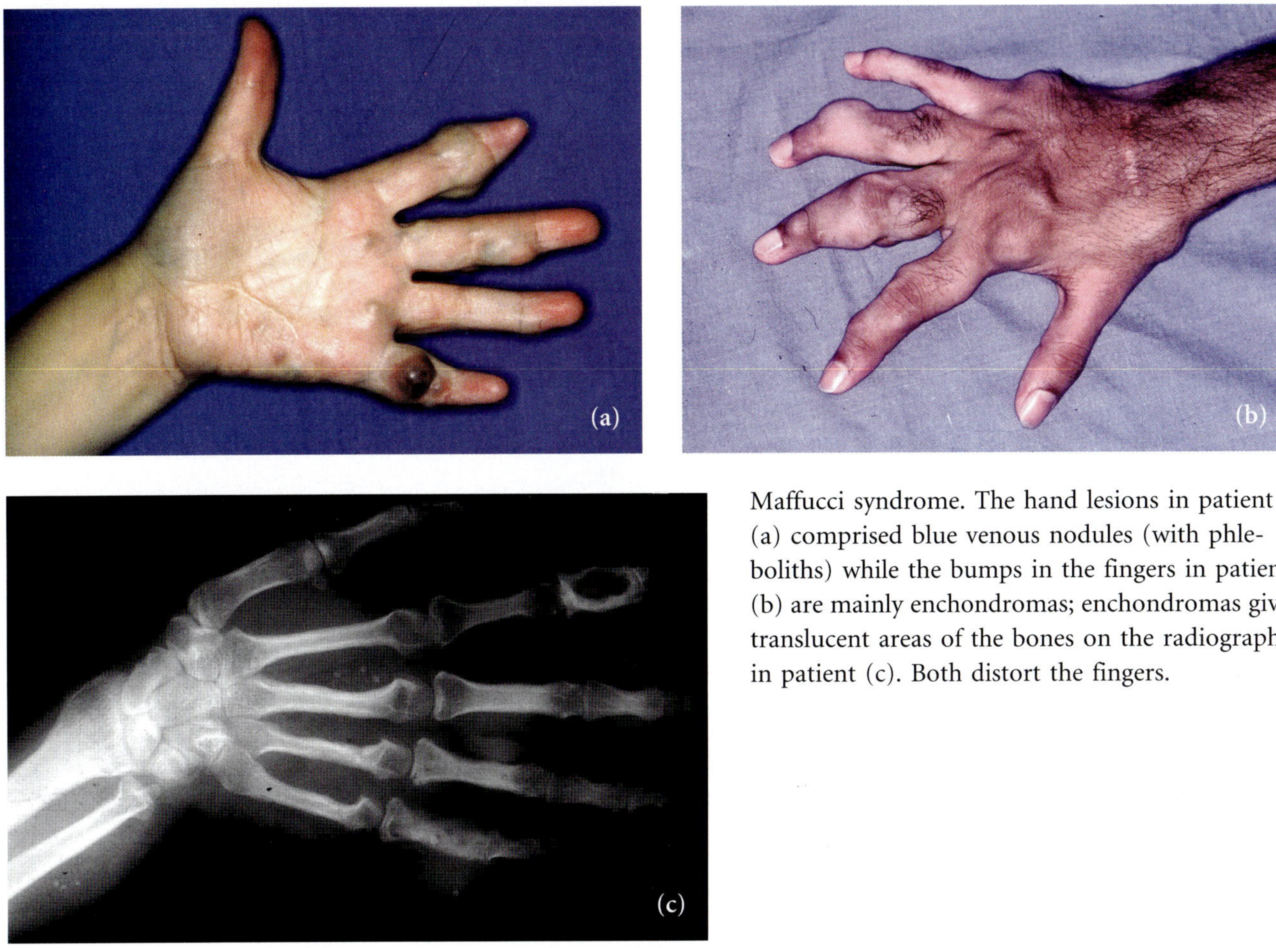

Maffucci syndrome. The hand lesions in patient (a) comprised blue venous nodules (with phleboliths) while the bumps in the fingers in patient (b) are mainly enchondromas; enchondromas give translucent areas of the bones on the radiograph in patient (c). Both distort the fingers.

References

1 Berenguer B, Burrows PE, Zurakowski D, Mulliken JB. Sclerotherapy of craniofacial venous malformations: complications and results. *Plast Reconstr Surg* 1999; **104**: 1–11; discussion 12–5.

2 Bigot JL, Iacona C, Lepreux A, Dhellemmes P, Motte J, Gomes H. Sinus pericranii: advantages of MR imaging. *Pediatr Radiol* 2000; **30**: 710–12.

3 Boon LM, Mulliken JB, Enjolras O, Vikkula M. Glomuvenous malformation (glomangioma) and venous malformation: distinct clinicopathologic and genetic entities. *Arch Dermatol* 2004; **140**: 971–6.

4 Boukobza M, Enjolras O, Guichard JP, Gelbert F, Herbreteau D, Reizine D et al. Cerebral developmental venous anomalies associated with head and neck venous malformations. *AJNR Am J Neuroradiol* 1996; **17**: 987–94.

5 Brouillard P, Boon LM, Mulliken JB, Enjolras O, Ghassibe M, Warman ML et al. Mutations in a novel factor, glomulin, are responsible for glomuvenous malformations ("glomangiomas"). *Am J Hum Genet* 2002; **70**: 866–74.

6 Brouillard P, Ghassibe M, Penington A, Boon LM, Dompmartin A, Temple IK et al. Four common glomulin mutations cause two thirds of glomuvenous malformations ("familial glomangiomas"): evidence for a founder effect. *J Med Genet* 2005; **42**: e13

7 Brouillard P, Vikkula M. Vascular malformations: localized defects in vascular morphogenesis. *Clin Genet* 2003; **63**: 340–51.

8 Burrows PE. *Treatment of sinus pericranii.* Communication in 15th ISSVA Workshop. Wellington, NZ. 22–25 February 2004.

9 Burrows PE, Laor T, Paltiel H, Robertson RL. Diagnostic imaging in the evaluation of vascular birthmarks. *Dermatol Clin* 1998; **16**: 455–88.

10 Burrows PE, Mason KP. Percutaneous treatment of low flow vascular malformations. *J Vasc Interv Radiol* 2004; **15**: 431–45.

11 Buxton N, Vloeberghs M. Sinus pericranii. Report of a case and review of the literature. *Pediatr Neurosurg* 1999; **30**: 96–9.

12 Cabrera J, Cabrera J Jr, Garcia-Olmedo MA. Sclerosants in microfoam. A new approach in angiology. *Int Angiol* 2001; **20**: 322–9.

13 Cabrera J, Cabrera J Jr, Garcia-Olmedo MA, Redondo P. Treatment of venous malformations with sclerosant in microfoam form. *Arch Dermatol* 2003; **139**: 1409–16.

14 Cabrera J, Redondo P, Becerra A, Garrido C, Cabrera J Jr, Garcia-Olmedo MA et al. Ultrasound-guided injection of polidocanol microfoam in the management of venous leg ulcers. *Arch Dermatol* 2004; **140**: 667–73.

15 Chapot R, Laurent A, Enjolras O, Payen D, Houdart E. Fatal cardiovascular collapse during ethanol sclerotherapy of a venous malformation. *Intervent Neuroradiol* 2002; **8**: 321–4.

16 Domini M, Aquino A, Fakhro A, Tursini S, Marino N, Di Matteo S et al. Blue rubber bleb nevus syndrome and gastrointestinal haemorrhage: which treatment? *Eur J Pediatr Surg* 2002; **12**: 129–33.

17 Dubois J, Garel L, Grignon A, David M, Laberge L, Filiatrault D et al. Imaging of hemangiomas and vascular malformations in children. *Acad Radiol* 1998; **5**: 390–400.

18 Dubois J, Soulez G, Oliva VL, Berthiaume MJ, Lapierre C, Therasse E. Soft-tissue venous malformations in adult patients: imaging and therapeutic issues. *Radiographics* 2001; **21**: 1519–31.

19 Dubois JM, Sebag GH, De Prost Y, Teillac D, Chretien B, Brunelle FO. Soft-tissue venous malformations in children: percutaneous sclerotherapy with Ethibloc. *Radiology* 1991; **180**: 195–8.

20 Enjolras O, Ciabrini D, Mazoyer E, Laurian C, Herbreteau D. Extensive pure venous malformations in the upper or lower limb: a review of 27 cases. *J Am Acad Dermatol* 1997; **36**: 219–25.

21 Enjolras O, Mulliken JB. Vascular tumors and vascular malformations (new issues). *Adv Dermatol* 1997; **13**: 375–423.

22 Ertem D, Acar Y, Kotiloglu E, Yucelten D, Pehlivanoglu E. Blue rubber bleb nevus syndrome. *Pediatrics* 2001; **107**: 418–20.

23 Gallo SH, McClave S. A Blue rubber bleb nevus syndrome: gastrointestinal involvement and its endoscopic presentation. *Gastrointest Endosc* 1992; **38**: 72–6.

24 Hammer FD, Boon LM, Mathurin P, Vanwijck RR. Ethanol sclerotherapy of venous malformations: evaluation of systemic ethanol contamination. *J Vasc Interv Radiol* 2001; **12**: 595–600.

25 Hein KD, Mulliken JB, Kozakewich HP, Upton J, Burrows PE. Venous malformations of skeletal muscle. *Plast Reconstr Surg* 2002; **110**: 1625–35.

26 Kassarjian A, Fishman SJ, Fox VL, Burrows PE. Imaging characteristics of blue rubber bleb nevus syndrome. *AJR Am J Roentgenol* 2003; **181**: 1041–8.

27 Lasjaunias P, Berenstein A. Endovascular treatment of craniofacial lesions. *Surgical Neuroangiography*. Vol. **2**. Berlin: Springer Verlag, 1987.

28 Mason KP, Michna E, Zurakowski D, Koka BV, Burrows PE. Serum ethanol levels in children and adults after ethanol embolization or sclerotherapy for vascular anomalies. *Radiology* 2000; **217**: 127–32.

29 Mazoyer E, Enjolras O, Laurian C, Houdart E, Drouet L. Coagulation abnormalities associated with extensive venous malformations of the limbs: differentiation from Kasabach–Merritt syndrome. *Clin Lab Haematol* 2002; **24**: 243–51.

30 Mounayer C, Wassef M, Enjolras O, Boukobza M, Mulliken JB. Facial "glomangiomas": large facial venous malformations with glomus cells. *J Am Acad Dermatol* 2001; **45**: 239–45.

31 Mulliken JB, Fishman SJ, Burrows PE. Vascular anomalies. *Curr Probl Surg* 2000; **37**: 517–84.

32 Paltiel HJ, Burrows PE, Kozakewich HP, Zurakowski D, Mulliken JB. Soft-tissue vascular anomalies: utility of US for diagnosis. *Radiology* 2000; **214**: 747–54.

33 Perkins P, Weiss SW. Spindle cell hemangioendothelioma. An analysis of 78 cases with reassessment of its pathogenesis and biologic behavior. *Am J Surg Pathol* 1996; **20**: 1196–204.

34 Puig S, Aref H, Chigot V, Bonin B, Brunelle F. Classification of venous malformations in children and implications for sclerotherapy. *Pediatr Radiol* 2003; **33**: 99–103.

35 Riche MC, Hadjean E, Tran-Ba-Huy P, Merland JJ. The treatment of capillary-venous malformations using a new fibrosing agent. *Plast Reconstr Surg* 1983; **71**: 607–14.

36 Siniluoto TM, Svendsen PA, Wikholm GM, Fogdestam I, Edstrom S. Percutaneous sclerotherapy of venous malformations of the head and neck using sodium tetradecyl sulphate (sotradecol). *Scand J Plast Reconstr Surg Hand Surg* 1997; **31**: 145–50.

37 Suh JS, Shin KH, Na JB, Won JY, Hahn SB. Venous malformations: sclerotherapy with a mixture of ethanol and lipiodol. *Cardiovasc Intervent Radiol* 1997; **20**: 268–73.

38 Vikkula M, Boon LM, Carraway KL 3rd, Calvert JT, Diamonti AJ, Goumnerov B et al. Vascular dysmorphogenesis caused by an activating mutation in the receptor tyrosine kinase TIE2. *Cell* 1996; **87**: 1181–90.

39 Waner M. Recent developments in lasers and the treatment of birthmarks. *Arch Dis Child* 2003; **88**: 372–4.

40 Wassef M, Enjolras O. Les malformations vasculaires superficielles, classification et histopathologie. *Ann Pathol* 1999; **19**: 253–64.

41 Yakes WF. Extremity venous malformations. *Semin Intervent Radiol* 1994; **11**: 332–9.

CHAPTER III.C

Lymphatic Malformations (LM)

III.C.1 Common Lymphatic Malformations

Introduction

Lymphatic malformation (LM) is a malformation of the lymphatic system, and it consists of small vesicles or large pouches filled with lymphatic fluid. The lymphatic system is an open-ended unidirectional system returning interstitial fluid, macromolecules and immune cells from the tissues to the blood circulatory system (34).

Microcystic LMs (also known as tissular LMs) infiltrate soft tissues including the skin and mucosa where they cause the emergence of clear or hemorrhagic vesicles, and they also can occupy visceral territories in the thorax or abdomen, and even bones.

Macrocystic LMs create large translucent lumps under normal skin, or are deeply located.

Combined micro- and macrocystic forms are relatively common, in all locations, superficially and internally.

LMs suddenly expand in the presence of regional inflammation or intralesional bleeding. Three quarters of LMs are clinically evident before 5 years of age (14). In the same series of 145 patients the most common location was the head and neck (36.5%) followed by the extremities and axilla (31%) and the trunk (24.1%), while visceral intrathoracic or abdominal lesions accounted for 8.2% of cases. In the group of 186 patients studied by Alqahtani et al. (2) 48% of lesions were in the head and neck and 42% were in the trunk or limbs, while 10% were internally located.

Ultrasonography detects intrauterine macrocystic LM ("cystic hygroma") as early as the late first trimester of pregnancy. Fetal hygroma colli cysticum are septated or nonseptated on sonography for morphological features, and they carry a risk of associated chromosomal abnormalities, particularly Turner syndrome and Trisomy 18 (36).

Clinical Aspects

Depending on their location both the microcystic and macrocystic LMs have distinctive effects and complications (11).

Microcystic LM

Long known as "lymphangioma circumscriptum," microcystic LM is a plaque-like ill-defined lesion involving the skin or visible on the mucous membranes. Clear, yellowish, or blood-filled and dark-red vesicles spread over the surface of a smooth area of swelling. Recurrent inflammation, bulging and bruises, or lymph and blood oozing, are regularly observed during the chronic course of this malformation. In childhood the surface occupied by vesicles is often minor compared to the true future visible extent of the lesion. This is why very often an early resection gives poor results, with vesicles later developing all around the surgical scar.

Macrocystic LM

In this condition (classically known as "cystic hygroma") the large cyst creates a soft lump under a normal or slightly bluish skin. A macrocystic LM in the mouth area may suddenly expand, usually during a nose or throat, viral or bacterial infection, or because there is dental caries or gingivitis. Whatever their location this sometimes sudden expansion results from intracystic spontaneous bleeding. As a consequence, the mass becomes inflammatory, red, firm on palpation, and tender.

Associated micro- and macrocystic LM is a common feature in the orbital area. Intraorbital and periorbital LM produces exophthalmos, and it has visual consequences (functional amblyopia, refraction abnormalities, mainly astigmatism and strabismus). Sudden orbital proptosis was observed in 45% of cases in a group of 42 children (16). In the same series one-half of the patients had both intraconal and extraconal involvement, and it was extraconal or intraconal in one-quarter. Visual loss may result from bleeding into orbital cysts encircling the optic nerve. In the group of 42 patients reported by Greene et al. (16) 40% of children had permanently diminished vision of multifactorial causes (amblyopia, exposure keratitis and corneal ulcer, congenital cataract, retinal detachment, and glaucoma), and three patients were blind in the affected eye.

Visceral LMs usually combine micro- and macrocystic cysts; however, microcystic infiltrating lesions preponderate in most patients. They occur in the thorax, abdomen, and buttocks and also involve bones. A number of the patients with visceral lesions endure a life-threatening disease, which begins usually by childhood or adolescence. It is frequently complicated by intralesional bleeding episodes because of chronic coagulopathy with elevated D-dimers and low fibrinogen.

Bony LMs have different presentations. In the trunk and limbs bone involvement is either benign with no symptoms and no progression (15) or it carries a risk of fracture in the affected bones, with possible neurological consequences when the spine is involved. In the cervicofacial region LM creates various patterns of osseous hypertrophy ending in widened interdental spaces, progressive maxillary deformity or mandibular distortion, increased mandibular height, class III malocclusion, anterior open bite, and prognathism (31).

Visceral LM with intestinal and pulmonary involvement is often called "lymphangiectasia." It results in pleural effusions, abdominal pain, protein-losing enteropathy, hypoalbuminemia and hypogammaglobulinemia, and lymphopenia. It often manifests during childhood or adolescence and has a bad prognosis and outcome. Intestinal lesions are managed by bowel rest and then a low-fat and medium-chain triglyceride diet. Various pharmacological agents, including interferon alpha, corticosteroids and vincristine, have usually been of no help. When there is a coexisting coagulopathy, protracted treatment with a low-molecular-weight heparin brings some improvement. There is one report of improved gastrointestinal symptoms with tranexamic acid (25), and another with the combination of corticosteroid and octreotide (a somatostatine analog).

Investigations

When clinical diagnosis for a macrocystic LM is unclear, the following techniques are all valuable:

ULTRASONOGRAPHY (US) AND US DOPPLER of a macrocystic LM show multiloculated anechoic cysts with no flow, while microcystic LM are heterogeneously hypoechoic with no flow.

CT SCANS With these cysts are hypodense.

MRI shows a septated mass, cystic spaces being hypointense on SE T1-sequences and usually there is no gadolinium contrast enhancement; cysts are of high signal intensity on SE T2-sequences with fat suppression.

DIRECT PUNCTURE of a macrocystic lesion permits liquid analysis, to rule out any other cystic lesion, in particular cystic malignancies. Direct iodinated contrast injection, under fluoroscopic control, better delineates the lesion before sclerotherapy.

Treatment

Sudden enlargement of a macrocystic LM is usually the result of intralesional bleeding or infection. Pain relief, antibiotics, and anti-inflammatory drugs (corticosteroids or nonsteroidal anti-inflammatory drugs) are prescribed. Rarely, incision and drainage are necessary. Some lesions may spontaneously regress after such an episode. Large cysts are treated with aspiration of the lymphatic fluid, followed by percutaneous intralesional injection of a sclerosing agent, under fluoroscopic guidance. Puig et al. (33) recommend the use of a double-needle to avoid elevation of pressure inside the lesion and to allow outflow of excess sclerosant and contrast. After the procedure erythema and swelling with variable pain are commonly observed: they require pain relief medication, and a few days of corticosteroid treatment. Complications of sclerotherapy include fistula with leakage of a mixture of the sclerosing agent, fibrin, and inflammatory cells, and consequently a scar. Partial regression of the cyst requires re-injection or excision. New cysts may develop months or years after apparently satisfactory sclerosing treatments.

Surgical resection of the macrocystic LM is proposed either as a second step after failure or incomplete results of sclerotherapy, or as first procedure (2, 16, 38). Recurrence after incomplete excision is not surprising and adequate management may be either a new surgical treatment or sclerotherapy. Post-operative complications include fistula with leakage of lymph fluid requiring drainage for weeks or months, infection, burst of vesicles on a previously apparently undamaged skin or mucosa, varying cosmetic damage with unaesthetic scarring, depending on the LM location, and lymphedema (32).

Nd-YAG and diode laser photocoagulation have been employed to reduce microcystic LM in two modalities: superficial, with or without continuous ice-cube surface cooling, or interstitial after puncture or the lesions, but large lesions tend to recur. Radiofrequency treatment is under evaluation for microcystic LM.

In extensive LM with lymphedema in the limbs, treatment will include compression with a pneumatic device, compressive bandaging, and adapted elastic support garments.

Macrocystic LM enlarges progressively during fetal life, but no prenatal intervention is required in the majority of cases (10). Prenatal MRI identifies the need for cesarean section. Massive lesions in the neck, tongue, and mouth areas may require tracheotomy after birth because of significant airway compromise, and a gastric tube may be necessary for feeding. Then various combined and multiple therapeutic procedures and operations will aim at restoring the airway and oropharyngeal function, and improving cosmesis (4).

III.C.2 Syndromic Lymphatic Malformations and Lymphedemas

III.C.2.1 LYMPHEDEMAS

The primary lymphedemas are usually divided into two categories, the rare congenital Milroy disease (OMIM 153100) and the more frequent late-onset Meige lymphedema (OMIM 153200).

Lymphedema can be associated with Turner and Noonan syndromes. In Turner syndrome acral congenital lymphedema of the extremities is a presenting manifestation as are the pterygium colli and redundant neck folds. They are sequels of altered lymphatic pathogenesis; when detected during pregnancy, rarely hygroma cysticum colli persists at birth; it usually resolves leaving the pterygium colli (24).

This subcutaneous swelling, lymphedema, is more common in the lower extremities, although it also occurs in the upper limbs, trunk, and even face. Aplasia or hypoplasia of lymph vessels results in clinical edema either at birth (early-onset forms) or later in life, until adulthood (late-onset forms).

Autosomal-dominant forms exist isolated or as part of a syndrome: primary congenital lymphedema (locus on 5q34–35, the mutated gene *FLT4 (VEGFR3)* is a tyrosine kinase receptor for vascular endothelial growth factor) (21), early-onset familial lymphedema of Milroy, late-onset familial lymphedema of Meige, lymphedema–distichiasis syndrome (with locus on 16q24.3, the mutated gene being *FOXC2*), and hypotrichosis–lymphedema–telangiectasia syndrome (locus on 20q, mutated gene *SOX18*)(7).

III.C.2.2 AAGENAES SYNDROME OR CHOLESTASIS–LYMPHEDEMA SYNDROME

This disease was identified in 1968 by Aagenaes (1) and half of the reported cases are of Norwegian origin. It combines a neonatal intrahepatic cholestasis that improves, and chronic severe lymphedema mainly in the lower extremities that worsens. Other features include: peripheral pulmonary stenosis, vertebral anomalies, and a distinctive facies. The gene has been located to chromosome 15q (8).

III.C.2.3 HENNEKAM SYNDROME

Hennekam syndrome was described in 1989 as an autosomal recessive disease comprising intestinal lymphangiectasia, lymphedema, facies anomalies, including downslanting palpebral fissures and epicanthal folds, and mental retardation (18). The phenotype was later expanded to other visceral anomalies (3).

III.C.2.4 GORHAM SYNDROME

Vanishing bone disease, the Gorham–Stout syndrome, or phantom bone, or vanishing bone syndrome is a sporadic progressive and spontaneous bone-destructive process. Numerous dilated blood or lymph vascular channels are present. They occupy the site of the vanished bones. The disease demineralizes and destroys the affected bones. On plain radiographs, radiolucency of the involved bones gives them a "licked stick of candy" appearance. Gorham syndrome causes death in 16% of cases. Phantom bone disorder can be associated with chronic coagulopathy and bleeding. An increase in osteoclast formation (from mononuclear precursors) and differentiation, promotes osteolysis (20). When the disease affects the spine and ribs it can cause chylothorax and paraplegia (40).

Figures

LYMPHATIC MALFORMATIONS
Pathology

The histological structure of LM is similar to VM. The malformed vessels can however be somewhat more round or open with less anastomosis. The lumen contain a clear fluid with rare macrophages.

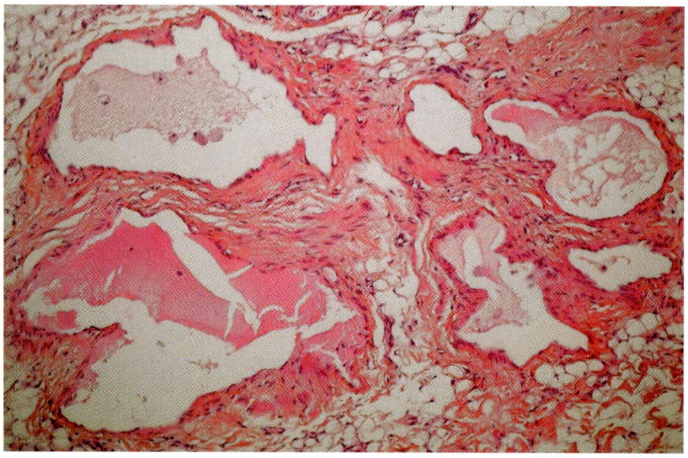

Some vessels have very thin walls and contain a clear fluid, sometimes with numerous intravascular lymphocytes. Aggregates of lymphocytes are also present in the tissue, closely associated to the malformed vessels. Inset: a vessel lumen containing lymphocytes, a macrophage, and red blood cells.

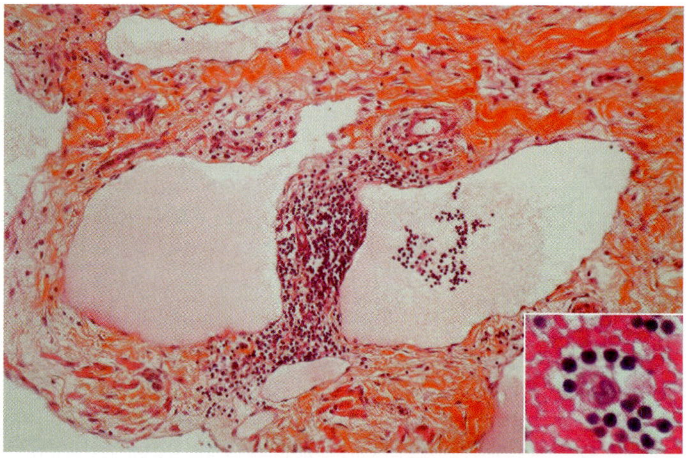

The dilated lymph vessels can be superficial and occupy and expand the papillae of the dermis or mucosa, covered with a thin epithelium. This is the pathological substratum to the vesicles that are present in some LM. Thin endothelial cell-covered fibrous projections, reminiscent of valves, are seen in the cavities.

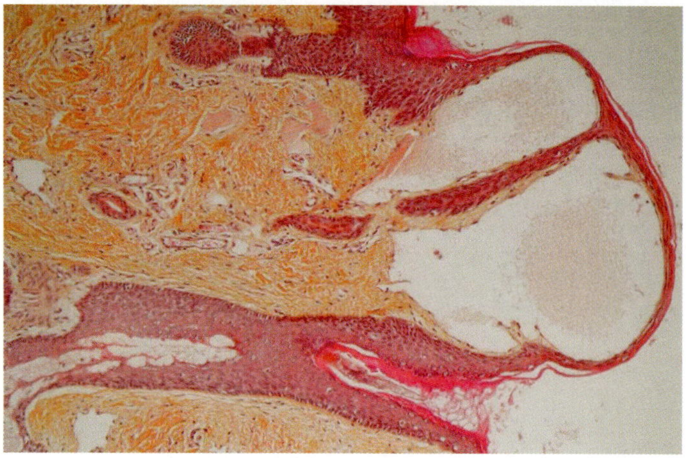

Pathology

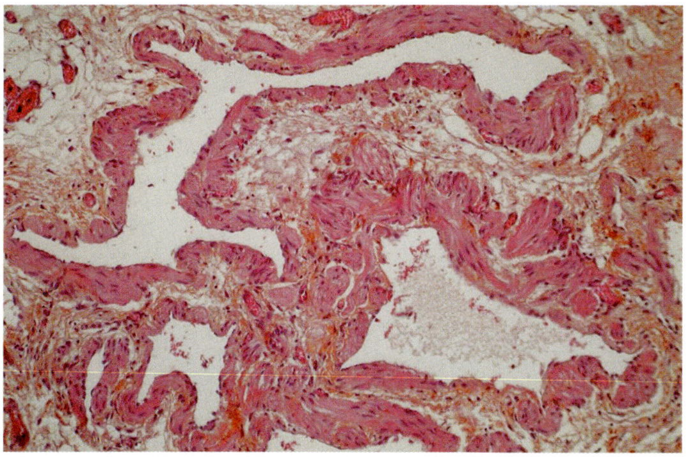

In other cases the wall of the malformed vessels comprises a thick muscular media. The muscle bundles are of uneven thickness and irregularly oriented.

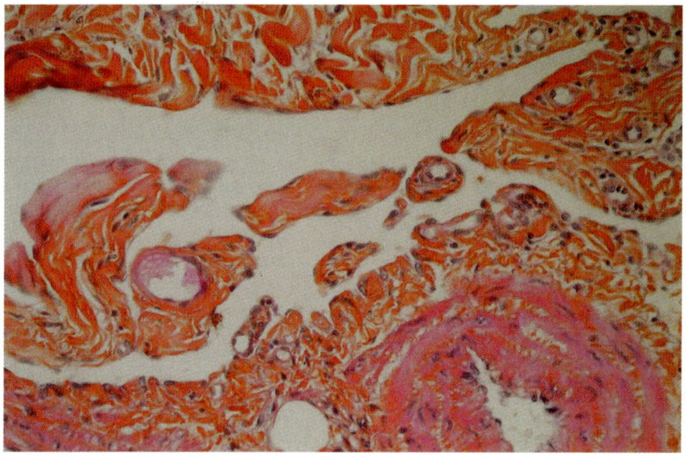

Some normal tissue elements (small nerves, arterioles, etc.) can be seen in the vascular lumen, completely surrounded by the abnormal cavities. This phenomenon is however rarer than in VM.

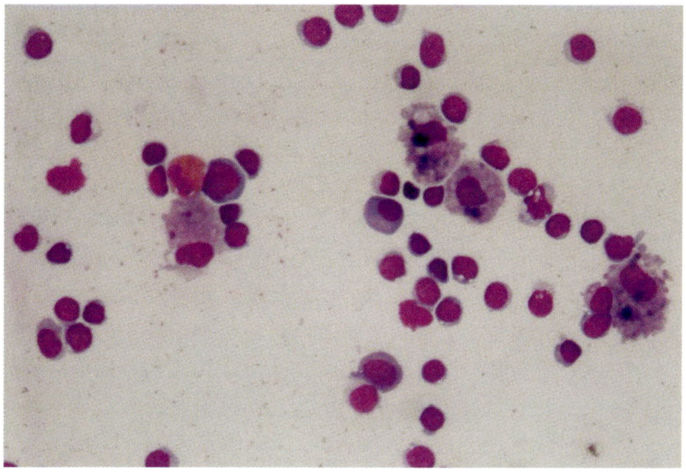

The cytological smears obtained after puncture of an LM contain numerous lymphocytes (sometimes with plasmacytoid features) and macrophages.
Some eosinophils may be present.

Pathology

The endothelial cells of LM express the lymphatic marker D2–40. This expression is however often heterogeneous and focal.

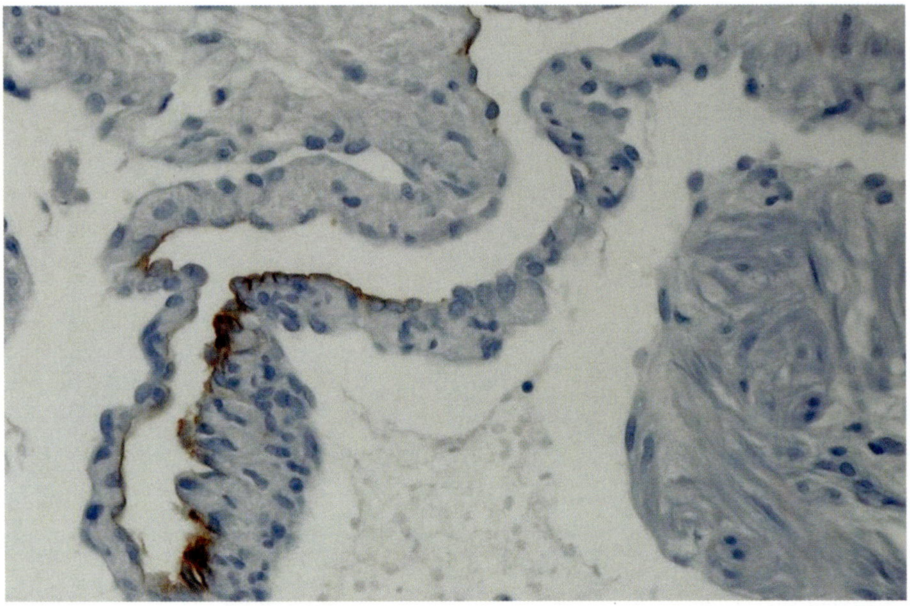

So-called benign lymphangioendothelioma (or acquired progressive lymphangioma) are made up of very-thin-walled lymphatic vessels dissecting through the collagen bundles of the dermis. Apart from the small size of the vessels, the appearance of the lesion is similar to other LM.

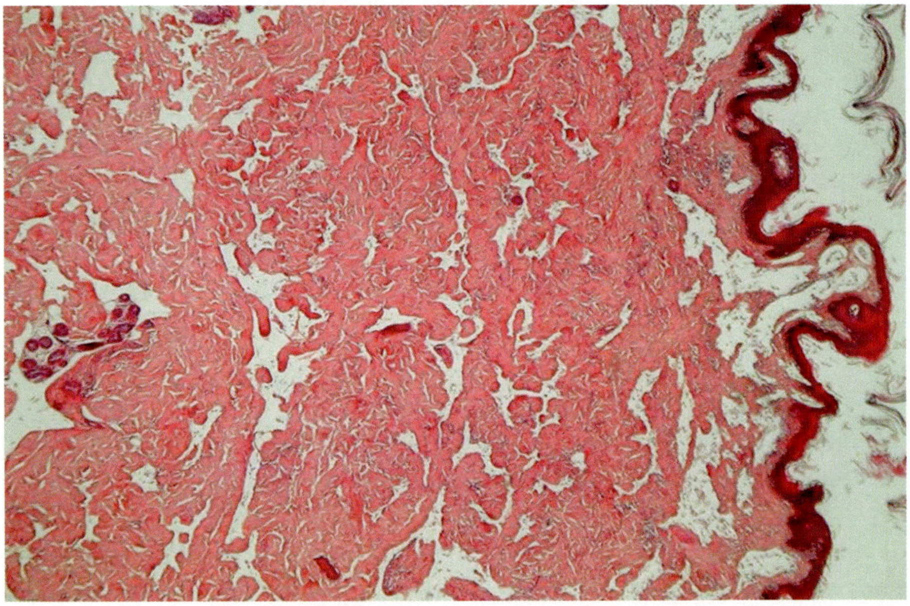

Specific Locations, Problems Created, Investigations, and Treatments

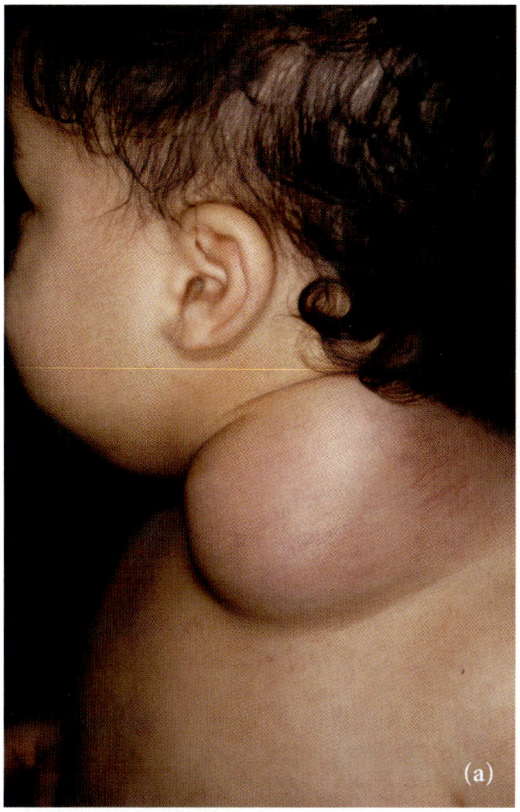

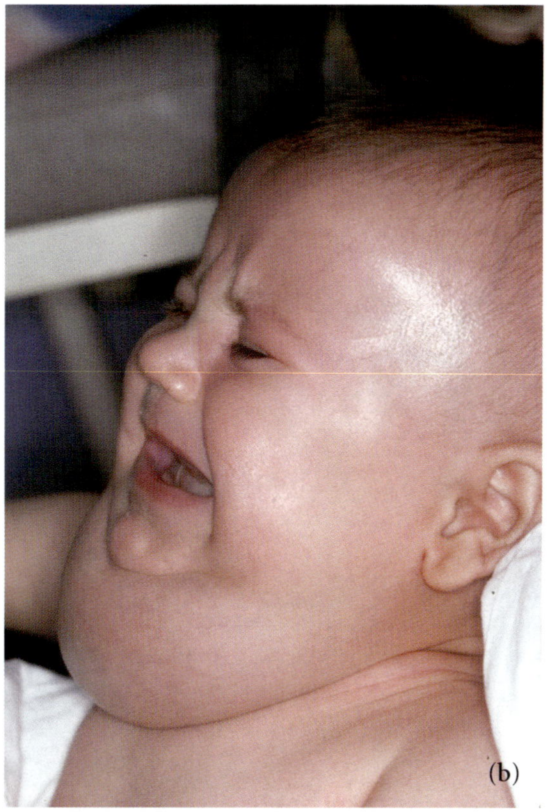

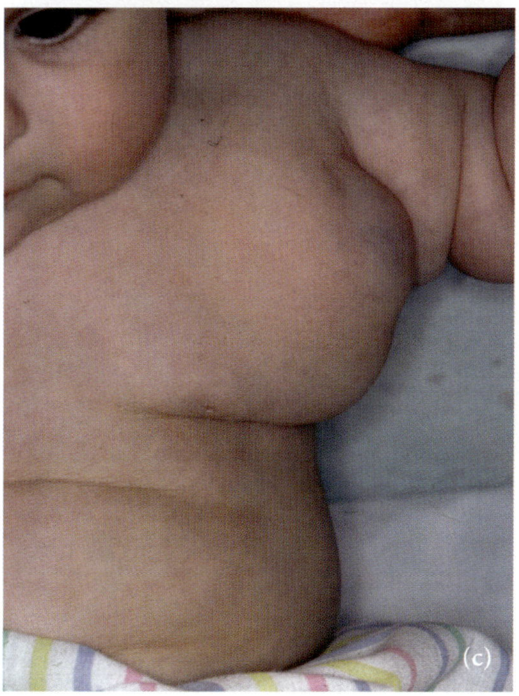

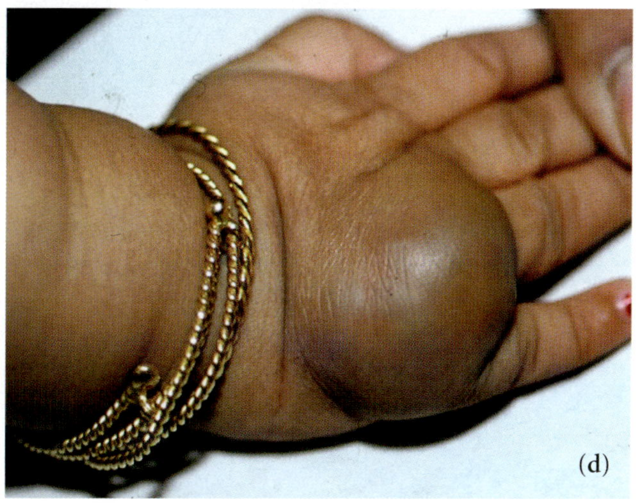

The most common location for a superficial macrocystic LM is the neck (a) (b) followed by the axillary region (c); limb lesions are less frequent (d).

Specific Locations, Problems Created, Investigations, and Treatments

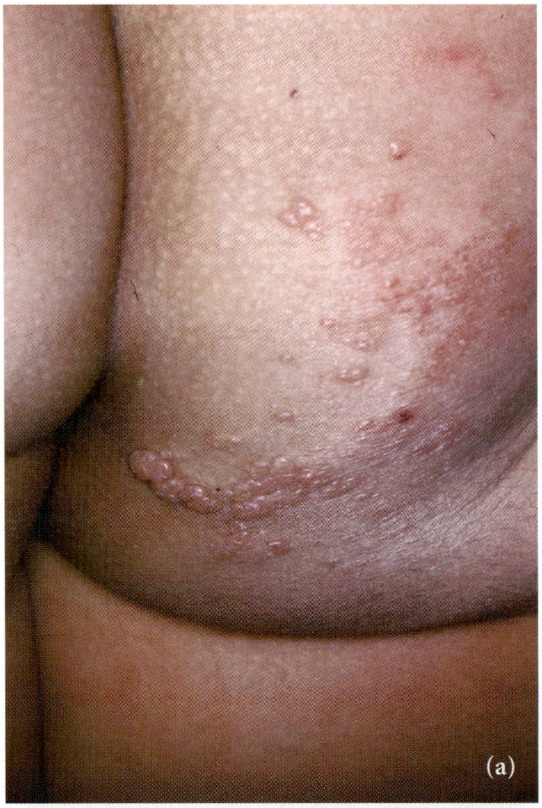

(a)

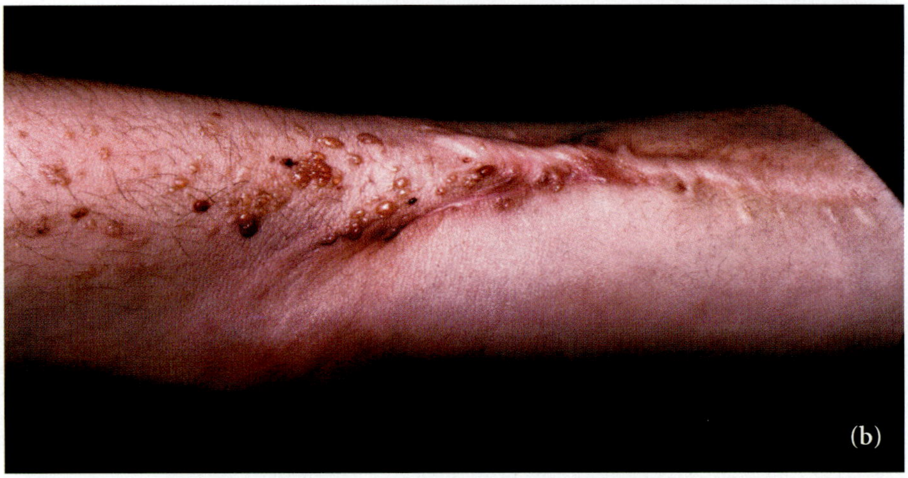

(b)

Microcystic LM consists of a collection of vesicles usually filled with clear colorless fluid (a), but periodically tinged with blood, giving them a color ranging from pink to dark red (b). An LM vesicle is a saccular dilatation bulging out from large dilated lymphatic vessels of the dermis and subcutis, occupying the dermal papilla and distending it, just beneath the epidermis. This explains why excision is often followed by recurrence, with new vesicles expanding along the scar (b).

Specific Locations, Problems Created, Investigations, and Treatments

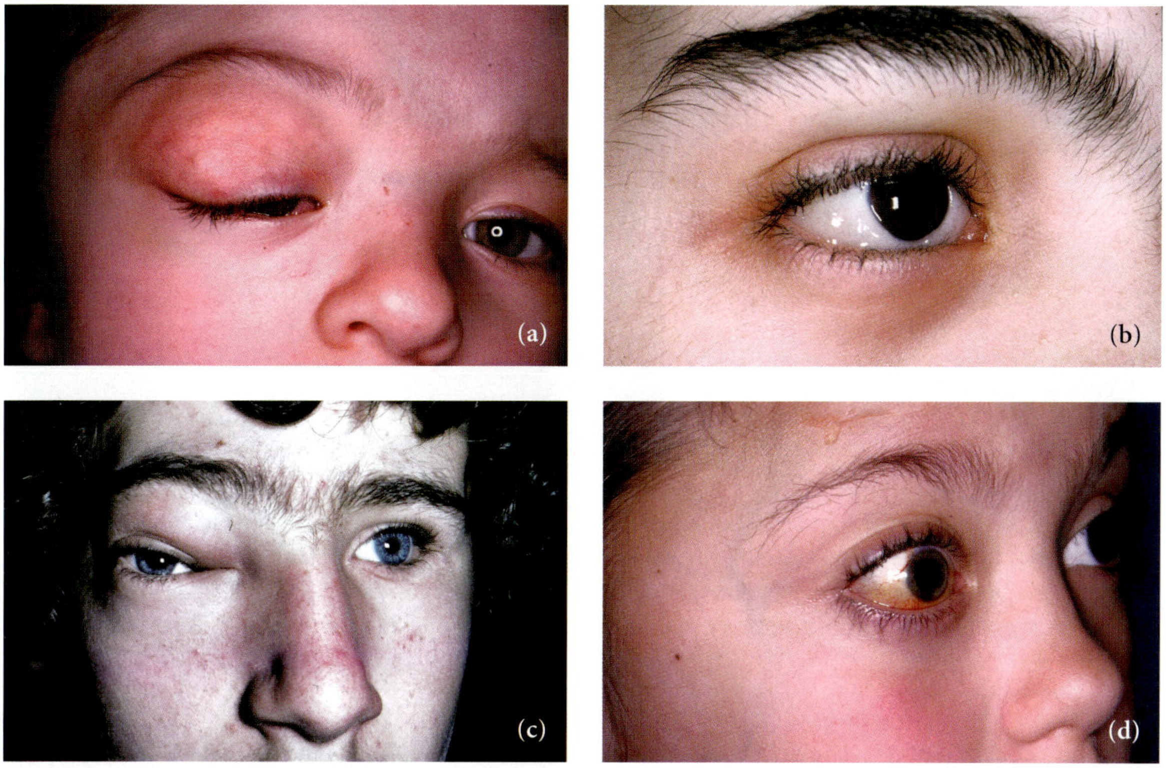

LM in the eyelid (a) creates soft tissue swelling with blepharoptosis and partial closure of the visual axis. Yellowish vesicles are sometimes noticed on the conjunctiva (b). Displacement of the eyeball, decreased ocular motility, diplopia, or strabismus happen frequently (c). Pain is a common complaint. Intraorbital and periorbital LMs produce exophthalmos (d), and they create various visual complications (functional amblyopia, refraction abnormalities, mainly astigmatism, strabismus, and even blindness).

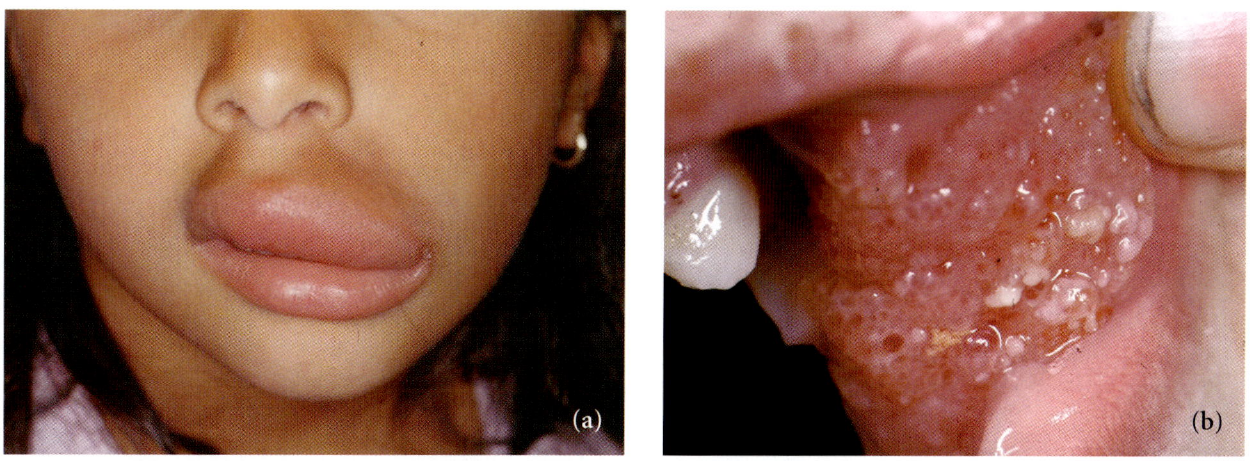

This microcystic LM of the lip creates a macrocheily; (a) on the mucosal aspect of the lip clear fluid-filled vesicles are present and they facilitate the diagnosis (b).

Specific Locations, Problems Created, Investigations, and Treatments

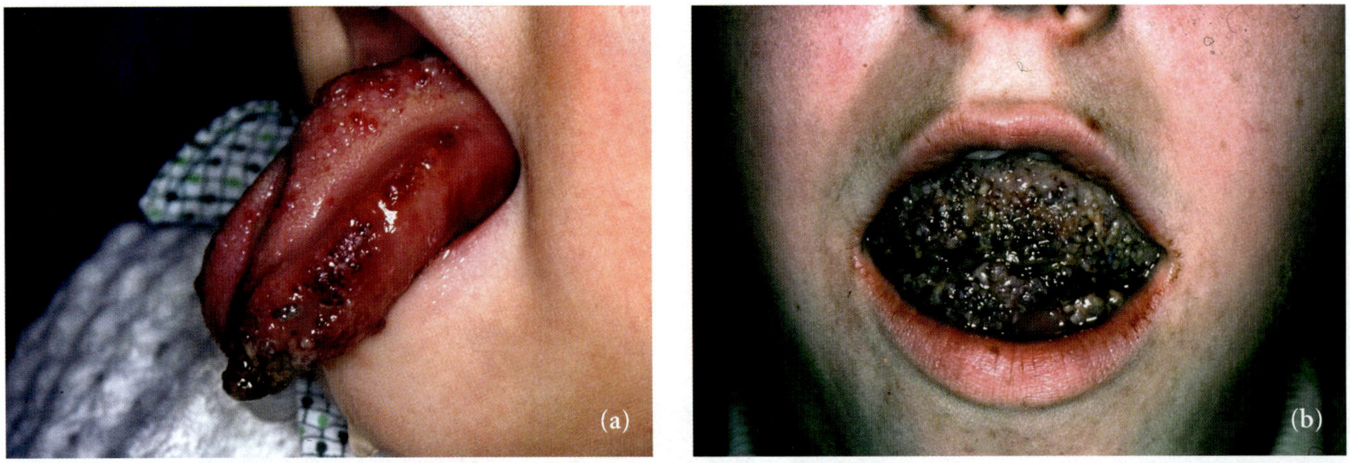

LM in the mouth area is frequently microcystic; vesicles are present on the tongue, and they frequently become hemorrhagic (a) and painful. Bulky LM of the tongue (b) impairs speech. Partial surgical resection of the anterior tongue limits its protraction. Patients with large LM of the tongue commonly experience episodes of infection and bleeding, with halitosis that has of psychological consequences. They also carry out aggressive caries with premature teeth loss. Hygiene of the mouth area is particularly important, even if it is difficult to carry out due to the fragility of the vesicles, ease of causing pain, and bleeding.

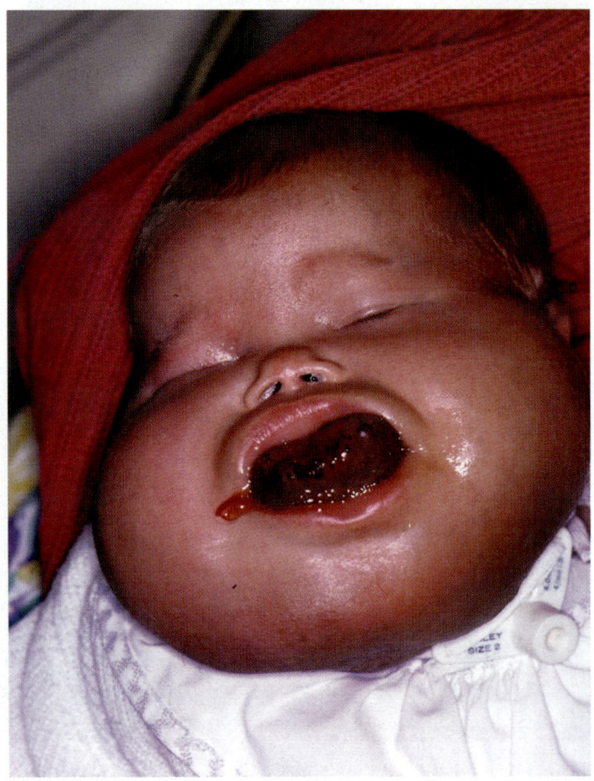

An infant with life-threatening LM of the face (cheeks, mouth, and neck) with swelling and hemorrhages of the tongue and respiratory distress (and the need for tracheotomy).

Specific Locations, Problems Created, Investigations, and Treatments

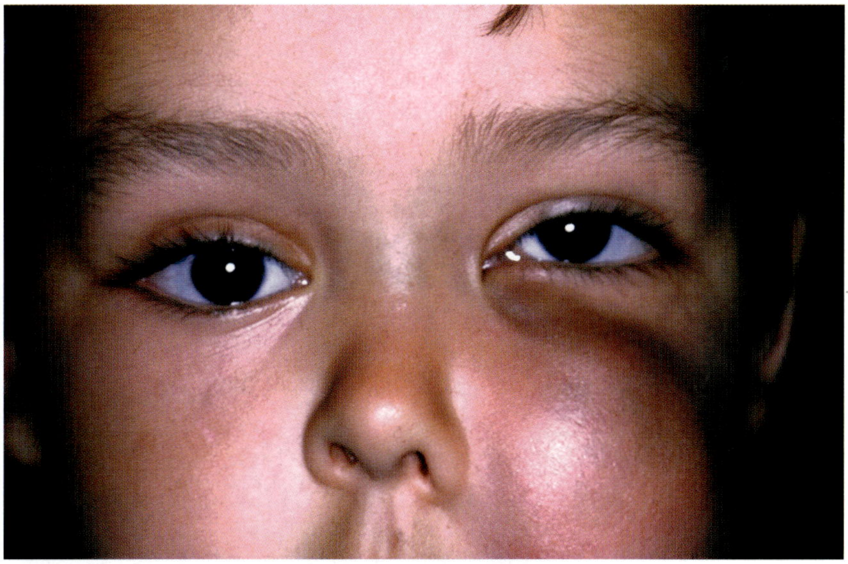

LM in the cheek is commonly both micro- and macrocystic causing asymmetry and distortion of facial features. Recurrent inflammation and swelling with bruising are regularly observed during the chronic course of the malformation.

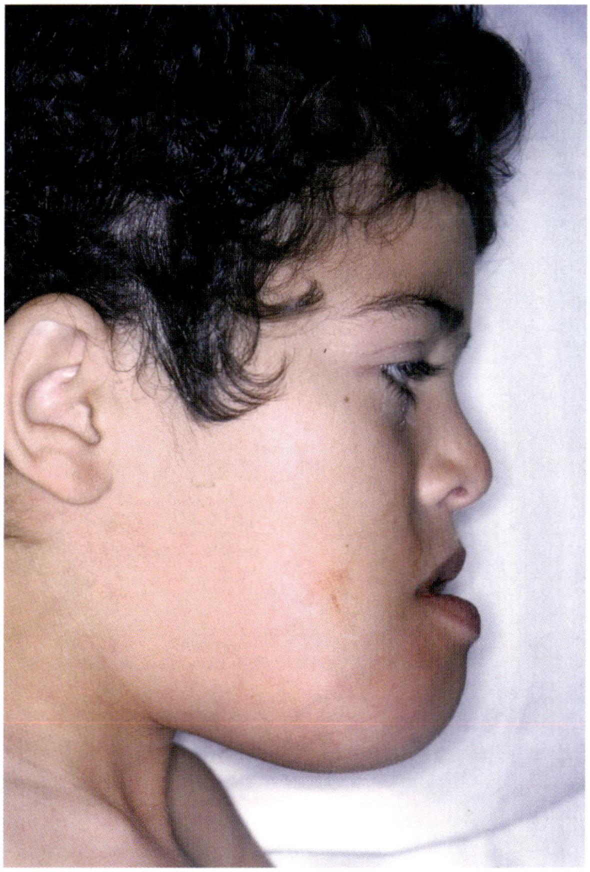

Bony overgrowth may occur in the mandible because the microcystic LM infiltrates the bone, enlarging it and creating a class III malocclusion. Not only enlargement but also distortion of the mandible occurs when the base of the tongue is involved in addition to the floor of the mouth and neck. Aggressive caries and loss of teeth impair feeding.

Specific Locations, Problems Created, Investigations, and Treatments

In the neck area, a diffuse LM creates airway obstruction, the most extensive cases necessitating tracheotomy on a lifelong basis (a, MRI showing the diffuse extent of a cervical and facial LM). LM in the trunk and axilla can invade the thorax (b), some of them encompassing recurrent pleural and pericardial effusion.

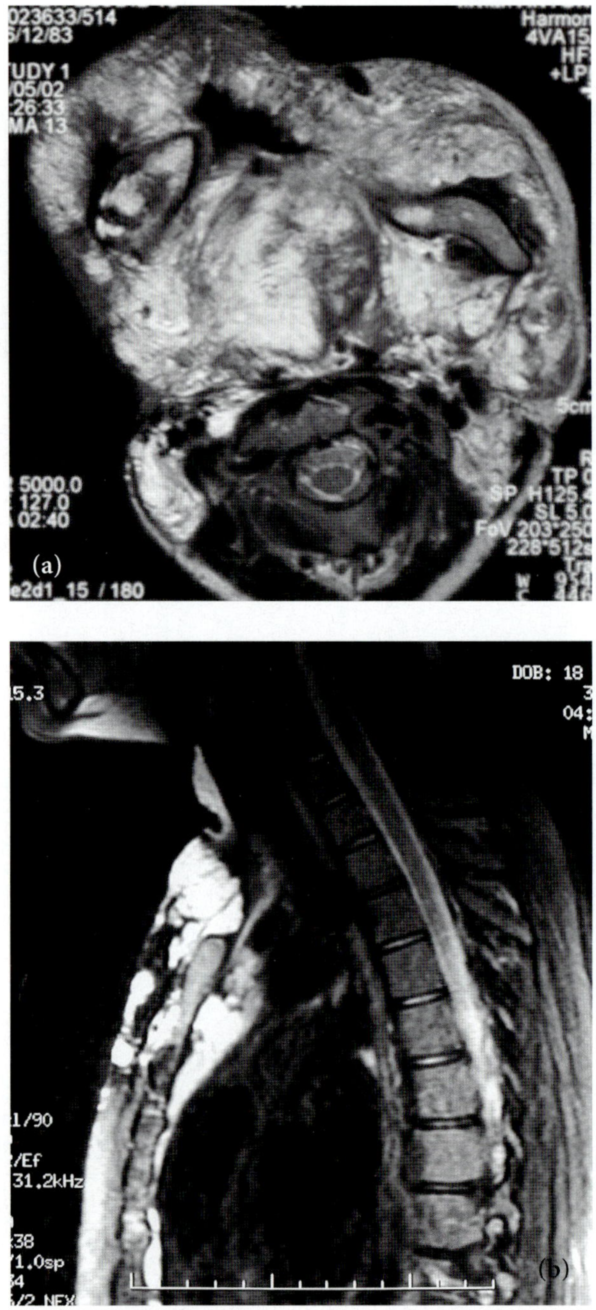

Specific Locations, Problems Created, Investigations, and Treatments

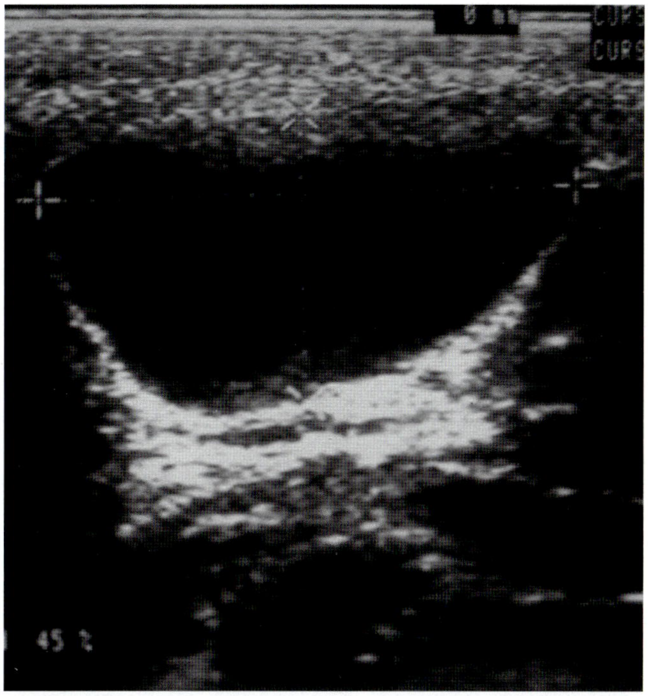

Ultrasonography (US) and US Doppler of a macrocystic LM show a multiloculated cystic mass with no flow; cysts are anechoic; fibrous septa split the liquid cavities. Microcystic LM will be heterogeneously hypoechoic with no flow, whatever the location, superficial or visceral.

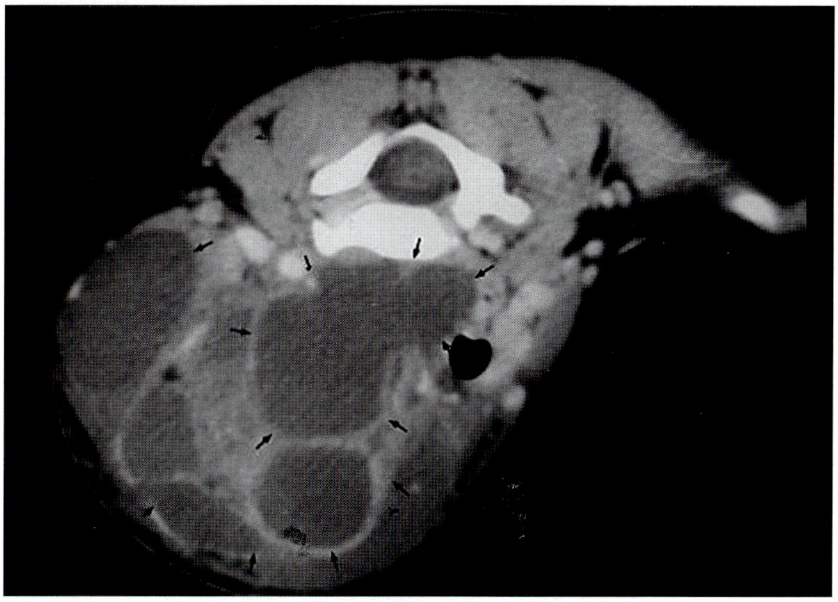

On CT cysts are hypodense and they are not enhanced after iodinated contrast injection.

Specific Locations, Problems Created, Investigations, and Treatments

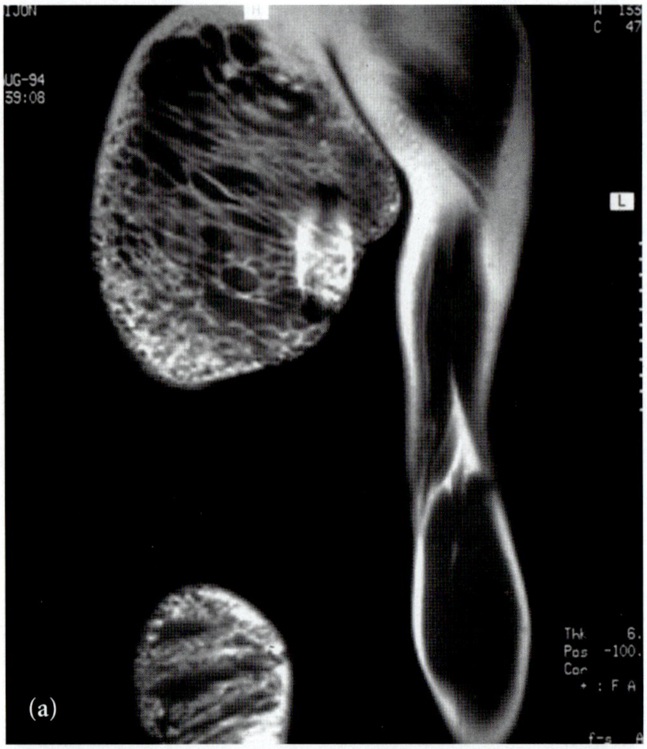

MRI is the most sensitive investigation (16). It shows a septated mass, cystic spaces being hypointense on SE T1-sequences ((a): LM in the thigh) and usually there is no gadolinium contrast enhancement. Cysts are of high signal intensity on SE T2-sequences with fat suppression ((b): LM in the upper neck).

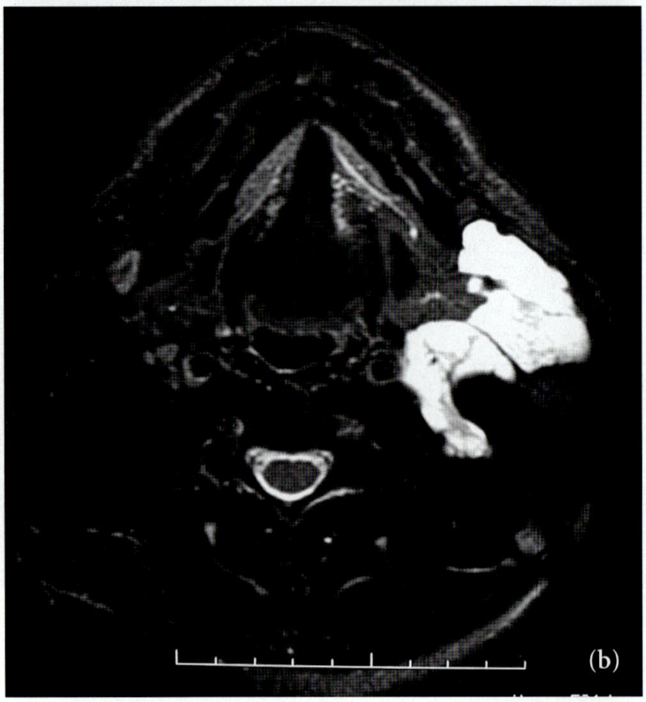

Specific Locations, Problems Created, Investigations, and Treatments

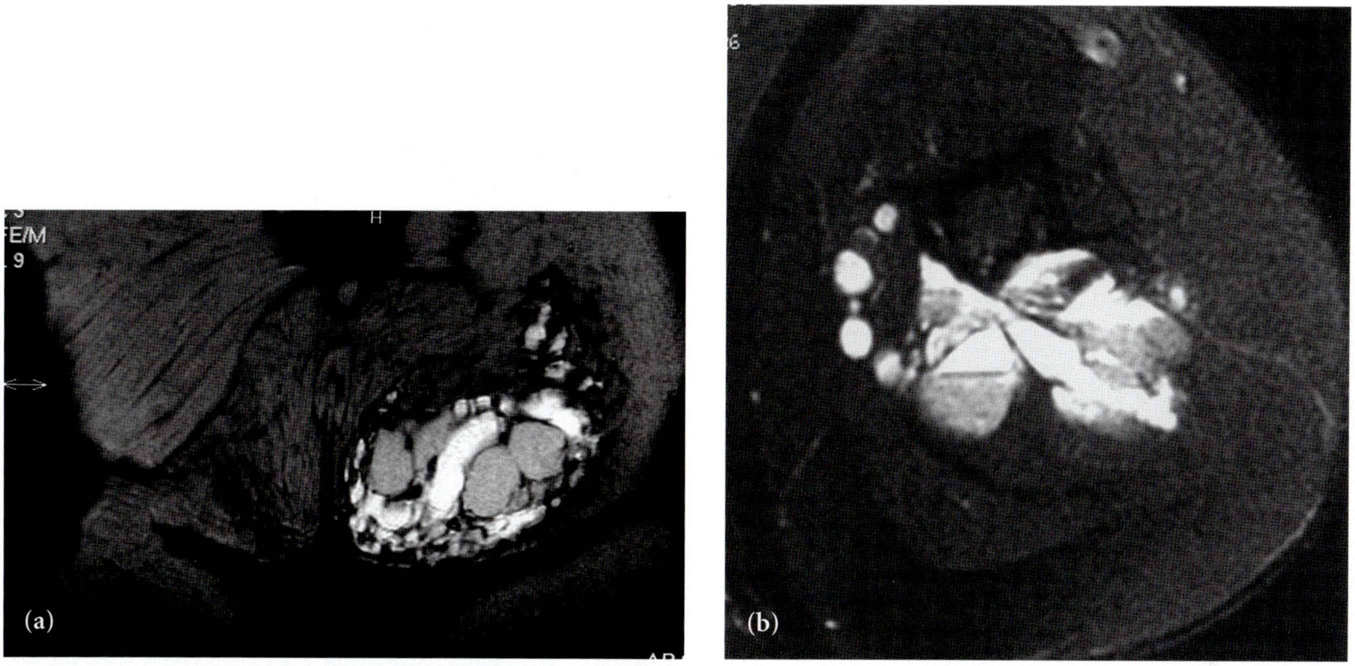

MRI may display variation in intensity of the signal (a) or fluid–fluid levels (b), particularly after intracystic bleeding (9, 12, 13).

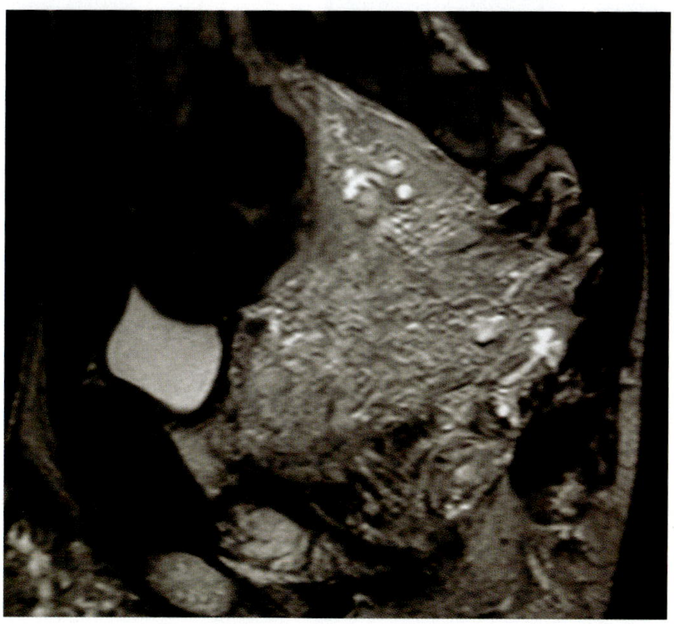

A microcystic LM is shown by MRI as a collection of hyperintense very small liquid cavities on T2: this pelvic LM is extremely invasive (courtesy of Dr. Metin Tovi, Karolinska Institute, Stockholm, Sweden).

Specific Locations, Problems Created, Investigations, and Treatments

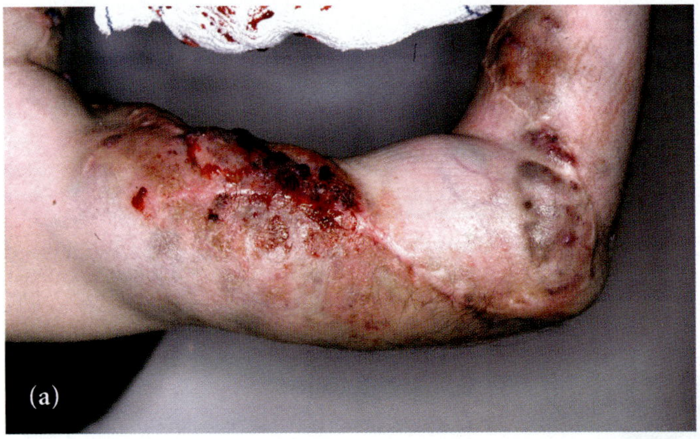

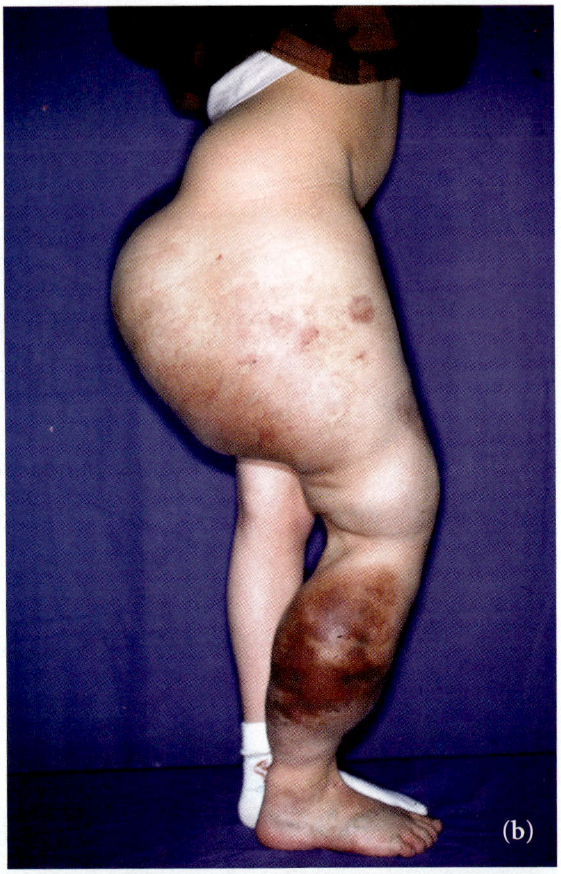

Chronic LIC, with hemorrhages, as seen in VM, also occurs in a number of patients with diffuse LM, particularly LM involving an entire extremity and internal organs. Oozing of skin vesicles and chronic lymphorrhea (a), or swelling and bruises (b) are observed. The patient with diffuse LM in limbs is at high risk of sepsis.

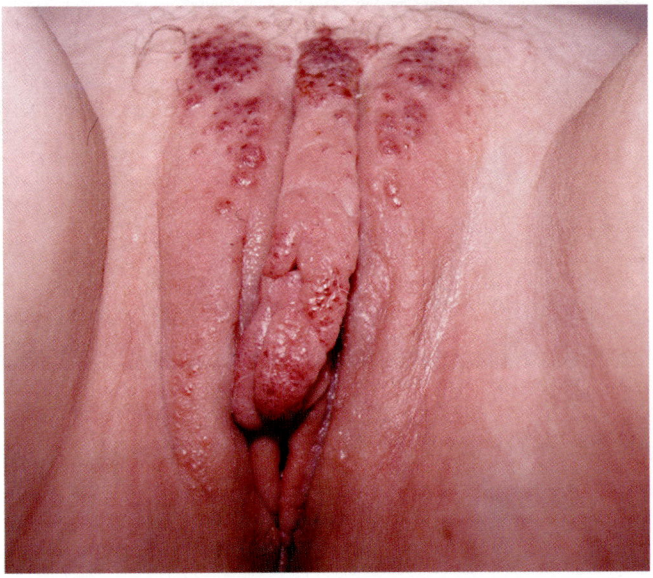

Pelvic LM sometimes manifests in females as vulvar lymphangiectasia and vaginal chylous discharge, even before puberty.

Specific Locations, Problems Created, Investigations, and Treatments

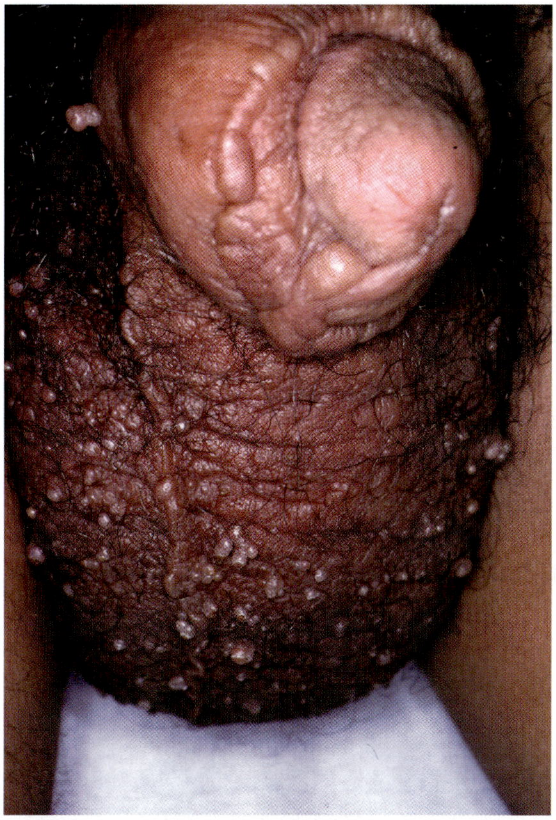

In males pelvic LM is revealed by scrotal and penis lymphedema with vesicles on top, or is discovered when an MR evaluation is performed because of abdominal pain.

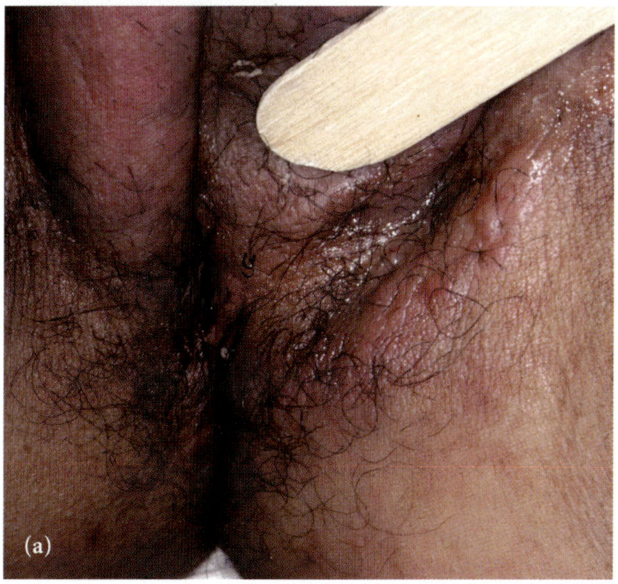

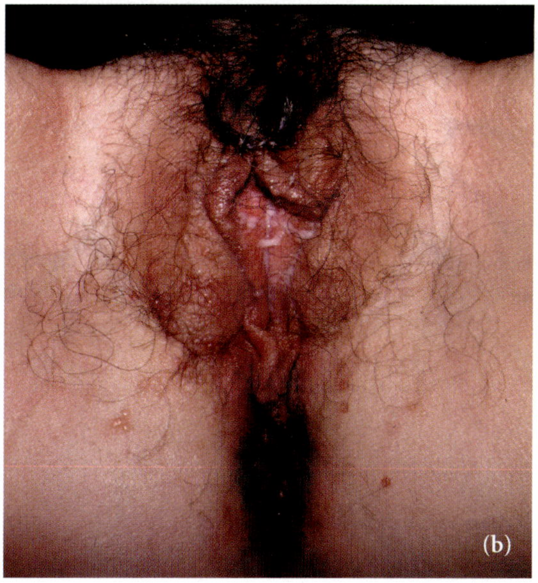

Lymphatic vesicles developing after acquired lymphatic obstruction secondary to radiotherapy for genital cancer (a), or lymphangiectasia occurring in the perineum of a female patient with Crohn disease (b) are indiscernible from microcystic vulvar LM (courtesy of Dr. M.Pelisse, Tarnier-Cochin Hospital, APHP Paris, France). And lymphatic vesicles resembling a congenital LM also develop on the lateral aspect of the thorax after mastectomy and radiotherapy for breast cancer (22).

Specific Locations, Problems Created, Investigations, and Treatments

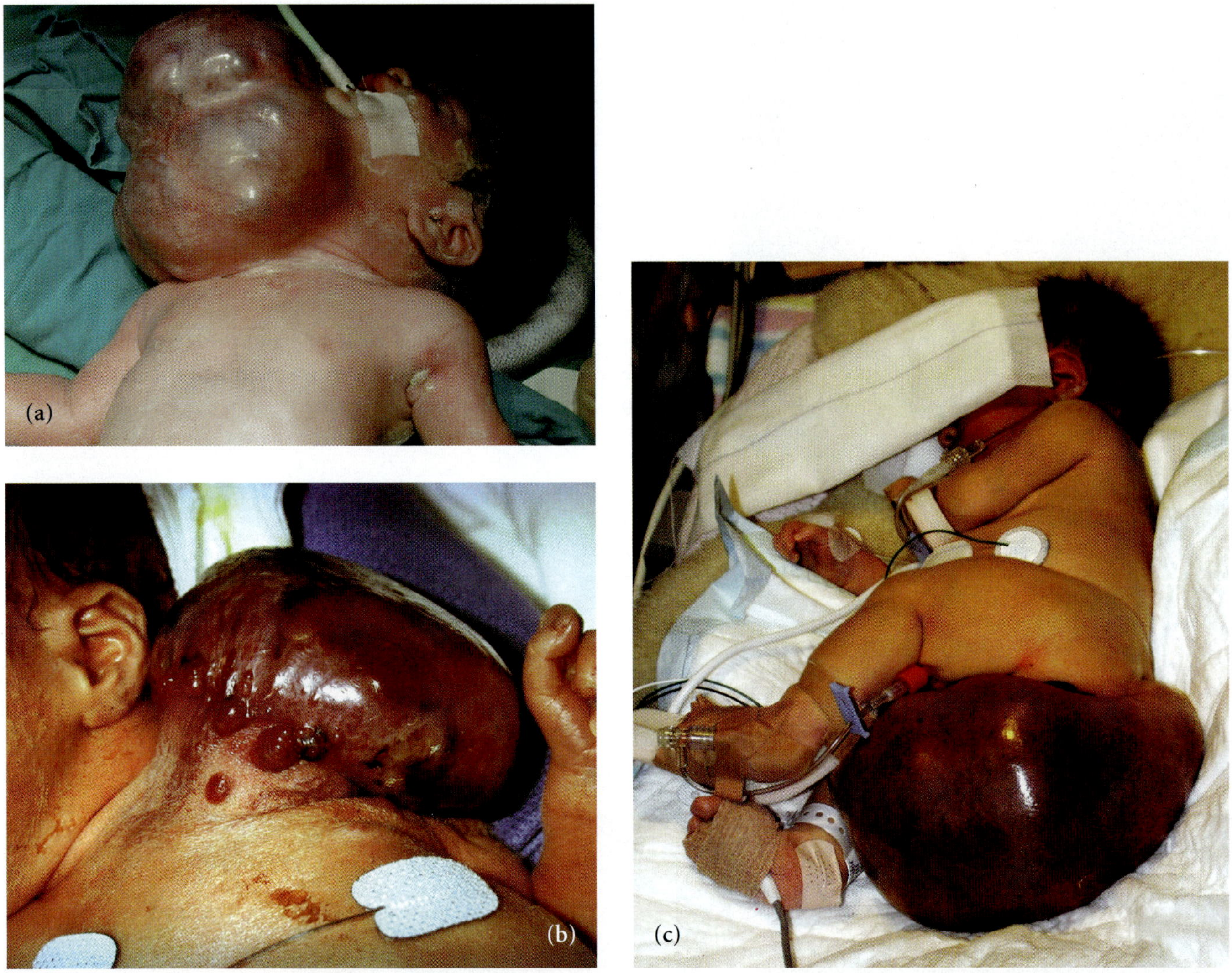

Macrocystic LM can present at birth with such large cysts that they are life-threatening. A compressive lesion was present in (a). Newborns with macrocystic LM in the neck area tend to have respiratory or feeding difficulties at birth (36). Hemorrhages can modify the appearance (b, c) and they result both from the obstetrical trauma and a neonatal consumption coagulopathy: these two lesions were resected with good outcome ((c) courtesy of Professor Maureen Rogers, Westmead Hospital, Sydney, Australia) ((b) courtesy of Dr. Metin Tovi, Karolinska Institute, Stockholm, Sweden).

Specific Locations, Problems Created, Investigations, and Treatments

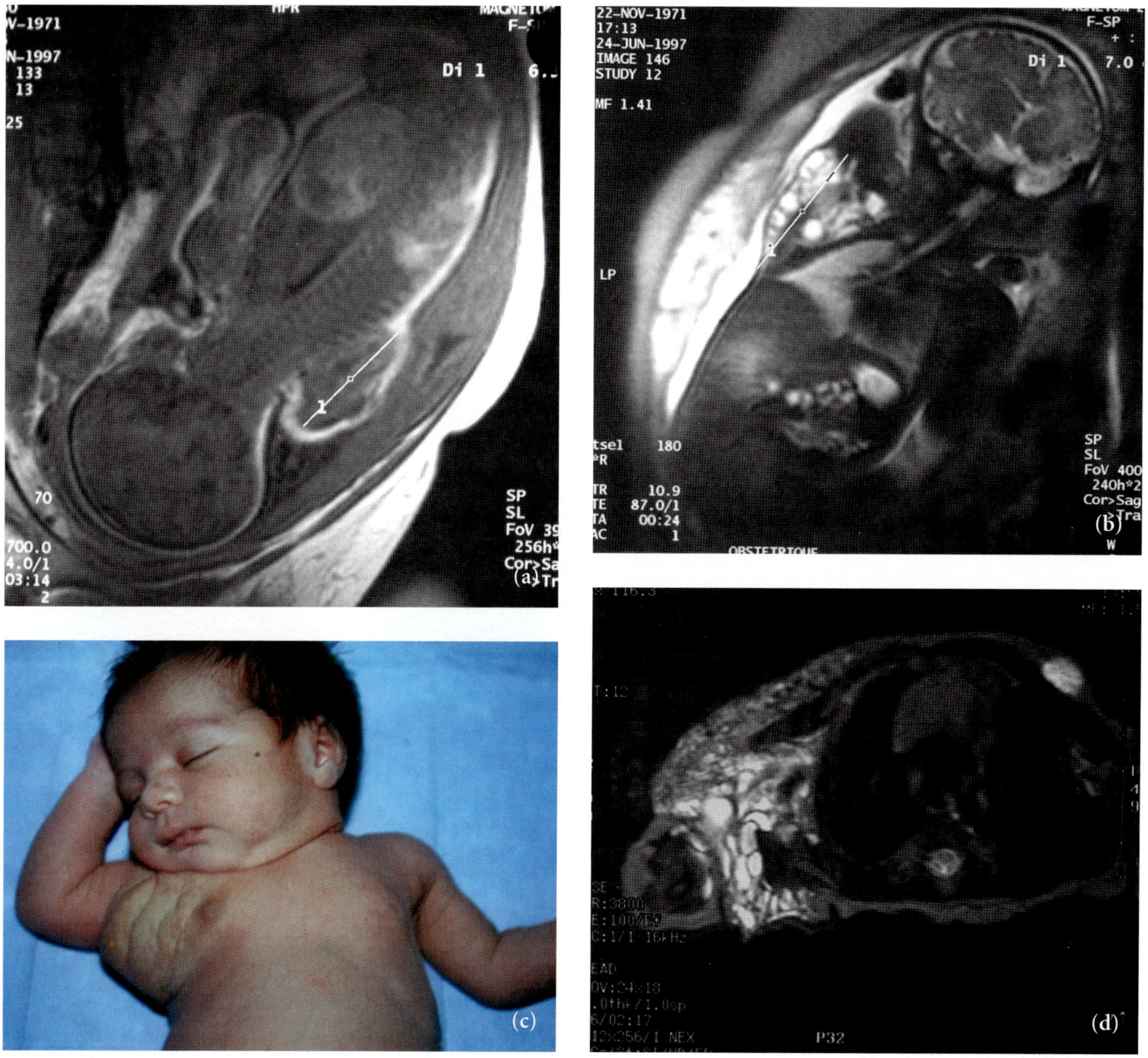

MRI performed in the third trimester of pregnancy provides prenatal complementary images of a cystic lymphatic malformation detected by US usually before the sixth month of the pregnancy. It allows the obstetrician to choose the best delivery technique and to plan neonatal management (30, 36). In this case prenatal MRI showed the large LM, both micro- and macrocystic, in the axilla (a, b), and the postnatal MRI of the truncal lesion (c) gave similar results (d).

Specific Locations, Problems Created, Investigations, and Treatments

Orbital LM either of intraconal and/or extraconal components, can have associated intracranial anomalies such as developmental venous anomalies (DVA) (23).

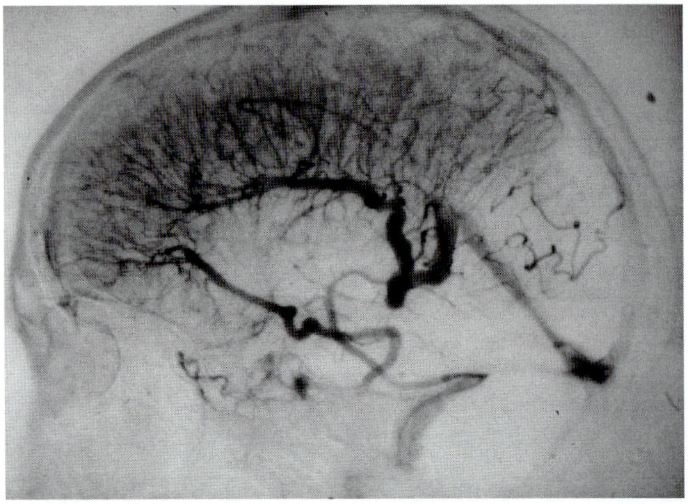

Dural arteriovenous malformation (with visual consequences as in this patient), cerebral cavernous malformation, or cerebral atrophy can occur in association with orbital LM (5).

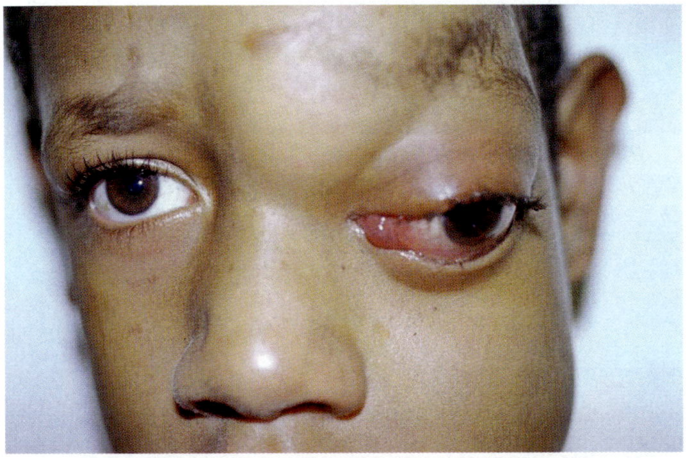

Benign lymphangioendothelioma is a rare benign vascular anomaly: a brownish or reddish skin patch appears on the extremities, trunk, or face. Intermittent bruising is possible and this child was referred to us with a suspicion of child abuse. The anastomosing dilated vascular structures in the dermis are considered to be different from classic microcystic LM (17).

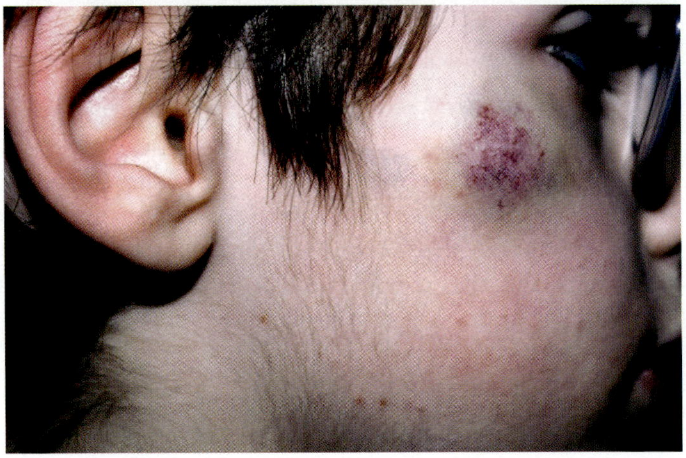

Specific Locations, Problems Created, Investigations, and Treatments

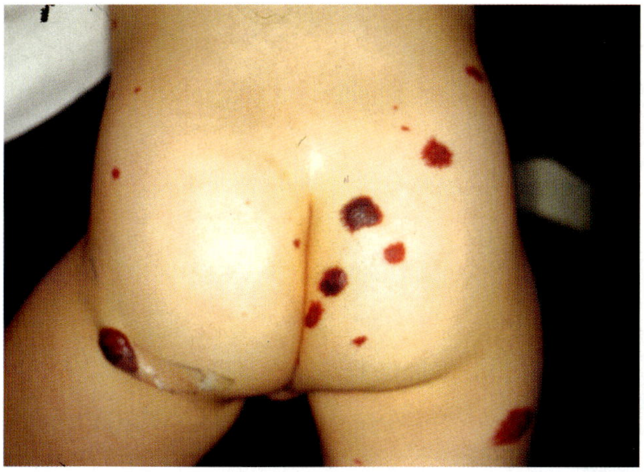

Multifocal lymphangioendotheliomatosis was identified in patients with unusual cutaneous and gastrointestinal tract vascular anomalies associated with thrombocytopenia (28). Multiple lesions, measuring between millimeters to several centimeters, were scattered over the skin, and of a bright red to burgundy color; they were made of dilated thin-walled vessels, lined by slightly hobnailed endothelial cells, and displaying intraluminal finger-like or tufted papillary projections; they stained for CD31 and for the lymphatic endothelial cell marker LYVE-1.

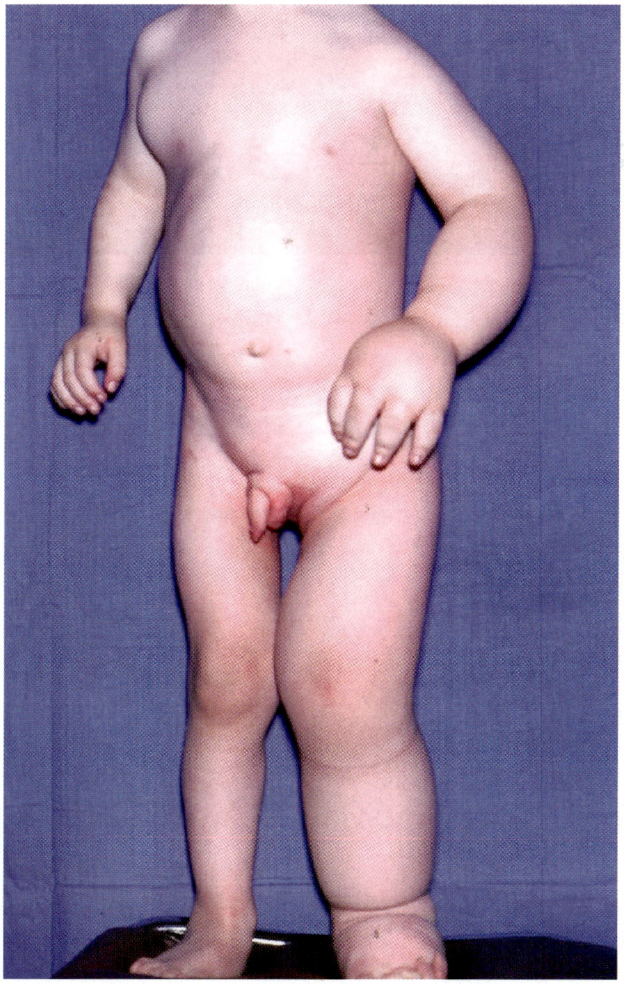

Lymphedema creating chronic swelling of the extremities is primary or secondary to a pathologic event. The most severe cases create limb elephantiasis with warty changes in the toes. Because bacterial infection easily propagates through the stagnant and malformed lymphatic system; erysipelas and lymphangitis recur and progressively worsen the local situation. Specific attention should be given to care and hygiene of the feet as well as disinfection of any wound in the area of the LM. Massage, lymphatic manual drainage, and adapted elastic garments are indispensable. Syndromic LM is either hereditary or sporadic. This child had combined lymphedema of the arm and leg on the left and macrocystic LM in the right axilla.

Specific Locations, Problems Created, Investigations, and Treatments

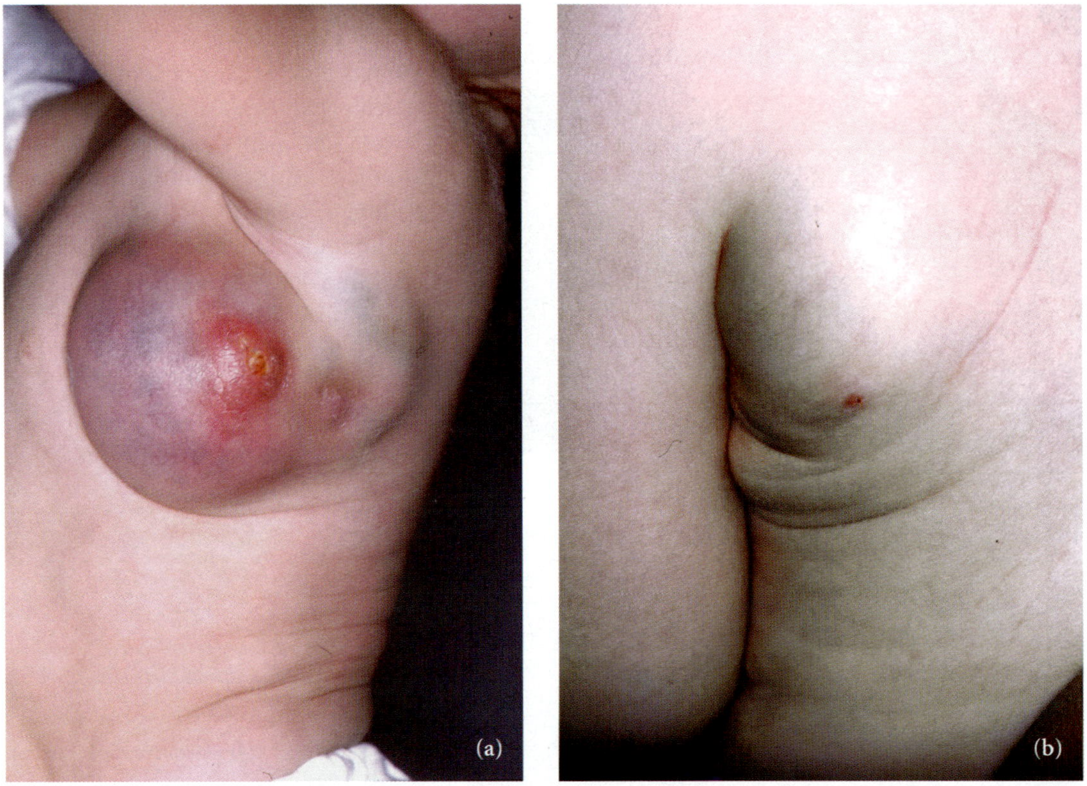

Sclerotherapy gives good results in more than half of the cases. Several sessions are usually required (16). A number of sclerosing substances have been used to create inflammation with subsequent shrinkage and fibrosis of the cysts, including doxycycline (27), Ethibloc®, ethanol, cyclophosphamide (39), bleomycin, dextrose, sodium morrhuate, sodium tetradecyl sulfate, and OK-432, a killed strain of group A *Streptococcus pyogenes* also known as Picibanil® (6, 29).

Ethibloc® is an alcoholic solution of zein: for Riché et al. (35) 8 out of 10 patients had excellent results; Martinot et al. (26) had excellent results in 12 out of 20 patients; for Dubois et al. (12) regression was excellent in 64% of 14 patients; and for Tovi et al. (37) regression was excellent in 57% of 52 patients. This sclerosant creates a local abscess and discharge in about 10% of patients with sometimes a need for incision and drainage, but the final scar is often negligible (19).

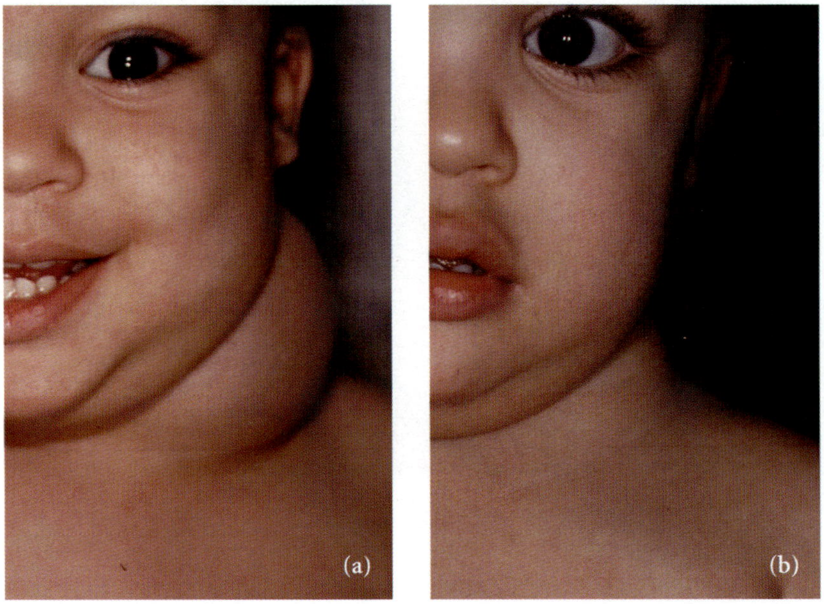

Specific Locations, Problems Created, Investigations, and Treatments

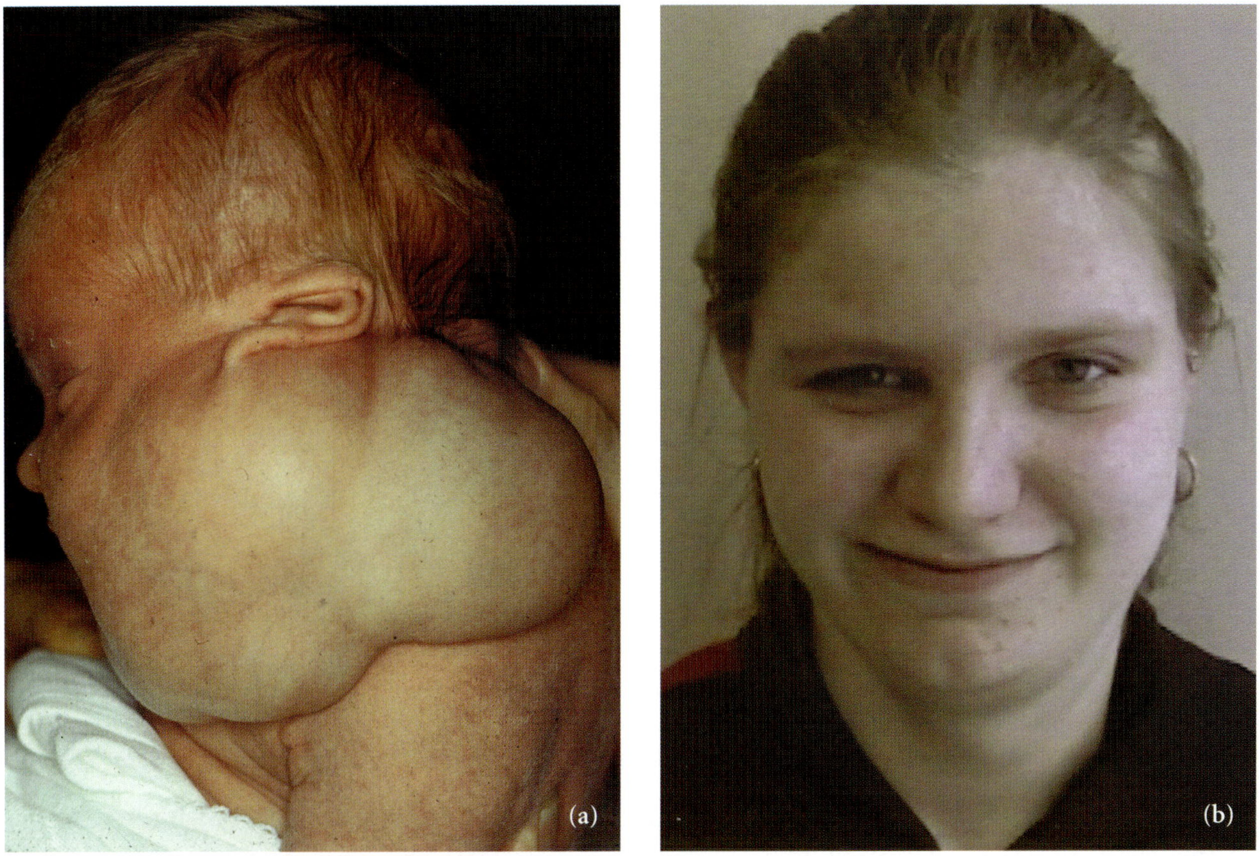

This huge cervical macrocystic LM (a) was diagnosed by prenatal US. After birth the first treatment option was sclerotherapy using Ethibloc®. The first procedure was performed at 1 month and five injections were carried out during the first year of life; she then had five additional procedures between 1 and 6 years. She had very good, long-standing improvement, as shown in picture (b) at 15 years of age (courtesy of Dr. GM Brevière, Hôpital Cardiologique, Lille, France).

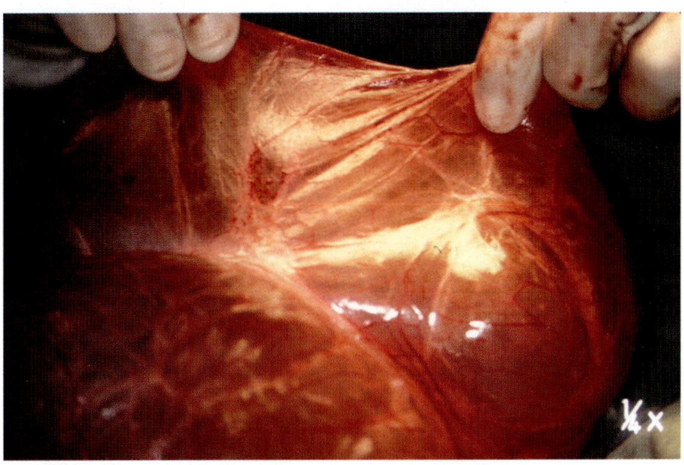

Per-operative view of a bulky macrocystic LM of the neck during surgical dissection (operator: Professor MP Vazquez, Hôpital Armand Trousseau, APHP, Paris, France).

Specific Locations, Problems Created, Investigations, and Treatments

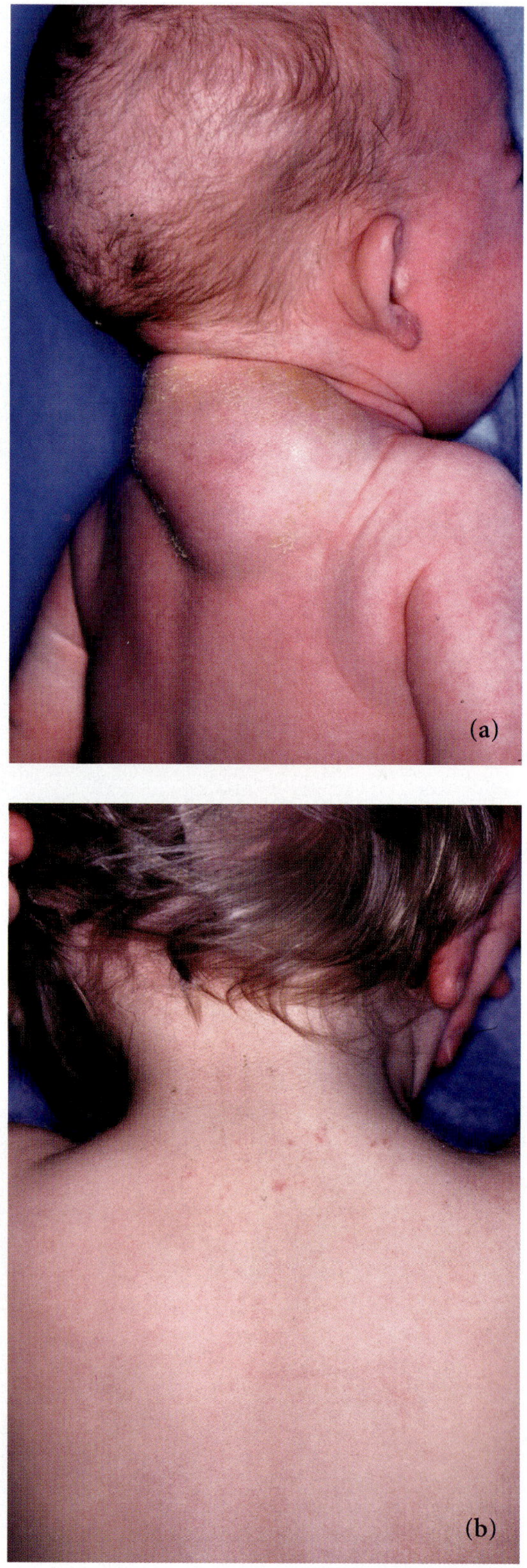

Rare example of spontaneous shrinking and cure of a congenital macrocystic LM of the nape of the neck, after spontaneous infection (courtesy of Professor MP Vazquez, Hôpital Armand Trousseau, APHP, Paris, France). Knowing of this rare observation, Ogita was the first to use killed bacteria as a "sclerosant" for LM (OK 432, later known as Picibanil®) (29), a pro-inflammatory injection helped secondary fibrosis and shrinking of the treated cysts.

Specific Locations, Problems Created, Investigations, and Treatments

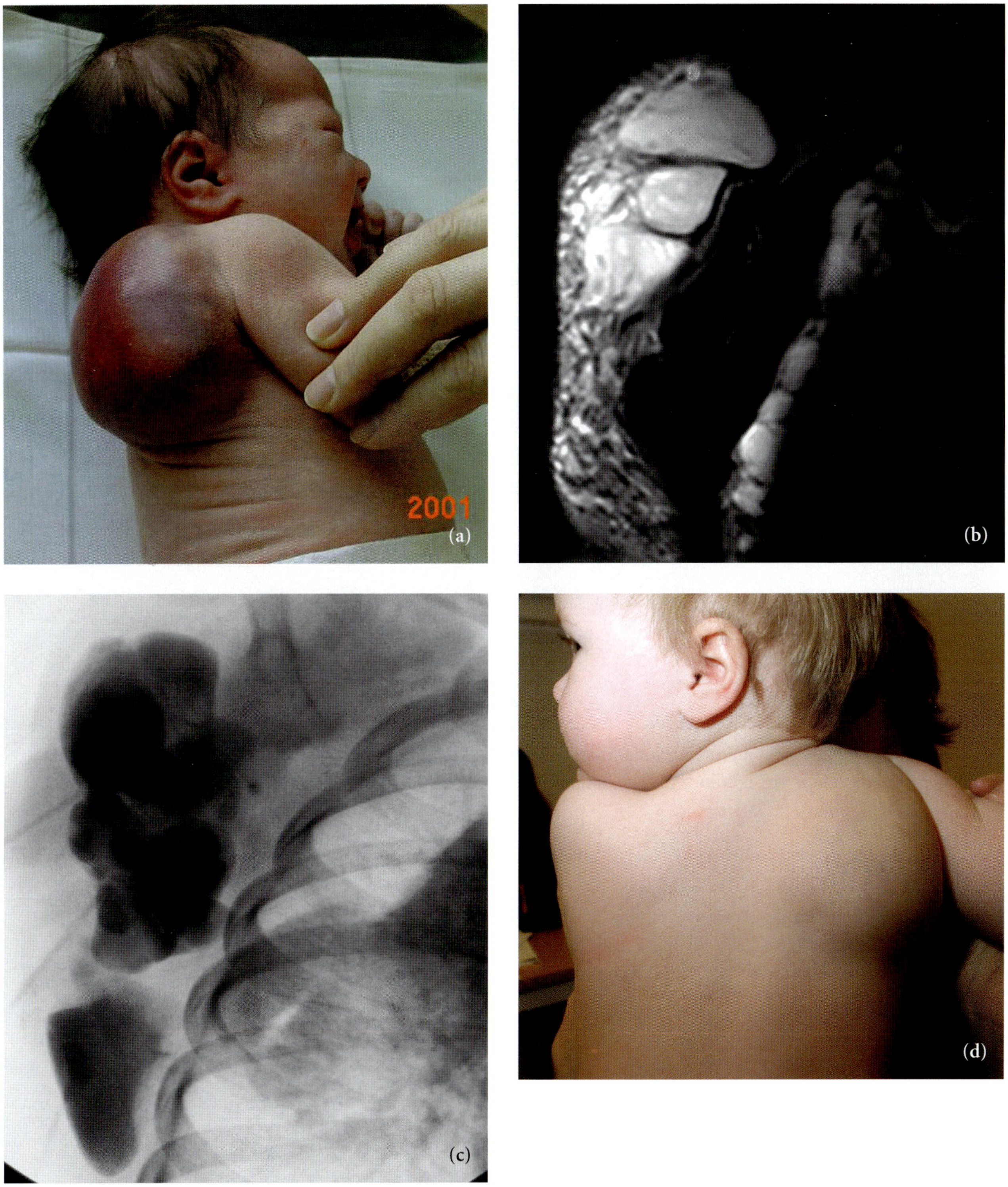

This newborn (a) had a large hemorrhagic mass at birth; MRI, T2-weighted sequence demonstrated large lymphatic cysts (b) and direct-puncture sclerotherapy was performed (c) with improvement (d) after two sessions over a year (courtesy: Dr. Metin Tovi, Karolinska Institute, Stockholm, Sweden).

Specific Locations, Problems Created, Investigations, and Treatments

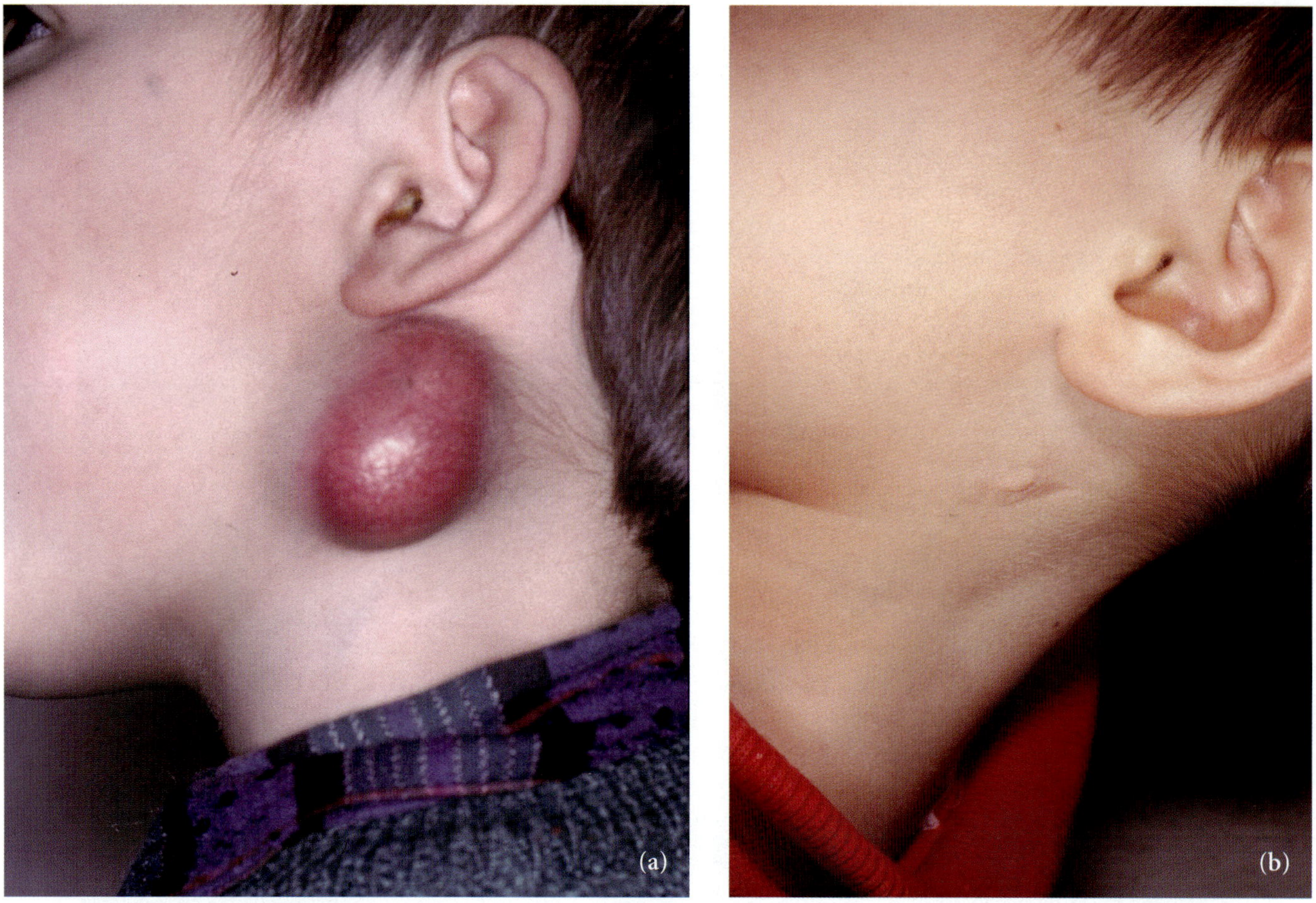

Ethibloc® sclerotherapy of LM gives an intense inflammatory reaction (a) with sometimes the need for incision and drainage, but in most cases the final scar (b) is minor and the clinical outcome is good.

References

1 Aagenaes O. Hereditary cholestasis with lymphoedema (Aagenaes syndrome, cholestasis–lymphoedema syndrome). New cases and follow-up from infancy to adult age. *Scand J Gastroenterol* 1998; **33**: 335–45.

2 Alqahtani A, Nguyen LT, Flageole H, Shaw K, Laberge JM. 25 years' experience with lymphangiomas in children. *J Pediatr Surg* 1999; **34**: 1164–8.

3 Angel B, Hersh JH. Expansion of the phenotype in Hennekam syndrome: a case with new manifestations. *Am J Med Genet* 1997; **71**: 211–14.

4 Azizkhan RG, Rutter MJ, Cohen A, Mason J, Lim L, Cotton RT. Lymphatic malformation of the tongue base: management and long-term outcome. Communication W21 in 15th ISSVA Workshop. Wellington, NZ. 22–25 February 2004.

5 Bisdorff A, Burrows P, Carrico J, Robertson R, Mulliken JB. Intracranial vascular anomalies in patients with fronto-orbital lymphatic malformation. Communiaction in 15th ISSVA Workshop. Wellington, NZ. 22–25 February 2004.

6 Brewis C, Pracy JP, Albert DM. Treatment of lymphangiomas of the head and neck in children by intralesional injection of OK-432 (Picibanil). *Clin Otolaryngol Allied Sci* 2000; **25**: 130–4.

7 Brouillard P, Vikkula M. Vascular malformations: localized defects in vascular morphogenesis. *Clin Genet* 2003; **63**: 340–51.

8 Bull LN, Roche E, Song EJ, Pedersen J, Knisely AS, van Der Hagen CB et al. Mapping of the locus for cholestasis-lymphedema syndrome (Aagenaes syndrome) to a 6.6-cM interval on chromosome 15q. *Am J Hum Genet* 2000; **67**: 994–9.

9 Burrows PE, Laor T, Paltiel H, Robertson RL. Diagnostic imaging in the evaluation of vascular birthmarks. *Dermatol Clin* 1998; **16**: 455–88.

10 Chen CP, Chen HC, Liu FF, Jan SW, Lin SP, Sheu JC et al. Progressive fetal axillary cystic lymphangioma with coexistent naevus flammeus. *Br J Dermatol* 1997; **136**: 102–4.

11 Davies D, Rogers M. Morphology of lymphatic malformations: a pictorial review. *Australas J Dermatol* 2000; **41**: 1–5.; quiz 6–7

12 Dubois J, Garel L, Abela A, Laberge L, Yazbeck S. Lymphangiomas in children: percutaneous sclerotherapy with an alcoholic solution of zein. *Radiology* 1997; **204**: 651–4.

13 Dubois J, Garel L, Grignon A, David M, Laberge L, Filiatrault D et al. Imaging of hemangiomas and vascular malformations in children. *Acad Radiol* 1998; **5**: 390–400.

14 Gimeno Aranguez M, Colomar Palmer P, Gonzalez Mediero I, Ollero Caprani JM. The clinical and morphological aspects of childhood lymphangiomas: a review of 145 cases. *An Esp Pediatr* 1996; **45**: 25–8.

15 Gomez CS, Calonje E, Ferrar DW, Browse NL, Fletcher CD. Lymphangiomatosis of the limbs. Clinicopathologic analysis of a series with a good prognosis. *Am J Surg Pathol* 1995; **19**: 125–33.

16 Greene AK, Burrows PE, Smith L, Mulliken JB. Periorbital lymphatic malformation: clinical course and management in 42 patients. *Plast Reconstr Surg* 2005; **115**: 22–30.

17 Guillou L, Fletcher CD. Benign lymphangioendothelioma (acquired progressive lymphangioma): a lesion not to be confused with well-differentiated angiosarcoma and patch stage Kaposi's sarcoma: clinicopathologic analysis of a series. *Am J Surg Pathol* 2000; **24**: 1047–57.

18 Hennekam RC, Geerdink RA, Hamel BC, Hennekam FA, Kraus P, Rammeloo JA et al. Autosomal recessive intestinal lymphangiectasia and lymphedema, with facial anomalies and mental retardation. *Am J Med Genet* 1989; **34**: 593–600.

19 Herbreteau D, Riche MC, Enjolras O, Lemarchand F, Brette MD, Laurian C et al. Cystic lymphatic malformations and their treatment. *J Mal Vasc* 1992; **17**: 54–6.

20 Hirayama T, Sabokbar A, Itonaga I, Watt-Smith S, Athanasou NA. Cellular and humoral mechanisms of osteoclast formation and bone resorption in Gorham–Stout disease. *J Pathol* 2001; **195**: 624–30.

21 Irrthum A, Karkkainen MJ, Devriendt K, Alitalo K, Vikkula M. Congenital hereditary lymphedema caused by a mutation that inactivates VEGFR3 tyrosine kinase. *Am J Hum Genet* 2000; **67**: 295–301.

22 Jappe U, Zimmermann T, Kahle B, Petzoldt D. Lymphangioma circumscriptum of the vulva following surgical and radiological therapy of cervical cancer. *Sex Transm Dis* 2002; **29**: 533–5.

23 Katz SE, Rootman J, Vangveeravong S, Graeb D. Combined venous lymphatic malformations of the orbit (so-called lymphangiomas). Association with noncontiguous intracranial vascular anomalies. *Ophthalmology* 1998; **105**: 176–84.

24 Lowenstein EJ, Kim KH, Glick SA. Turner's syndrome in dermatology. *J Am Acad Dermatol* 2004; **50**: 767–76.

25 MacLean JE, Cohen E, Weinstein M. Primary intestinal and thoracic lymphangiectasia: a response to antiplasmin therapy. *Pediatrics* 2002; **109**: 1177–80.

26 Martinot V, Descamps S, Fevrier P, Patenotre P, Breviere JM, Piette F et al. Evaluation of the treatment of cystic lymphangioma by percutaneous injection of Ethibloc in 20 patients. *Arch Pediatr* 1997; **4**: 8–14.

27 Molitch HI, Unger EC, Witte CL, vanSonnenberg E. Percutaneous sclerotherapy of lymphangiomas. *Radiology* 1995; **194**: 343–7.

28 North PE, Kahn T, Cordisco MR, Dadras SS, Detmar M, Frieden IJ. Multifocal lymphangioendotheliomatosis with thrombocytopenia: a newly recognized clinicopathological entity. *Arch Dermatol* 2004; **140**: 599–606.

29 Ogita S, Tsuto T, Deguchi E, Tokiwa K, Nagashima M, Iwai N. OK-432 therapy for unresectable lymphangiomas in children. *J Pediatr Surg* 1991; **26**: 263–8; discussion 268–70

30 Ogura T, Hamada H, Obata-Yasuoka M, Watanabe H, Okuno S, Fujiki Y et al. Antepartum assessment of fetal cystic lymphangioma by magnetic resonance imaging. *Gynecol Obstet Invest* 2002; **53**: 237–9.

31 Padwa BL, Hayward PG, Ferraro NF, Mulliken JB. Cervicofacial lymphatic malformation: clinical course, surgical intervention, and pathogenesis of skeletal hypertrophy. *Plast Reconstr Surg* 1995; **95**: 951–60.

32 Paradies G, Leggio S, Leggio A. The treatment of lymphangioma. Surgery versus sclerotherapy. *Eur J Pediat Dermatol* 2001; **11**: 23–8.

33 Puig S, Aref H, Brunelle F. Double-needle sclerotherapy of lymphangiomas and venous angiomas in children: a simple technique to prevent complications. *Am J Roentgenol* 2003; **180**: 1399–401.

34 Rafii S, Skobe M. Splitting vessels: keeping lymph apart from blood. *Nat Med* 2003; **9**: 166–8.

35 Riche MC, Lemarchand-Venencie F, Enjolras O, Hadjean E, Merland JJ, Laurian C. Nonsurgical treatment of cystic lymphangioma. *Ann Otolaryngol Chir Cervicofac* 1986; **103**: 67–70.

36 Tanriverdi HA, Hendrik HJ, Ertan AK, Axt R, Schmidt W. Hygroma colli cysticum: prenatal diagnosis and prognosis. *Am J Perinatol* 2001; **18**: 415–20.

37 Tovi M, Herbreteau D, Enjolras O, Merland JJ. 52 patients with cystic lymphatic vascular malformations. Percutaneous sclerotherapy – simple, fast and repeatable. *Lakartidningen* 1998; **95**: 643–7.

38 Tunc M, Sadri E, Char DH. Orbital lymphangioma: an analysis of 26 patients. *Br J Ophthalmol* 1999; **83**: 76–80.

39 Turner C, Gross S. Treatment of recurrent suprahyoid cervicofacial lymphangioma with intravenous cyclophosphamide. *Am J Pediatr Hematol Oncol* 1994; **16**: 325–8.

40 Van der Horst CMAM. Gorham Stout syndrome. A rare complication of lymphatic malformation. Communication DC1 in 15th ISSVA Workshop. Wellington, NZ. 22–25 February 2004.

CHAPTER III.D

Arteriovenous Malformations (AVM)

III.D.1 Common Arteriovenous Malformations

Introduction

An arteriovenous malformation (AVM) is a hemodynamically active, fast-flow vascular malformation. The "nidus" is made of arterial feeders and enlarged draining veins directly connecting through micro- and macro-fistulas. AVMs are rare and they occur both superficially and viscerally. Most of them are present at birth but some only become evident around puberty. They never regress. In a series of 200 consecutive cases of superficial AVMs, seen by one of us (OE), 34% were visible at birth although in a somewhat equivocal presentation, 21% became evident during childhood and 8.5% at puberty, while only 21.5% were undetectable before adulthood (9). When fully developed, an AVM is warm, with pulsations, there is a bruit and sometimes a thrill, and usually a superficial cutaneous faint blush or a stain of varying hues of red. The head and neck is the most common location (70%); however, they can occur in any location. Some AVMs are included in complex syndromes, e.g. the Parkes Weber syndrome in the extremities, with staged multiple arteriovenous fistulas and gigantism of the affected limb; the Cobb syndrome at the trunk and spinal cord level; the Bonnet–Dechaume–Blanc syndrome or Wyburn-Mason syndrome in the cephalic region.

Clinical Features

An AVM is commonly misdiagnosed in infancy and childhood as an involuting hemangioma or capillary malformation (CM, port-wine stain) because it is not yet obviously fast-flow and warm with pulsations. It usually evolves and become clinically evident in the second or third decade of life (12, 13). In the majority of patients puberty and trauma trigger the growth of an AVM, and then its fast-flow nature manifests: redness increases as well as local warmth, a thrill and a bruit point to a fast-flow anomaly. As an AVM gets worse, draining veins become obvious and then tortuous, tense, and large.

AVM worsens at any time of the life but particularly at puberty and with trauma. Skin alterations, secondary to a capillary steal syndrome, develop, including modification of skin color, pigmentary changes, skin atrophy, ulcers with intractable pain, sudden life-threatening hemorrhage, or recurrent, intermittent bleeding. In the limbs skin changes resembling purple plaques of Kaposi sarcoma may expand. All of these are rare in childhood, and they arise by adolescence or later (14).

A facial AVM localized to the skin and/or facial bones leads to facial asymmetry, gingival hypertrophy, unstable teeth and periodontal bleeding, and skin or mucosal ulcers with secondary infection. The ear is a quite common location in the head and neck. A nasal AVM causes epistaxis. Ischemia of the tips of the fingers or toes complicates an extremity distal AVM; it is linked to arterial steal and venous hypertension, with a lack of normal blood supply to the skin. AVM in a finger or a toe gradually narrows the distal phalanx, causing purple necrotic skin changes; chronic adhesive crusts arise, and there is a progressive miniaturization of the nail. Bony AVM creates osteolysis, sometimes due to the venous drainage through the bones of an adjacent AVM. Shunting through the fistulas in large AVMs can cause congestive heart failure, but this occurs in less than 2% of cases, and in two situations: soon after birth in infants with massive AVM, and later in life, often in young adults, in patients with a large rapidly worsening AVM of an extremity or trunk (9).

SCHOBINGER STAGING is a severity scoring system for AVMs: stage I is the quiescent stage when the AVM mimics a capillary malformation or an involuting hemangioma; stage II is expansion: the lesion becomes warmer, bigger, throbbing, with a thrill and a bruit; stage III is destruction, with all the symptoms above plus ulcers, hemorrhages, and bony lytic lesions; stage IV is rare and is comprised of all of above plus congestive cardiac failure with increased cardiac output and left ventricle hypertrophy (9, 13).

Radiological Investigations

ULTRASONOGRAPHY COMBINED WITH COLOR DOPPLER documents the AV shunting. An AVM exhibits low-resistance high-velocity arterial flow, above the baseline, with high diastolic flux, and pulsatile venous flow below the baseline. Vessels are tortuous.

PULSED DOPPLER measures the arterial output (of carotid, humeral or femoral arteries) on the affected side as compared with the normal side. This is an excellent and reliable noninvasive technique to follow the course of an AVM or to monitor the stability of the results of a treatment.

Computed tomography (CT) with iodinated contrast demonstrates soft tissue involvement, a highly enhancing lesion, and dilated feeding and draining vessels, but it cannot definitely differentiate between hemangioma, VM and AVM.

CT angiography gives interesting representation and 3-D reconstruction of the vascular network in AVMs.

MRI of an AVM shows a collection of vascular flow voids (black tubular structures), corresponding to fast-flow vessels, in all sequences (spin–echo T1- and T2-weighted sequences) and there is no contrast parenchymal enhancement (no tumor aspect). Some signal abnormalities may exist in relation to a fibrofatty matrix (4, 17).

Magnetic resonance angiography (MRA) shows the anomalous vascular network. MRA can replace an arteriogram in the work-up when a treatment is not considered (for example in the case of a quiescent AVM in a child or an elderly patient) and for follow-up of AVM, but is not yet discussed for therapy.

Digital arteriography remains an indispensable tool to depict the angio-architecture of the AVM, prior to the discussion about therapy, and prior to therapeutic embolization; it demonstrates the dilated, lengthened and often tortuous feeding arteries, localizes the nidus, and detects the early venous drainage through enlarged veins (6).

Treatment

An AVM is usually not treated in its quiescent stage I, except for example when complete resection is possible without conspicuous cosmetic damage; however, early embolic and/or surgical treatment of a quiescent AVM remains controversial. Partial excision leads to transient improvement, then the AVM inevitably re-expands over time. Ligature or proximal closure by embolization of arterial feeding vessels is contraindicated, as incomplete surgical treatment is not recommended. After a period of apparent benefit, a vascular recruitment phenomenon occurs, new collateral arteries supply the nidus, intense capillarogenesis spreads out, while the residual lesion regrows and progresses. Treatment of an AVM is always challenging, and is either palliative (arterial embolization) to control a complication (ulcer, bleeding, and bone lytic lesion with a risk of fracture) or aims at being curative (embolization followed by wide surgical resection and reconstruction) (5, 15, 25). Therapeutic intervention becomes necessary whenever local (Schobinger stage III) and/or cardiac complications (Schobinger stage IV) develop. Long-term post-treatment follow-up is indispensable to ensure the permanent results.

III.D.2 Syndromic Arteriovenous Malformations

III.D.2.1 BONNET–DECHAUME–BLANC SYNDROME OR WYBURN-MASON SYNDROME

These are the two names for a sporadic syndrome with AVM involving the face, retina, and brain (2, 23). The most extensive cases result in distortion of facial features, recurrent epistaxis, gingival bleeding, blindness and cerebral hemorrhage. The facial AVM occupies the mid-face (the nose, forehead, and lip) or is hemifacial. In a retrospective study of 15 patients the most common presenting sign was reduced acuity or visual field, and a cutaneous lesion was present in only four patients; 14 had orbital involvement, and the neurologic involvement includes the optic nerve (in 13/15), the retina (in 11/15), the thalamus (in 9/15), and the chiasm/hypothalamus (in 9/15); two patients also had a maxillofacial AVM (1). In a series of 10 patients from our department (personal communication, Dr. Monique Boukobza, Department of Neuroradiodiagnostics, Hôpital Lariboisière, Paris, France) facial and cerebral involvement was present in all. The syndrome is hypothesized to be the result of a somatic mutation in the region of the neural crest, taking place before the cell migrations occur (thus, before the fourth week of embryo development) to produce this cerebrofacial arteriovenous metameric syndrome (CAMS) (1).

III.D.2.2 COBB SYNDROME

This is another sporadic arteriovenous metameric syndrome at the trunk level, linking the spinal cord to a skin AVM in the same metamere. Symptoms related to the spinal cord AVM usually appear in late childhood and they occur suddenly or progressively. They include pain, sensory and motor deficit, and loss of control of sphincters. Depending on the level of the spinal lesion, the patient may also have AVM in the arm or leg. In a series of 155 patients with spinal cord arteriovenous malformations or fistulae, 10 had Cobb syndrome (18).

Table 16 Parkes Weber syndrome: characteristics, course, and management.

Location	*Lower or upper extremity*
Skin aspect	Stained red by large mascules (pseudo port-wine stains)
Capillarogenesis	Increasing over the years, and after incomplete treatment
Veins	Enlarging and becoming tortuous, with a thrill
Arteries	Enlarging, possibly aneurysms
Lymphedema	Common, localized, or diffuse
Limb length	Increasing during the growth of the child, possibly ending in limb length discrepancy of several centimeters
Limb girth	Augmented in most patients
Bones	Possibly bone alterations (osteolysis)
Skin lesions (vascular steal syndrome)	Pigmentation, pseudo Kaposi sarcoma skin changes, ulcers, hemorrhages, pain, distal elephantiasis
General consequences	Cardiac failure (high output) in about 2% of patients
Work-up	Ultrasonography, doppler evaluation, including arterial output determination, CT and/or MRI/MRA, digital angiography
Treatment	Superselective arterial embolization, surgical resection with adequate margins, and reconstructive surgical procedures

III.D.2.3 PARKES WEBER SYNDROME

This syndrome is usually sporadic although rare familial cases have been observed. It affects the upper or lower limbs. The full disease spectrum consists of progressive overgrowth of the affected extremity during childhood (discrepancy in girth and length compared to the normal limb), lymphedema, red congenital cutaneous stain (pseudo CM), excess cutaneous warmth, and arteriovenous fistulas along the extremity (see Table 13 page 129, and Table 16). Commonly, during infancy the AV shunting may be indiscernible on the angiogram, which only detects a diffuse hypervascularization. Later in childhood on follow-up angiogram the AV fistulas become noticeable. These lesions are triggered by puberty and trauma (8).

III.D.2.4 ARTERIOVENOUS FISTULAS (AVF) AND AVM IN RENDU–OSLER–WEBER DISEASE

Rendu–Osler–Weber disease or hereditary hemorrhagic telangiectasia (HHT) is characterized by multiple telangiectasia developing on the skin (lips, fingers, etc.)

and mucosa. Bleeding (epistaxis, GI tract bleeding) causes anemia. There are two known genotypes: HHT1 linked to mutations of *endoglin*, and HHT2 linked to mutations of *ALK 1*. In both cases AVF and AVM can develop, particularly in the liver, the lungs (thus creating a loss of the pulmonary filter for bacteria, with a risk of brain abscess), and brain. In patients with HHT a work-up is necessary to detect them; lung AVFs are usually amenable to endovascular treatment (see also pages 134–5).

III.D.2.5 CM–AVM SYNDROME

A newly identified familial vascular syndrome associates CM and AVM: CM–AVM syndrome caused by mutations of *RASA 1* (7). In an affected family some members have multiple small pink to brownish macules of CM scattered over the body, with ill-defined border and often a thin pale halo, and usually one member of the family has an AVM, including possible Parkes Weber syndrome in an extremity, or a visceral AVM, in addition to the multiple small CMs.

III.D.2.6 AVM IN COWDEN SYNDROME

Cowden syndrome is the consequence of germline mutations of *PTEN.* Patients develop benign and malignant tumors of the skin, breast, thyroid, and GI tract. They can also have multiple AVMs (20).

III.D.2.7 AVM IN EHLERS–DANLOS TYPE IV SYNDROME

A rare and very severe familial syndrome with possible multiple AVF and AVM is Ehlers–Danlos syndrome type IV, the vascular type: patients have a dysmorphic face, thin fragile and translucent skin with a too visible venous network, vessels and internal organs burst. The disease is linked to a mutation of COL3A1 and these patients are at a very high risk of arterial dissection and arterial rupture during endovascular investigation including a diagnostic angiography.

Figures

ARTERIOVENOUS MALFORMATIONS
Pathology

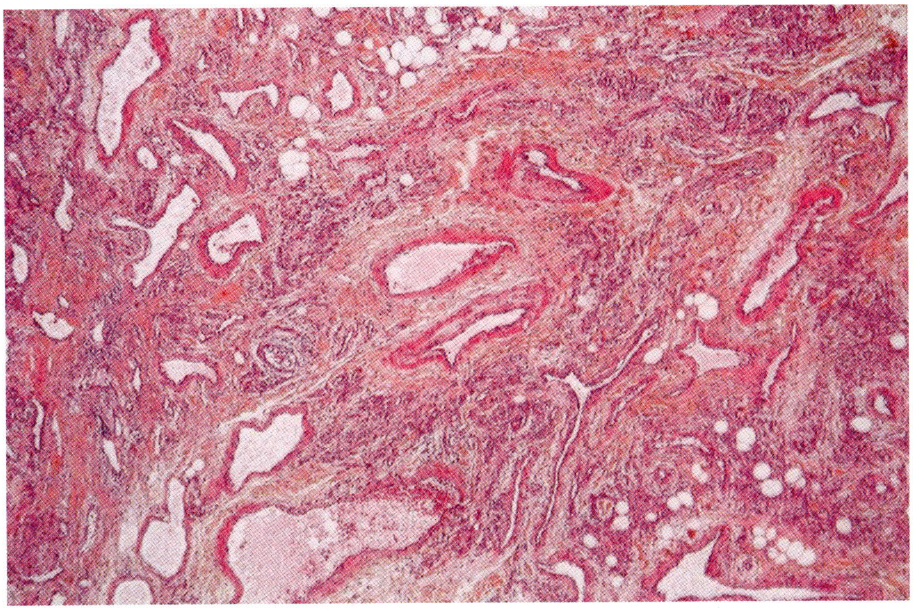

The lesion comprises vessels of various caliber evenly distributed in the tissues, with relatively thick walls. The walls of some vessels are of uneven thickness.

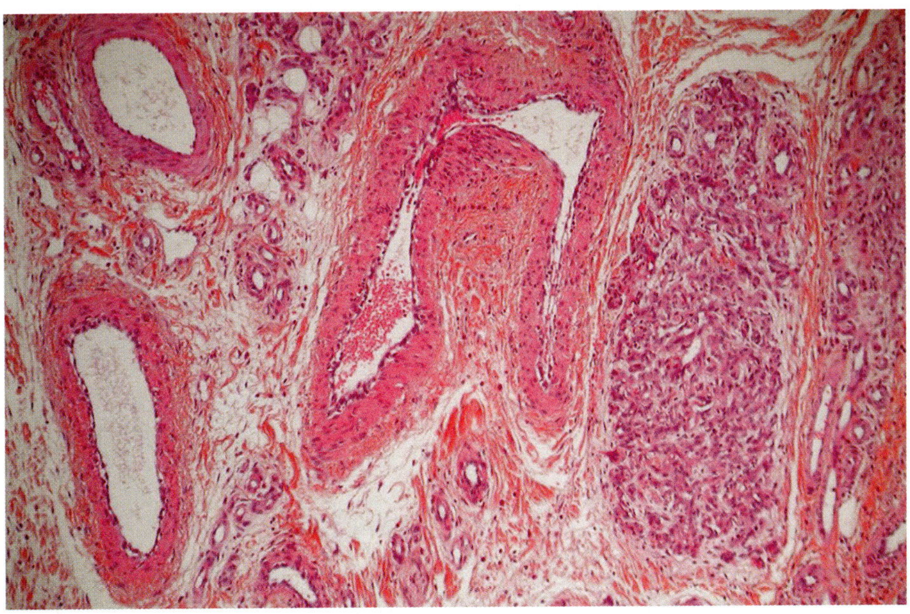

The vessels are arteries, veins, and numerous vessels of intermediate or undefined type. A capillary component is often present, randomly distributed or grouped in lobules as in this figure.

Pathology

In this case of AVM, the capillary component dissects between the skeletal-muscle cells, respecting the borders of the fascicle.

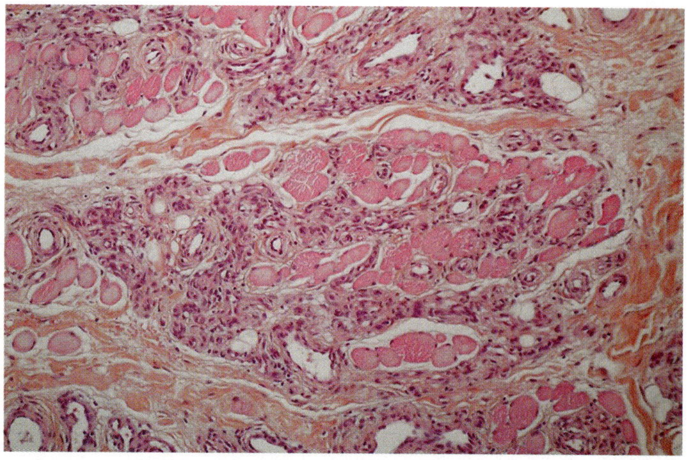

On elastic tissue (orcein) staining, the architecture of the malformed vessels is better seen. Some are veins with thickened elastic fibers (upper vessel), some are arteries of normal structure (middle), and others lack any elastic component (lower right) being a malformed vessel without features of an artery or of a vein.

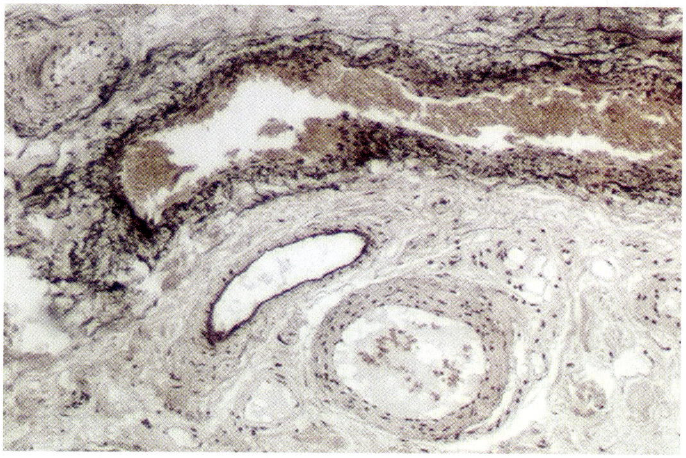

Orcein staining also highlights the presence of direct arteriovenous communications (fistulae) between an artery with thick undulating internal elastic lamina (upper left) and a venous-type vessel (lower right).

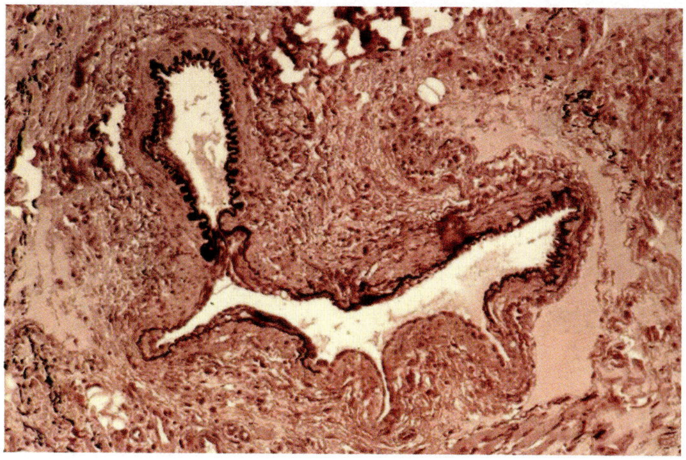

Specific Locations, Problems Created, Investigations, and Treatments

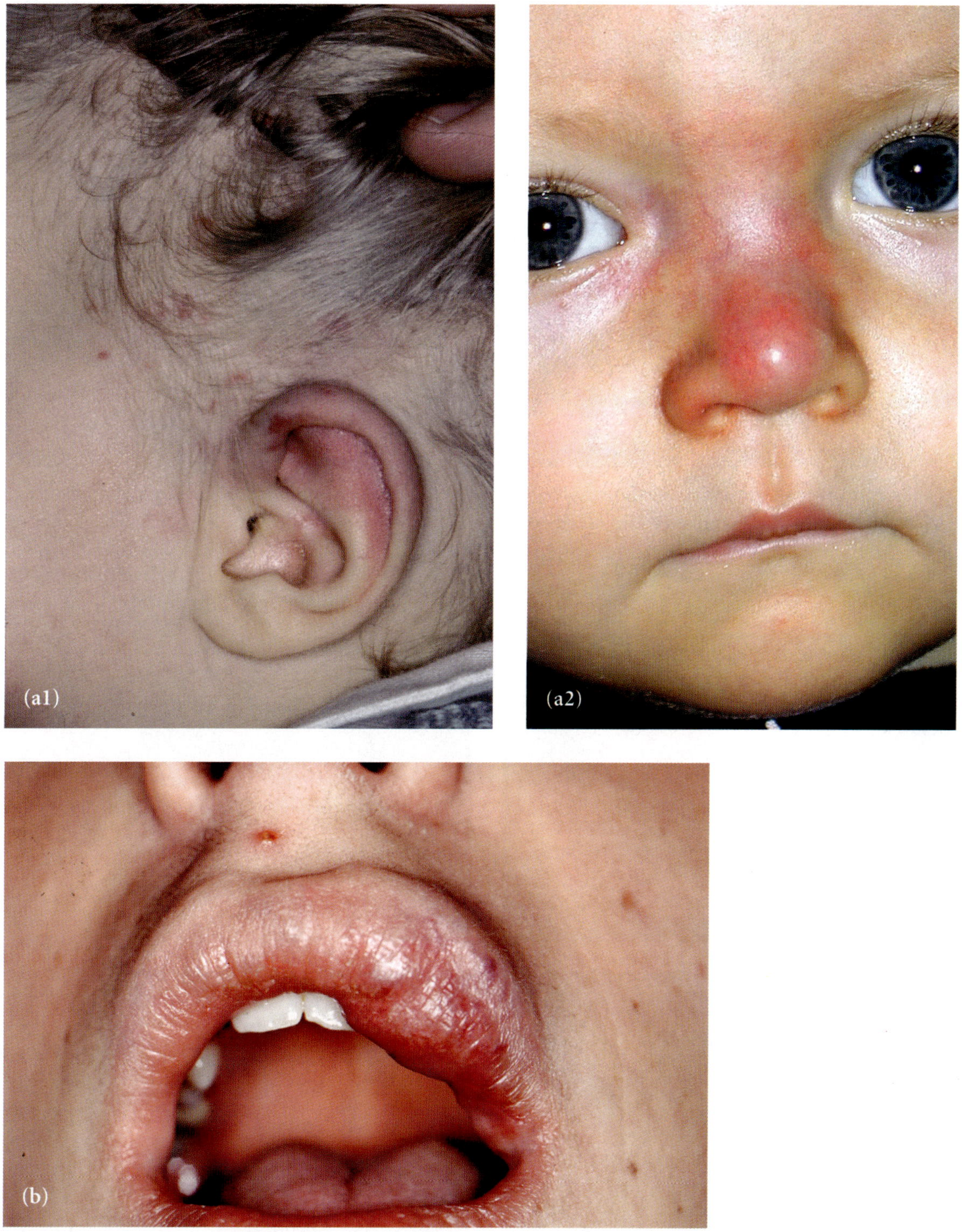

Schobinger staging of AVMs, based on clinical signs/symptoms, gives an indication of the evolution: stage I is the quiescent initial period with blush, stain, and local warmth. The vascular lesion may be misdiagnosed in infancy as CM (a1, a2) and later as involuting hemangioma (b).

Specific Locations, Problems Created, Investigations, and Treatments

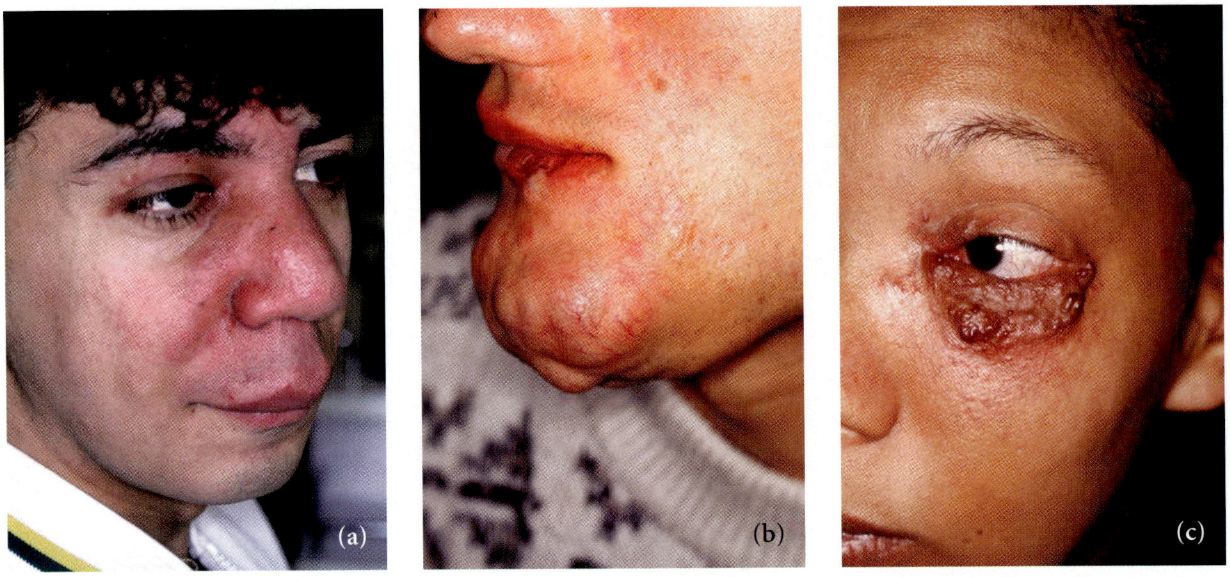

Stage II is the time when the vascular fast-flow lesion expands, with increased red color, thickening, increased size, evident bruit and thrill. This may be the results of ill-advised treatment: in (c) the AVM clearly expanded after several sessions of pulsed dye laser treatment.

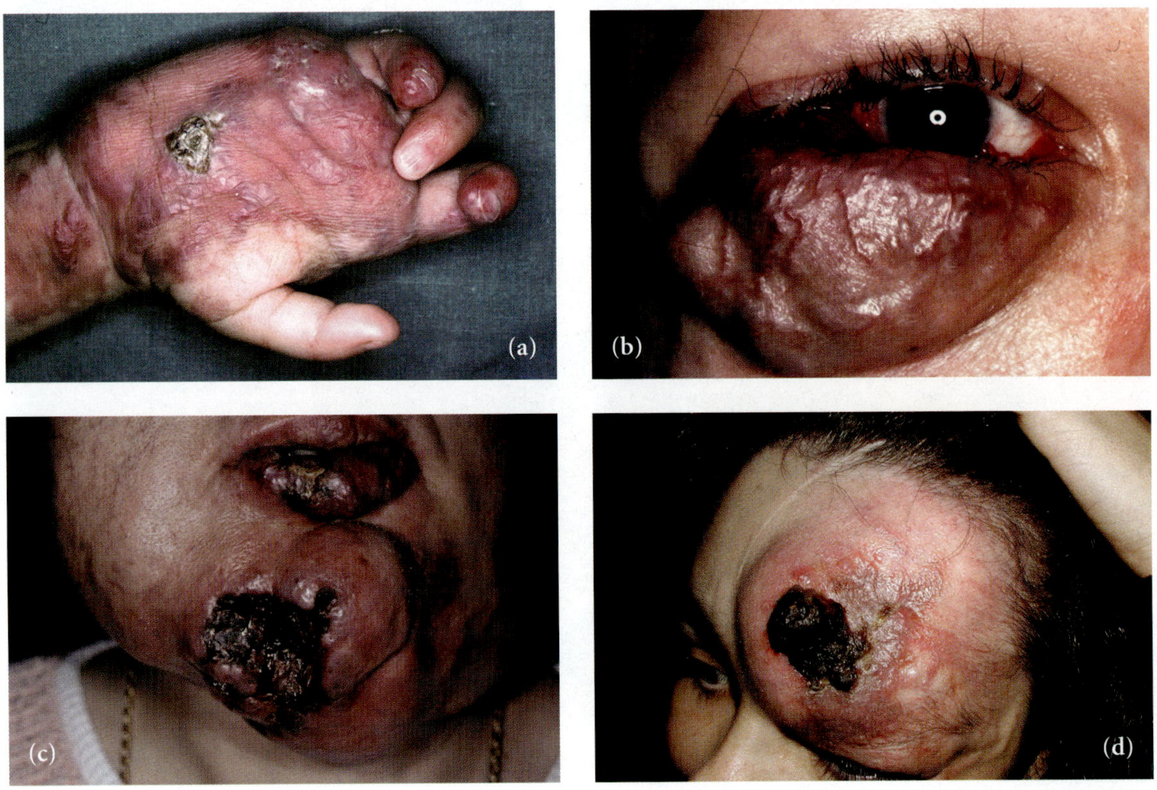

During stage III the AVM not only expands but it damages the tissues; crusts, chronic ulcerations, acute pain, bleeding, and even life-threatening hemorrhages appear. This stage is rare in childhood (a), and usually it is the result of ill-advised treatments.

Specific Locations, Problems Created, Investigations, and Treatments

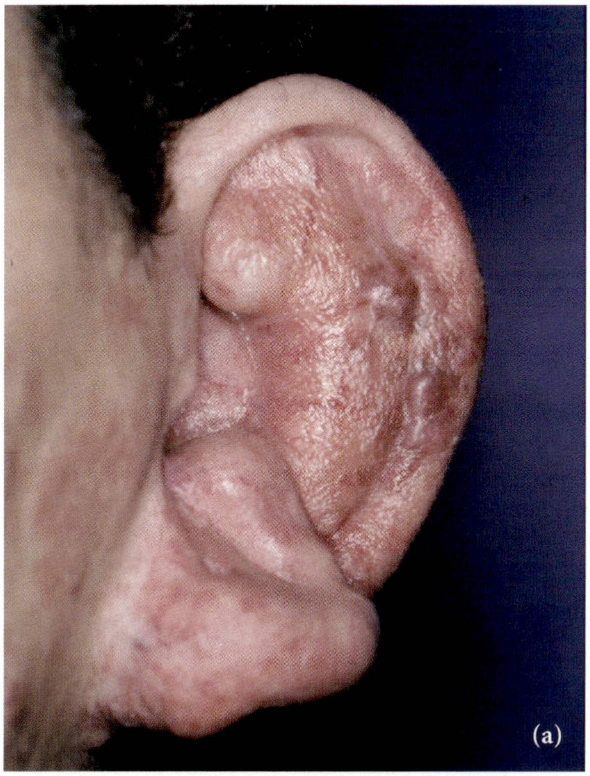

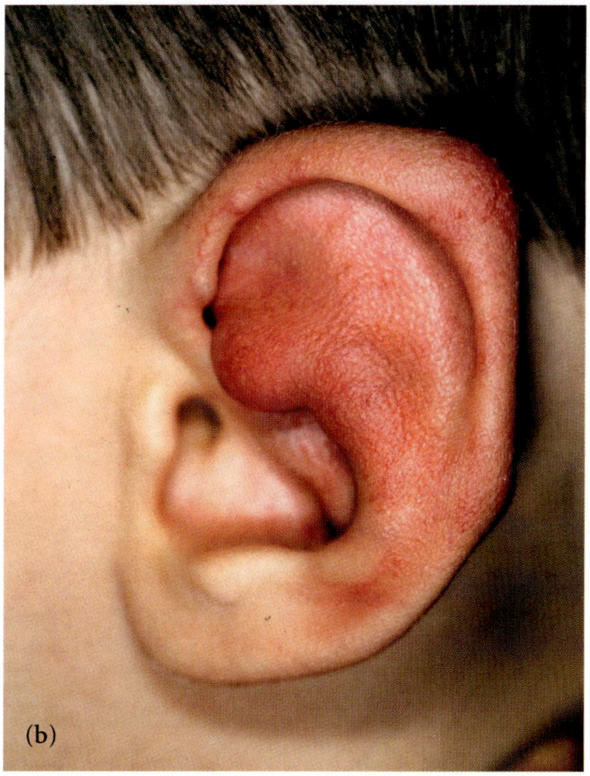

When an ear AVM involves clinically only part of the auricle (b), it is usually the upper part and the lobe is spared; the full auricle (a) is involved in other patients. With time and progressive worsening an apparently partial involvement may extend to the entire external ear. In fact in these patients an angiogram performed in early Schobinger stages (I–II) would have demonstrated a more diffuse involvement than clinically suspected. Macrotia (a) is a common feature in ear AVM, and pulsations, pain, and buzzing are frequently reported by patients (22).

Specific Locations, Problems Created, Investigations, and Treatments

The ear is the second most common location of head and neck AVMs after the face. In a series of 49 patients with ear AVM 65.9% had a congenital auricular vascular lesion (a); most patients recorded expansion of the AVM during puberty and pregnancy (b), while only 7 out of 49 worsened before 5 years of age; 78% had extra-auricular involvement, mainly anterior to the auricle in the cheek, or posterior to the auricle in the neck and scalp areas; the middle and inner ear was not involved (22).

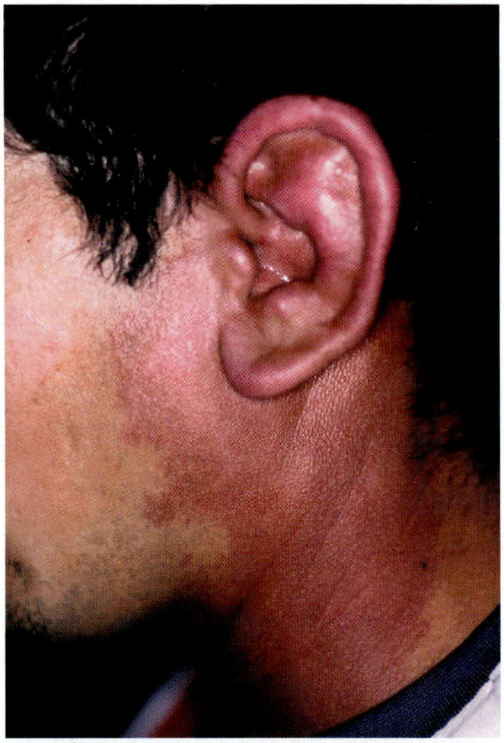

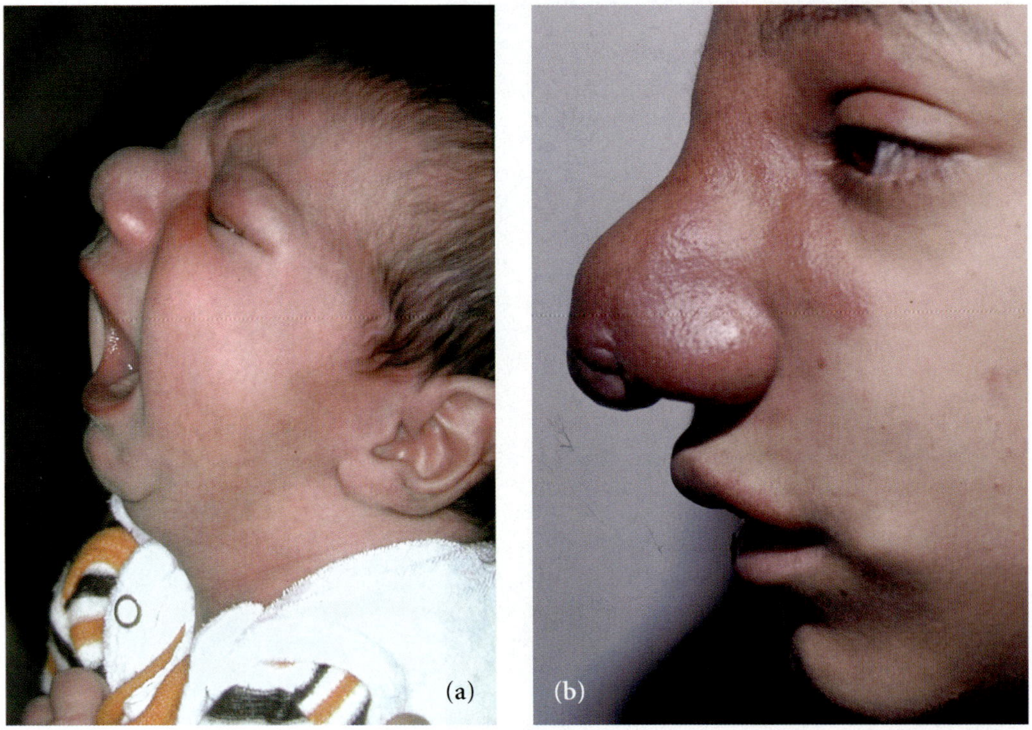

The progressive worsening of a mid-facial (nose, upper lip, and mid-forehead) AVM between birth (a) and puberty (b), at which time uncontrolled life-threatening nasal bleeding occurred, requiring embolization and partial nasal amputation.

Specific Locations, Problems Created, Investigations, and Treatments

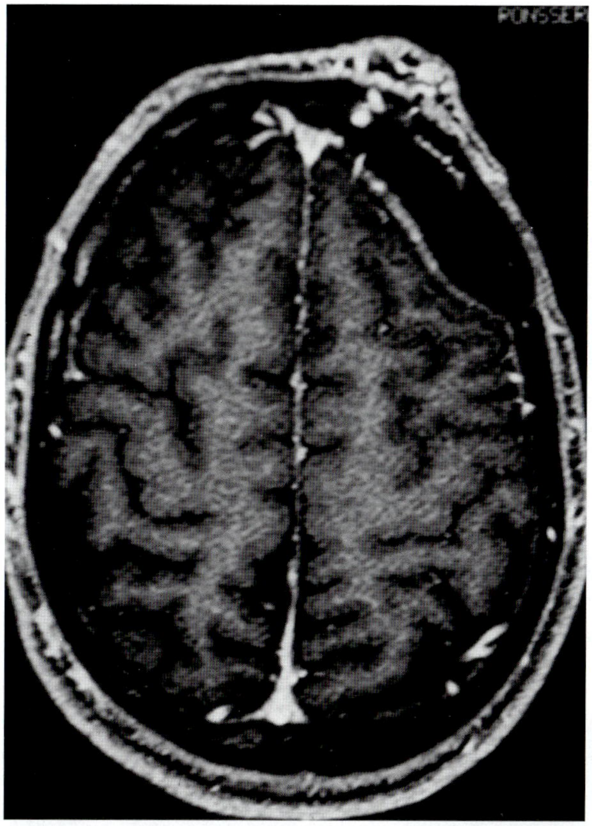

MRI in this patient demonstrates flow-voids and thickening of the cranial bone, an indication of the AVM located within the skin of the forehead, with intradiploic extension.

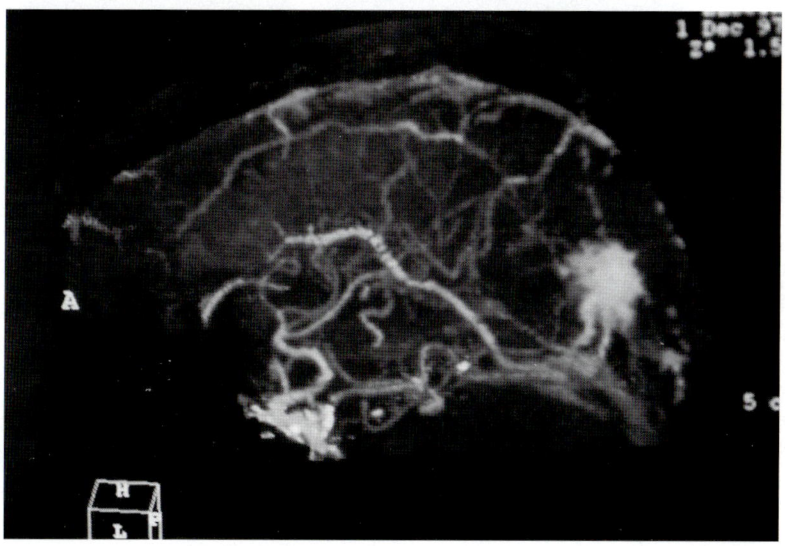

This 65-year-old woman affected with arterial hypertension and hyperlipidemia had a late occurrence of a scalp AVM creating a pulsatile bump under a normally colored and hairy scalp; her lesion did not cause major signs or symptoms and therefore no treatment was considered: in her case an angio-CT scan gave enough information on the blood supply, and replaced the angiogram (arteriography in an atheromatous patient might dislodge a plaque of atheroma and be potentially dangerous).

Specific Locations, Problems Created, Investigations, and Treatments

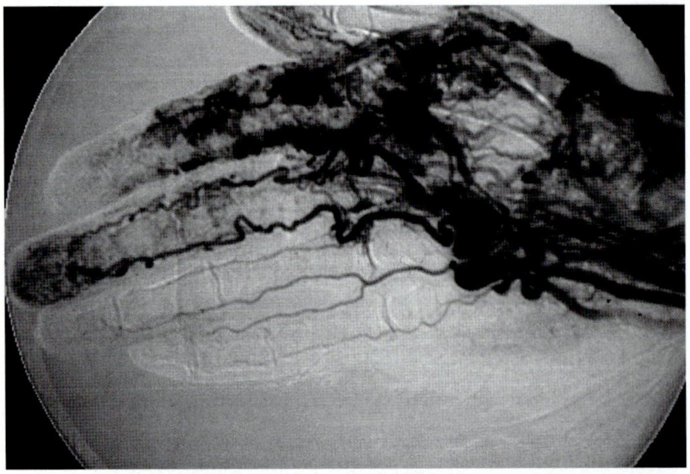

This patient had noticed worsening of the hand AVM. Arteriography remains the best investigative tool to depict the arterial feeders, the AVM nidus and the venous drainage, and decide if endovascular embolization is an appropriate therapeutic option.

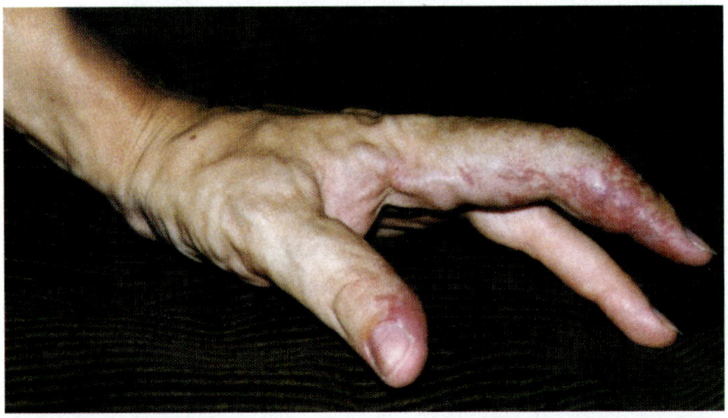

A patient with distal AVM of the upper extremity at the beginning of Schobinger stage III AVM, with recent discoloration of the second finger, an indication of ischemia, and progressively enlarging distorted draining veins.

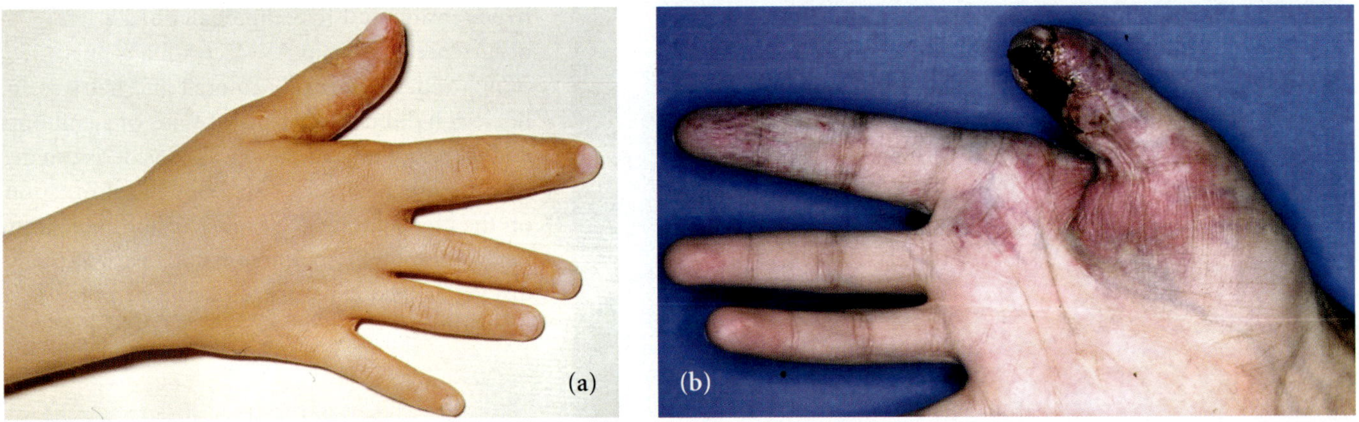

Six years of progression of an AVM involving the first and second fingers (a). No relief was provided by palliative embolizations. Puberty occurred during this six-year period and seemed to have triggered the expansion. Distal necrotic skin changes in the thumb, with ulcer, infection, bleeding, and intense pain occurred (b). It was impossible to reverse miniaturization of the nail and distal phalanx by arterial embolization, and phalanx amputation was the final outcome. Superselective arterial embolization, to eradicate the nidus of an extremity AVM, has been considered the treatment

Specific Locations, Problems Created, Investigations, and Treatments

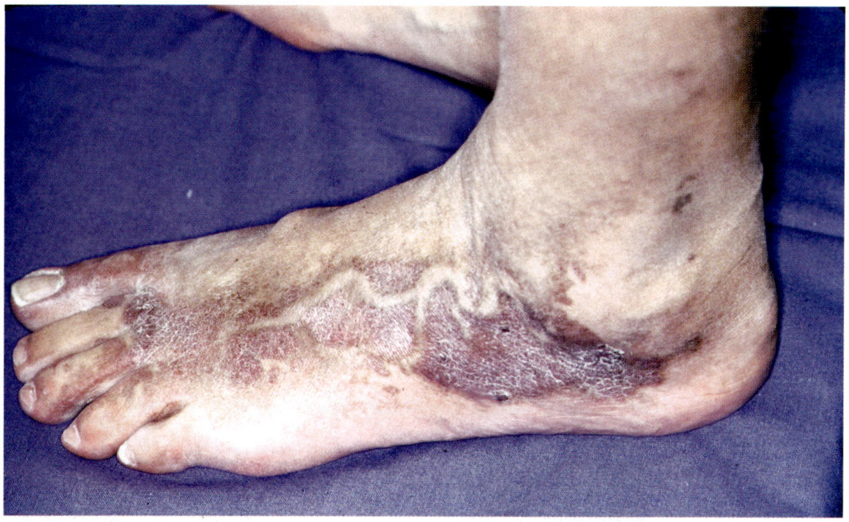

Pseudo Kaposi sarcoma skin changes, with purple infiltrated plaques may develop early in adulthood with distal AVM of the leg (14). In this patient with stage II–III AVM, red infiltrated plaques resembling Kaposi sarcoma appeared in the skin of the foot and ankle, and slowly extended, but only in the affected extremity, a major clinical difference from Kaposi sarcoma; in addition, there were dilated veins giving a thrill on palpation due to the fast-flow vascular anomaly.

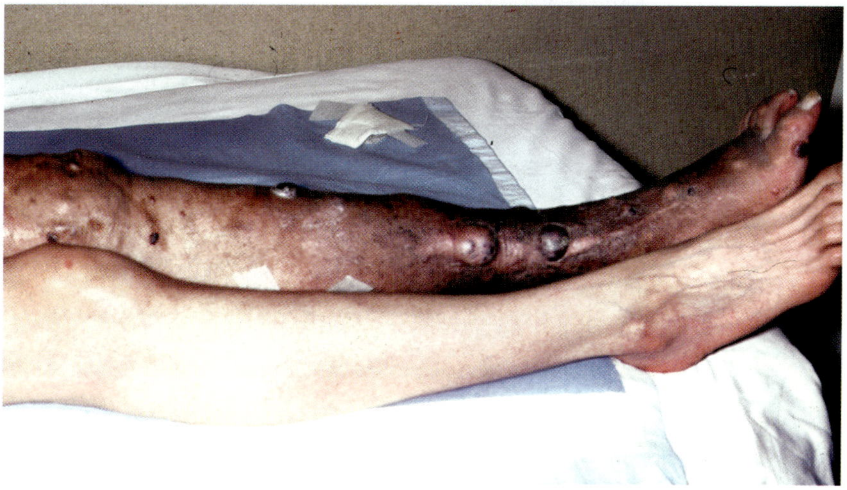

AVM with multiple AVF fistulae along the lower extremity, in Parkes Weber syndrome, may progressively create severe skin complications, pigmentary changes, bulges in the draining veins, and ulcers.

offering the highest level of success, thanks to advances in instrumentation (19). Good initial angiographic results are frequent. However, long-term follow-up is required because of possible recanalization and recruitment of new arterial feeders to the nidus. Complications of these procedures include tissue necrosis and nerve injury.

Specific Locations, Problems Created, Investigations, and Treatments

This young man has Parkes Weber syndrome with multiple arteriovenous fistulas of the lower extremity. Knee cartilage artery embolization was used in childhood to try to slow down the excess growth of the limb, but was only of transient and partial benefit. His leg length discrepancy being more than 5 cm he had epiphyseodesis with epiphyseal stapling of the knee. Afterwards the AVM worsened severely around the knee joint, with large venous channels draining the nidus (a), and he distally developed lymphedema and skin alterations in the toes (b). In patients with Parkes Weber syndrome, when epiphyseodesis is considered it should be the least invasive possible (percutaneous epiphyseodesis with minimal incision and minimal invasive technique) to avoid boosting the fast-flow lesions (8, 11).

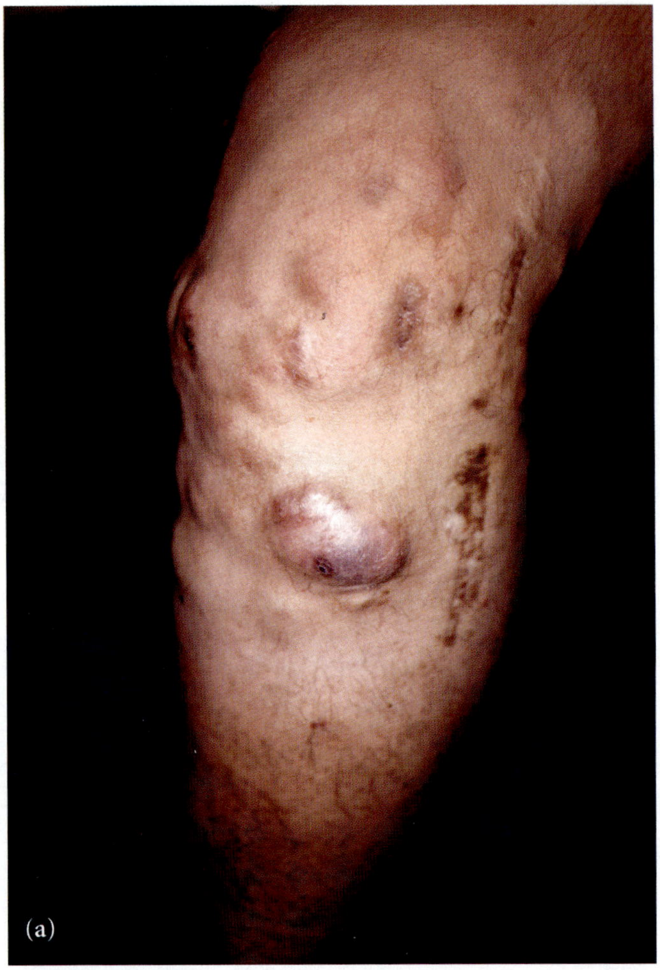
(a)

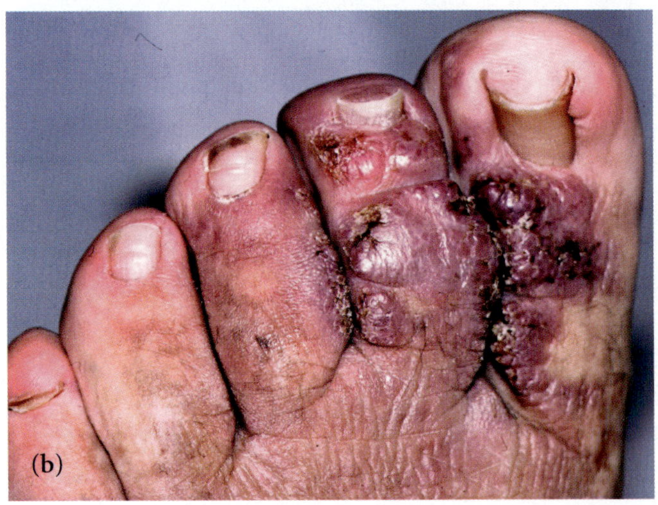
(b)

Specific Locations, Problems Created, Investigations, and Treatments

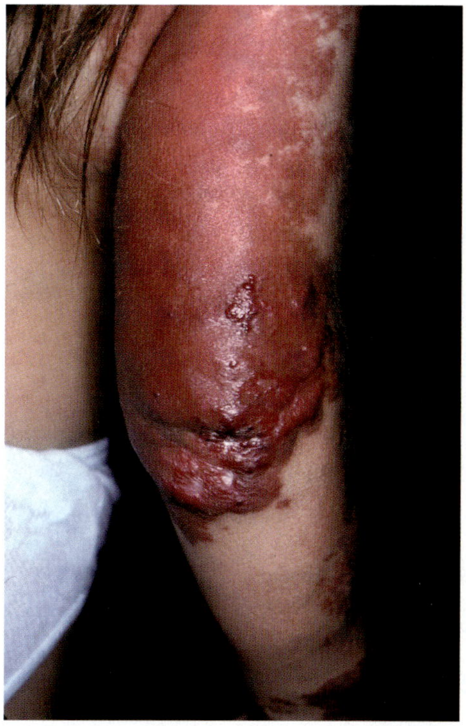

Parkes Weber syndrome of the arm with cardiac failure. This is a rare situation observed in less than 2% of patients with AVMs in our experience but when this complication develops it may be uncontrolled and lethal (9, 10). Tolerance of the heart to the high flow is sometimes surprising when the AVM has gradually worsened in a slow protracted course over childhood and adolescence. It is not uncommon to see a patient with diffuse lower limb AVM, who has a femoral output 10 times higher in the affected extremity than in the normal one, as measured by pulsed Doppler, and who has a relatively good cardiac tolerance of the malformation, with acceptable cardiac output as measured with a Doppler probe, and moderate hypertrophy of the left ventricle.

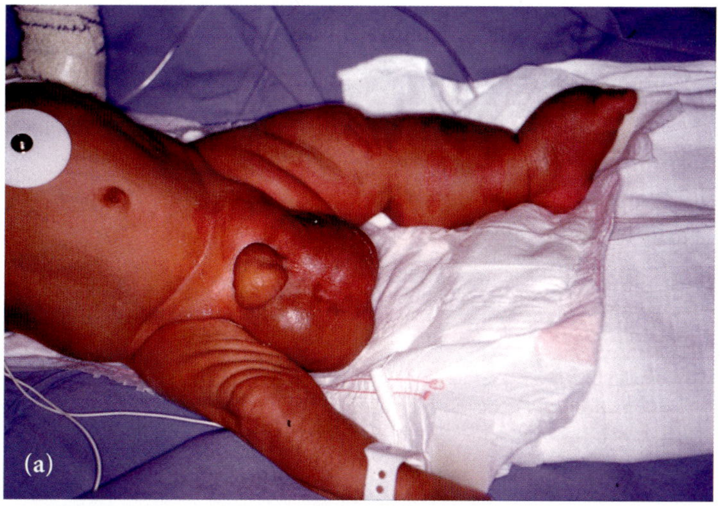

(a)

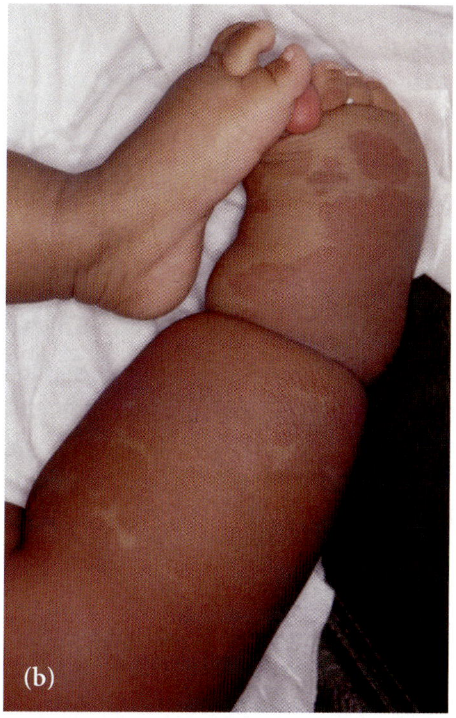

(b)

Parkes Weber syndrome in these two infants was manifest at birth. In both cases lymphedema of the lower extremity, large red cutaneous stains and abnormal warmth of the limb were present; AV fistulas were shown by US/Doppler. One infant (a) had cardiac failure at birth: a palliative embolization reduced the cardiac output.

Specific Locations, Problems Created, Investigations, and Treatments

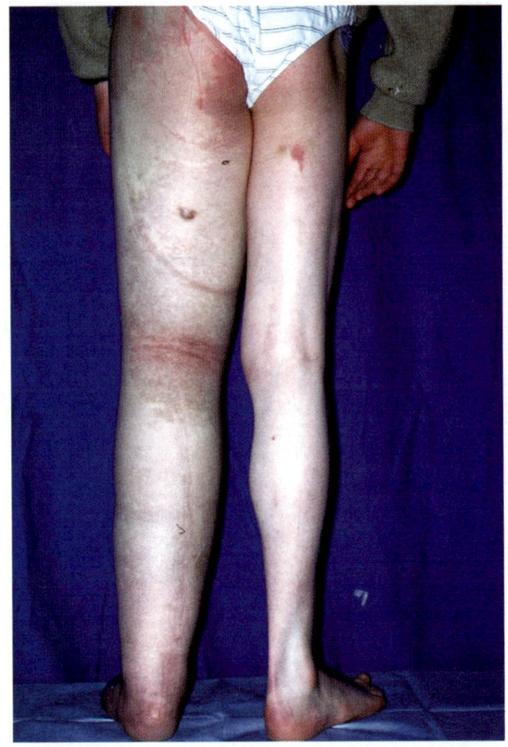

In patients with AVM of the lower extremity the association of arteriovenous fistulas and lymphedema is quite common. Elastic stockings are indispensable, limiting the lymphedema, providing pain relief and reducing the flow through the AV fistulas. However, they need to be carefully tailored: in this patient the elastic garments are too tight in the popliteal fold with redness and a risk of wound and infection. Manual lymphatic draining massage is also useful before adapting the compressive garments.

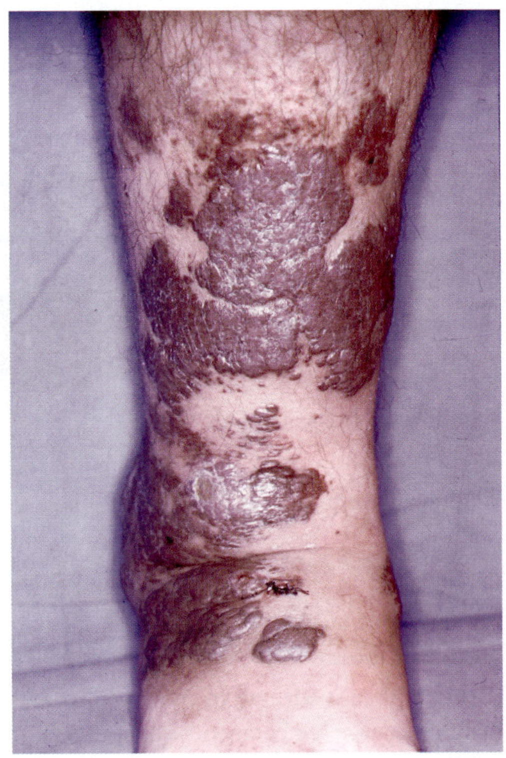

Pseudo Kaposi sarcoma skin changes are particularly extensive in the leg of this patient with arteriovenous malformation, some degree of lymphedema and the absence of elastic garments controlling the edema might have facilitated the skin complication.

Specific Locations, Problems Created, Investigations, and Treatments

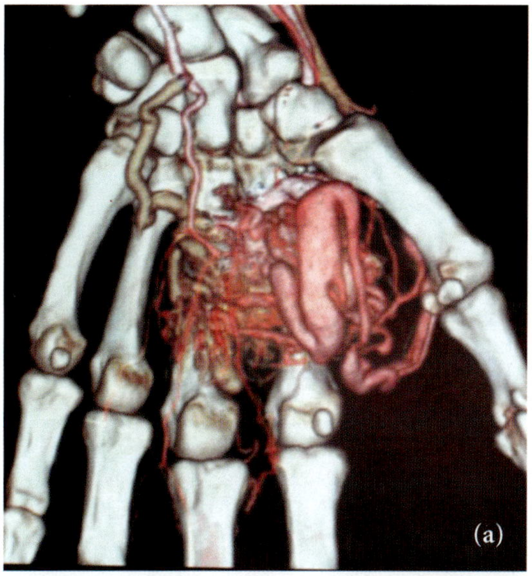

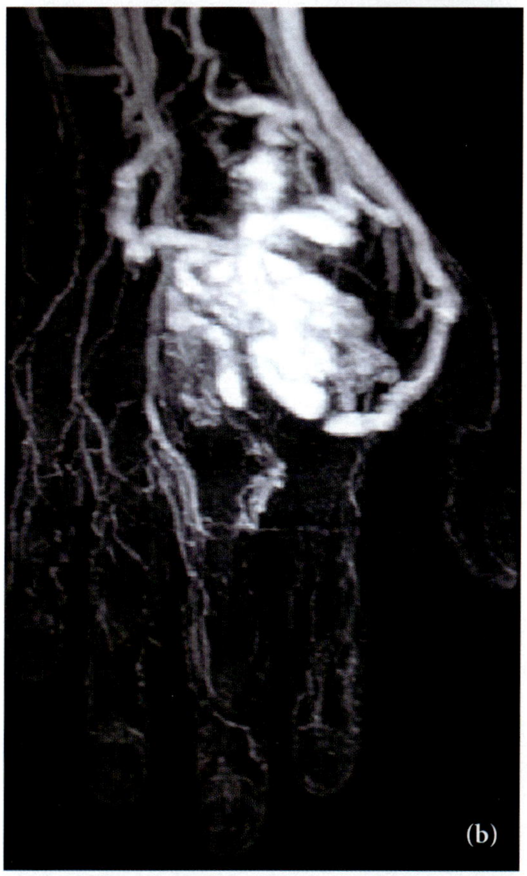

Angio-CT scans and MRA scans were performed in this man who has a mass of AVM in the middle of the hand, with increased warmth and a thrill, but normal skin overlying the AVM. A non-invasive work-up was first preferred to angiography to clarify the symptoms: increasing pain and sensory and motor disturbances by EMG evaluation. In this case the scans detect both AVM nidus and aneurysm.

Specific Locations, Problems Created, Investigations, and Treatments

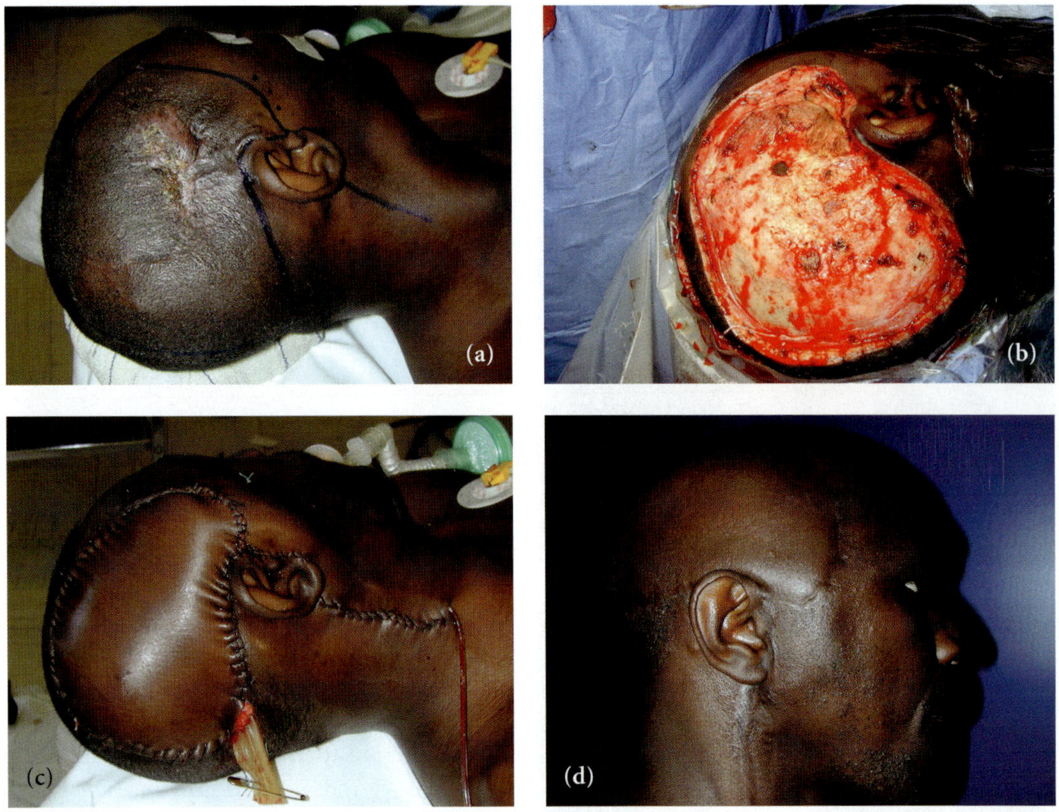

This man had an AVM of the scalp, previously treated 10 years ago by a combination of embolization and excision with local plasty. The recurrence was highly hemorrhagic (a) and not controlled by arterial endovascular treatment.The AVM was draining through the parietal bone to the contralateral venous sinus. The treatment consisted of embolization by both arterial and direct puncture routes. The large surgical wound (b) was reconstructed using a free skin-and-muscle flap transfer, from the latissimus dorsalis, microanastomozed to the cervical arteries (c). The cosmetic results was excellent and stable during the 44 months of follow-up (d) (operator: Dr. Didier Salvan, Hôpital Lariboisière, Paris, France).

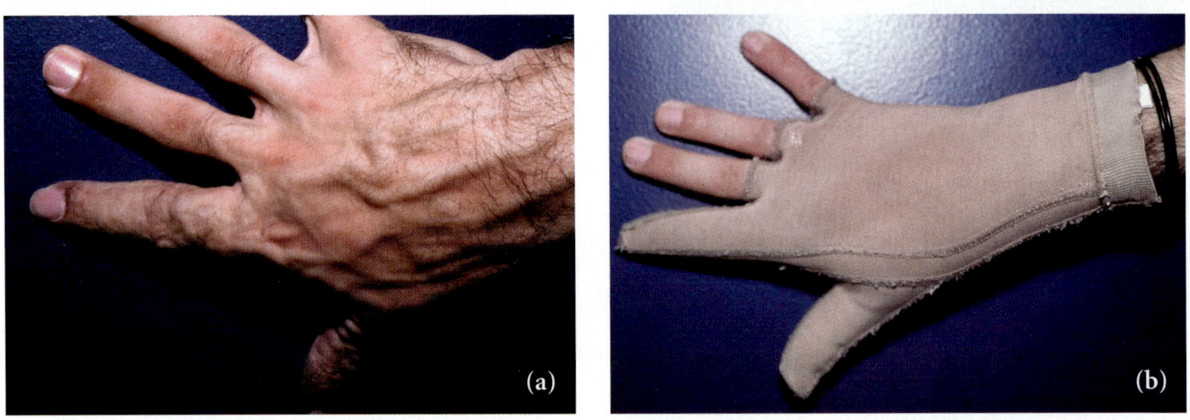

An elastic glove protects the hand from trauma and reduces the flow through the AV fistulas in this young man with stage II hand AVM; this helps prevent progression to stage III (21).

Specific Locations, Problems Created, Investigations, and Treatments

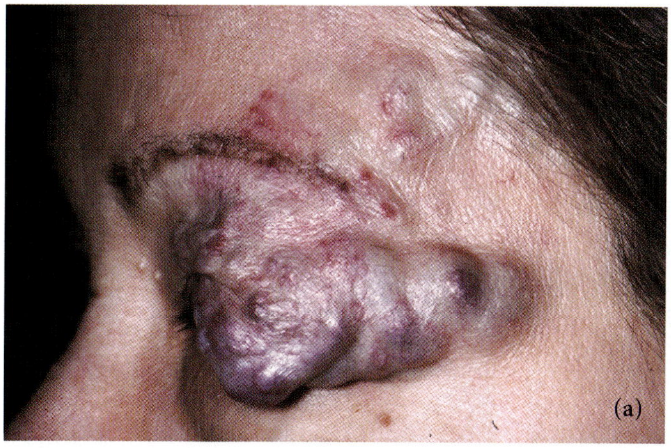
(a)

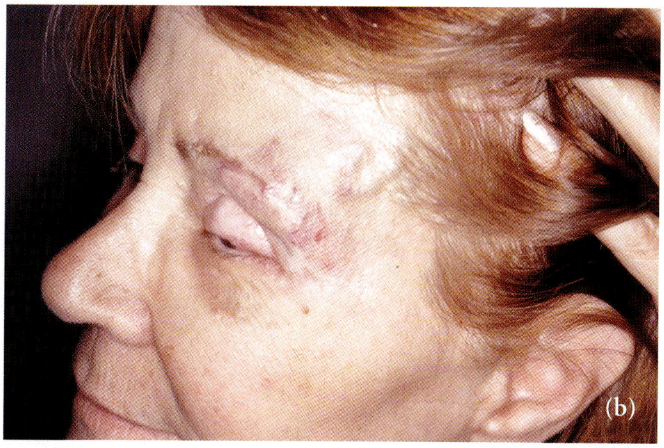
(b)

This woman had from birth a red stain of the upper eyelid. Growth of the AVM progressively occluded the visual axis. Excision, after embolization, was performed, with a graft to reconstruct the unit (operators: Dr. Dominique Deffrennes and Dr. Didier Salvan, Hôpital Lariboisière, Paris, France). Pre-operative embolization is always delicate in this location as the ophthalmic artery is also feeding the AVM nidus.

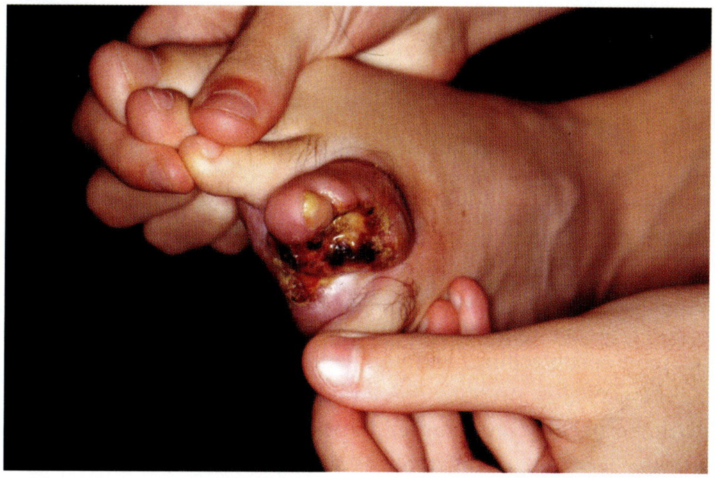

This painful arteriovenous malformation of the foot received palliative arterial embolization, to deliver an ablative embolic material (absolute ethanol) to the nidus and try to occlude it. However, inadvertent migration of ethanol and embolization of adjacent tissue during the procedure resulted in local complications: necrosis developed and the patient underwent amputation of two toes. Ethanol embolization for ablating AVM involves similar complications to those described for VM sclerotherapy, and complications are more frequent than with VM, due to the rapid flow. In a series of 450 patients (2055 procedures) with either slow-flow or fast-flow lesions, according to Yakes and Yee, minor local complications included blistering (8.2%), infection (2.2%), and temporary or permanent loss of sensation (1.1%); major local complications were facial nerve weakness (0.2%), decreased motor strength in an extremity (0.5%), amputation (0.1%), tissue injuries (0.36%), and cardiopulmonary arrest (0.06%); however, the conclusion of this report is that, to be safe, the procedure requires experienced operators and dedicated facilities (25). In a group of 61 patients (232 procedures) Burrows et al. (3) found a much higher rate of complications (minor and self-limited in 36.06%, and severe in 32.78% of patients) for ethanol embolization of AVM.

Specific Locations, Problems Created, Investigations, and Treatments

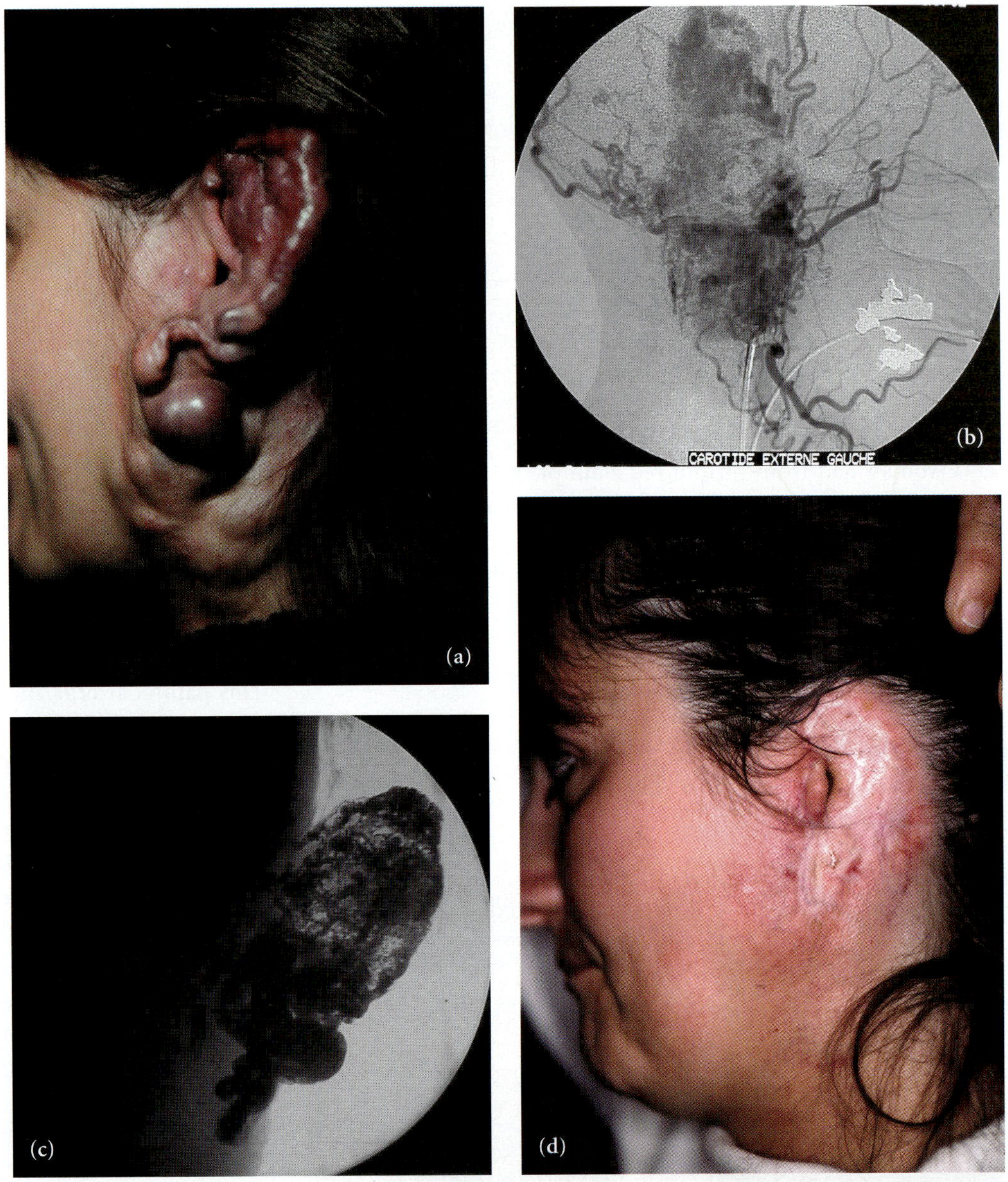

Stage III AVM, with macrotia, pain and bleeding, and very large draining veins (a). This clinical situation led to auriculectomy, after preoperative embolization to minimize intraoperative bleeding (b, c). Embolization was achieved with in situ injection of an acrylic glue filling both arteries and veins. The large draining veins shrank to normal size after amputation of the ear (d) and resection of the AVM nidus (operator: Dr. Benoit Faucon, Hôpital Lariboisière, Paris, France). Depending on the size of the resection (the ear only or the ear plus adjacent skin) the surgical wound is closed either by direct closure, or a skin graft, or a flap transfer. Arterial embolization alone, even ethanol embolization as close as possible to the AVM nidus (24, 25) cannot cure a ear AVM. In our experience it gives some transient relief of the symptoms, which is helpful in young patients, then re-expansion occurs (22). Two to five years after ear amputation, in a stable patient, ear reconstruction may be considered (16) or a prosthetic ear can be offered.

Specific Locations, Problems Created, Investigations, and Treatments

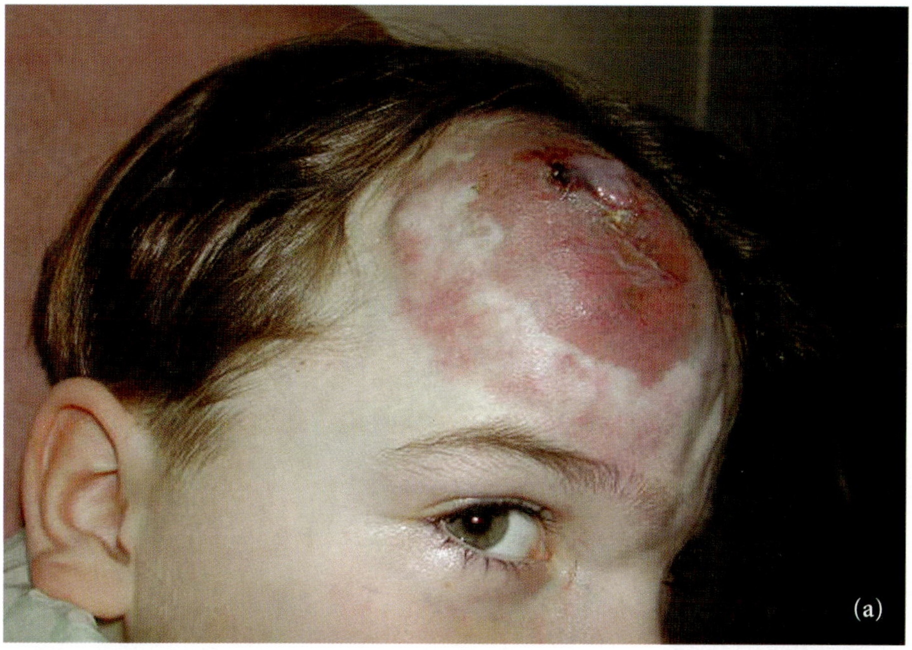

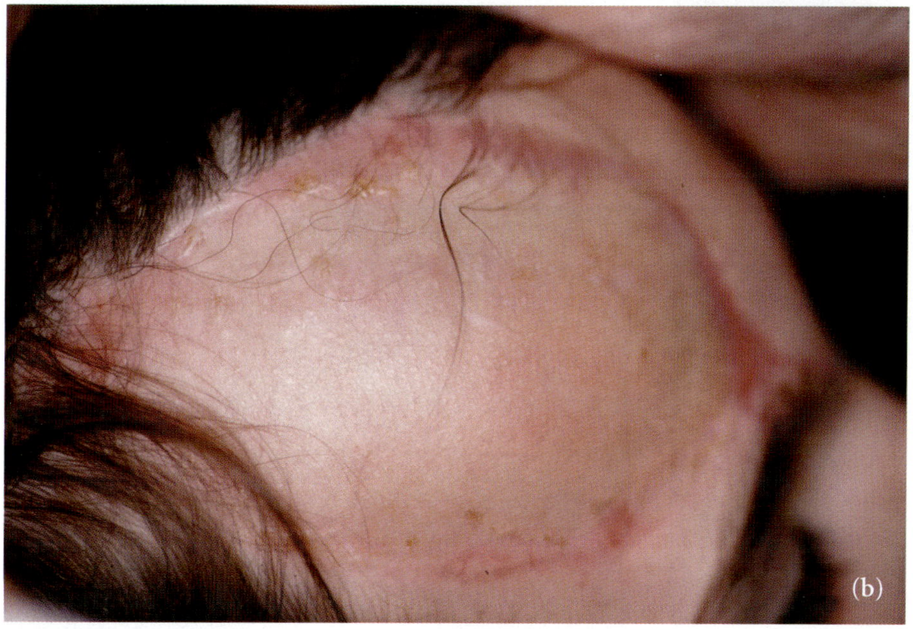

Stage III AVM is rare in childhood: in this eight-year-old boy (a) hemorrhages necessitated curative treatment, combining pre-operative embolization and large resection. A skin graft (b) was preferred for reconstruction because of the young age of the patient (operator: Dr. Didier Salvan, Hôpital Lariboisière, Paris, France). The post-operative course is assessed once a year by clinical examination, US and color Doppler screening of the scar, and pulsed Doppler evaluation of both carotid outputs. Long-term follow-up is mandatory to monitor absence of recurrence.

Specific Locations, Problems Created, Investigations, and Treatments

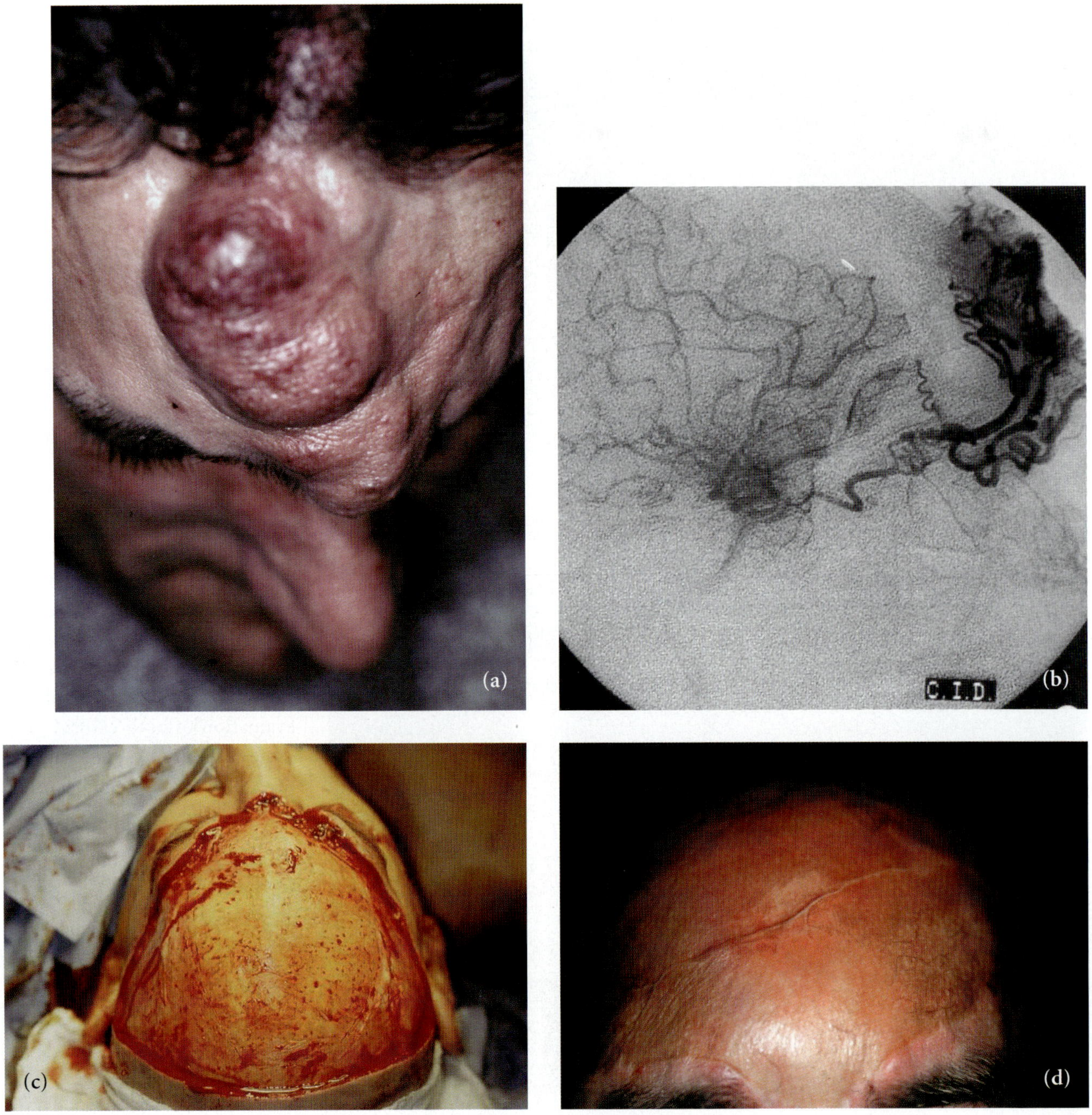

AVM of the mid-forehead in an adult man creating a large mass with pulsations and intermittent bleeding from minor necrotic areas. The AVM was fed by both facial arteries and one ophthalmic artery; embolization was achieved by puncture of the primary intranidus vein and injection of acrylic glue that diffused retrogradely into the distal portion of all feeders. After pre-operative embolization, resection of the full forehead unit and glabella including the vascular lesion was achieved. Reconstruction used the transfer of a free muscle flap (latissimus dorsalis), anastomosed to the external carotid artery, and covered with a thin skin graft, for better cosmetic results (a better color than with a full skin-and-muscle flap) (operators: Dr. Didier Salvan and Dr. Emmanuel Racy, Hôpital Lariboisière, Paris, France). (a) Pre-operative aspect, (b) pattern on arteriogram (internal carotid feeding of the AVM), (c) is the appearance after resection, and (d) is the scar 18 months later.

Specific Locations, Problems Created, Investigations, and Treatments

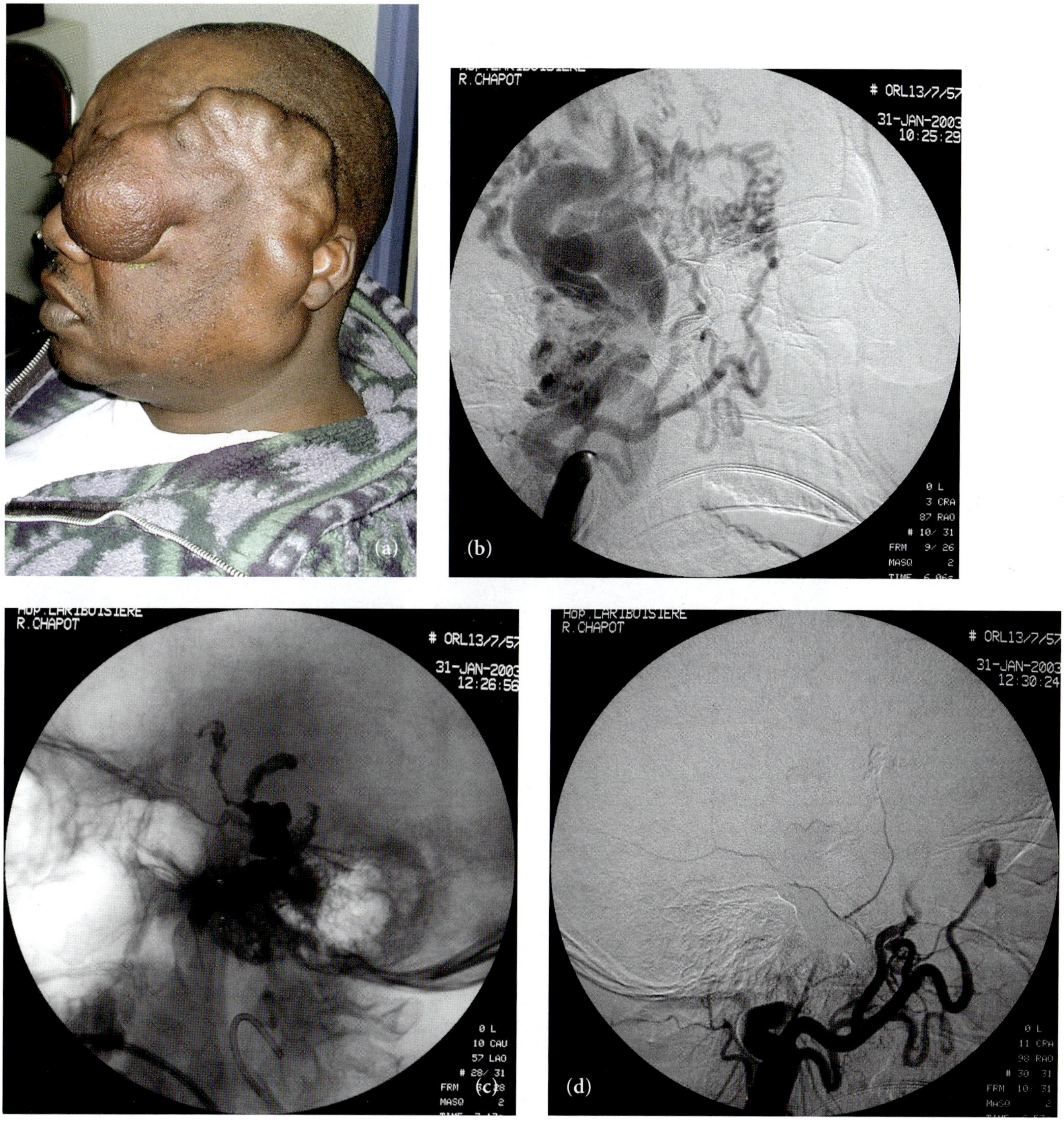

A transverse facial artery fistula gives this 49-year-old African man a facial mass made of enlarged tortuous and throbbing vessels (a). Angiography found a single AV shunt that was occluded with coils and glue (b, c), allowing complete angiographic cure (d). Clinically, progressive shrinkage of the vascular mass was noted.

Specific Locations, Problems Created, Investigations, and Treatments

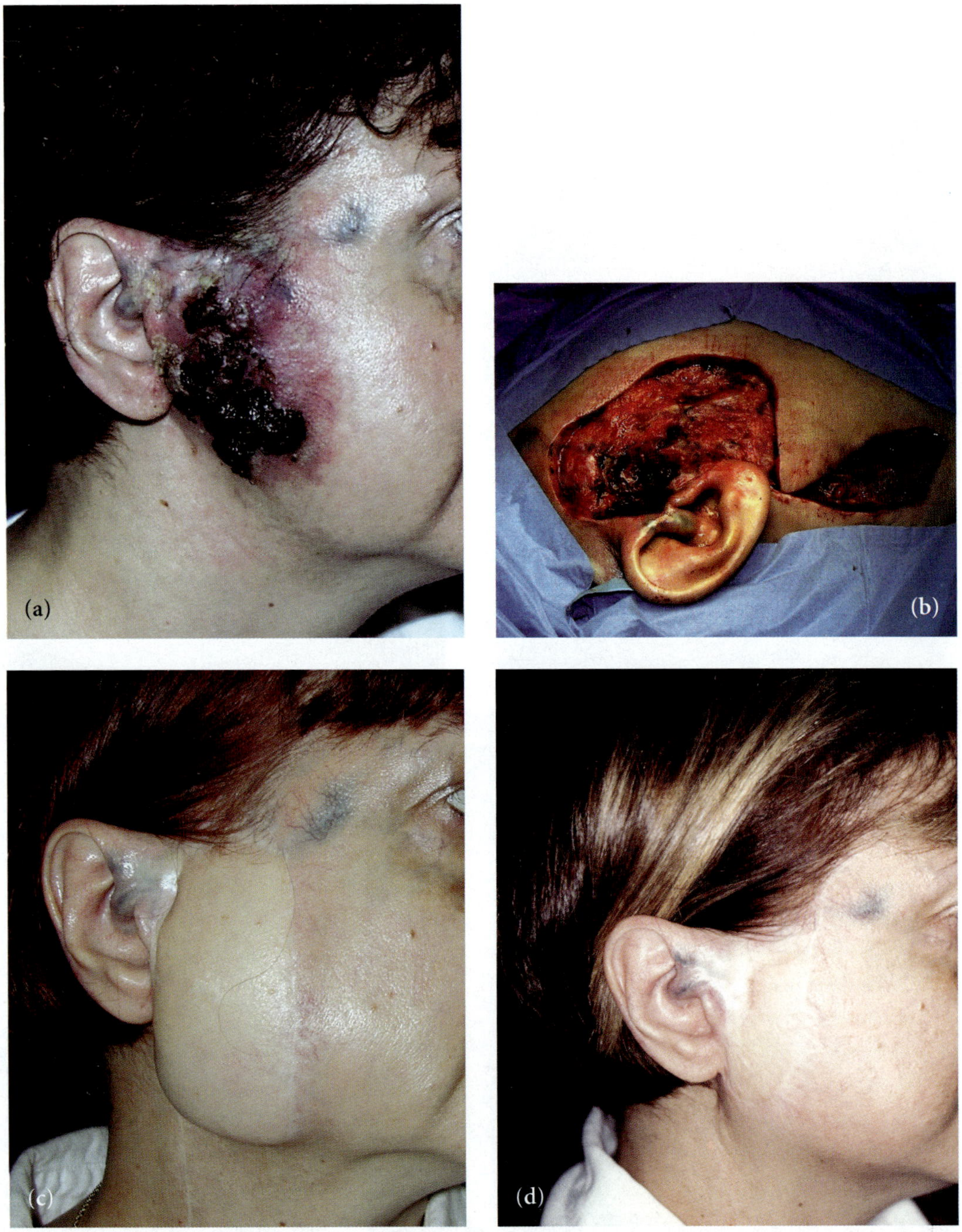

This stage III AVM in the parotid area was necrotic. Significant hemorrhages required treatment (a). Healing was not obtained despite various embolization procedures. Consequently, total excision was decided on. Pre-operative embolization with particles was performed. Then the full lesion and the superficial part of the parotid gland were excised (b). Reconstruction used an anastomosed skin-and-muscle flap transfer from the latissimus dorsalis (c). The flap was thick; when the post-therapeutic vascular situation was stable, the size of the flap was reduced 34 months later. At four years of follow-up (d) the results were good; there was no facial palsy, and no vascular recurrence was noted by US/Doppler scan (operators: Dr. Didier Salvan and Dr. Emmanuel Racy, Hôpital Lariboisière, Paris, France).

Specific Locations, Problems Created, Investigations, and Treatments

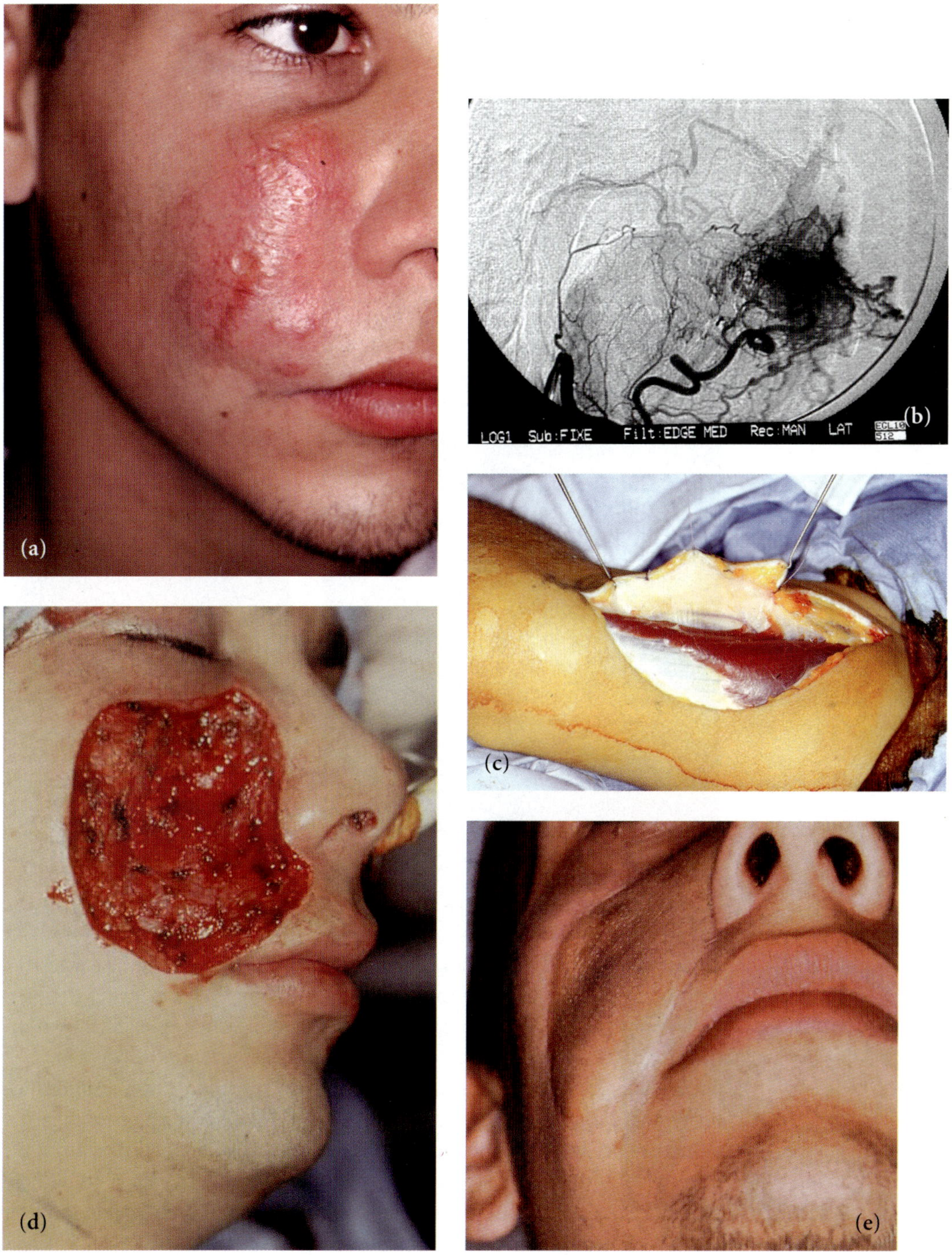

This adolescent with AVM in the cheek had, at 16 years, embolization and excision with direct closure; 18 months later the AVM regrowth was obvious (a); the large nidus (b) fed by the facial and internal maxillary arteries was embolized to minimize intraoperative bleeding, and a second surgical treatment was performed, including total resection of the cheek (c). Reconstruction required a free flap (brachial flap) anastomosed to the facial artery (operator: Dr. Didier Salvan, Department of ENT and Plastic Surgery, Hôpital Lariboisière, Paris, France). At two years of follow-up the results were stable (d).

Specific Locations, Problems Created, Investigations, and Treatments

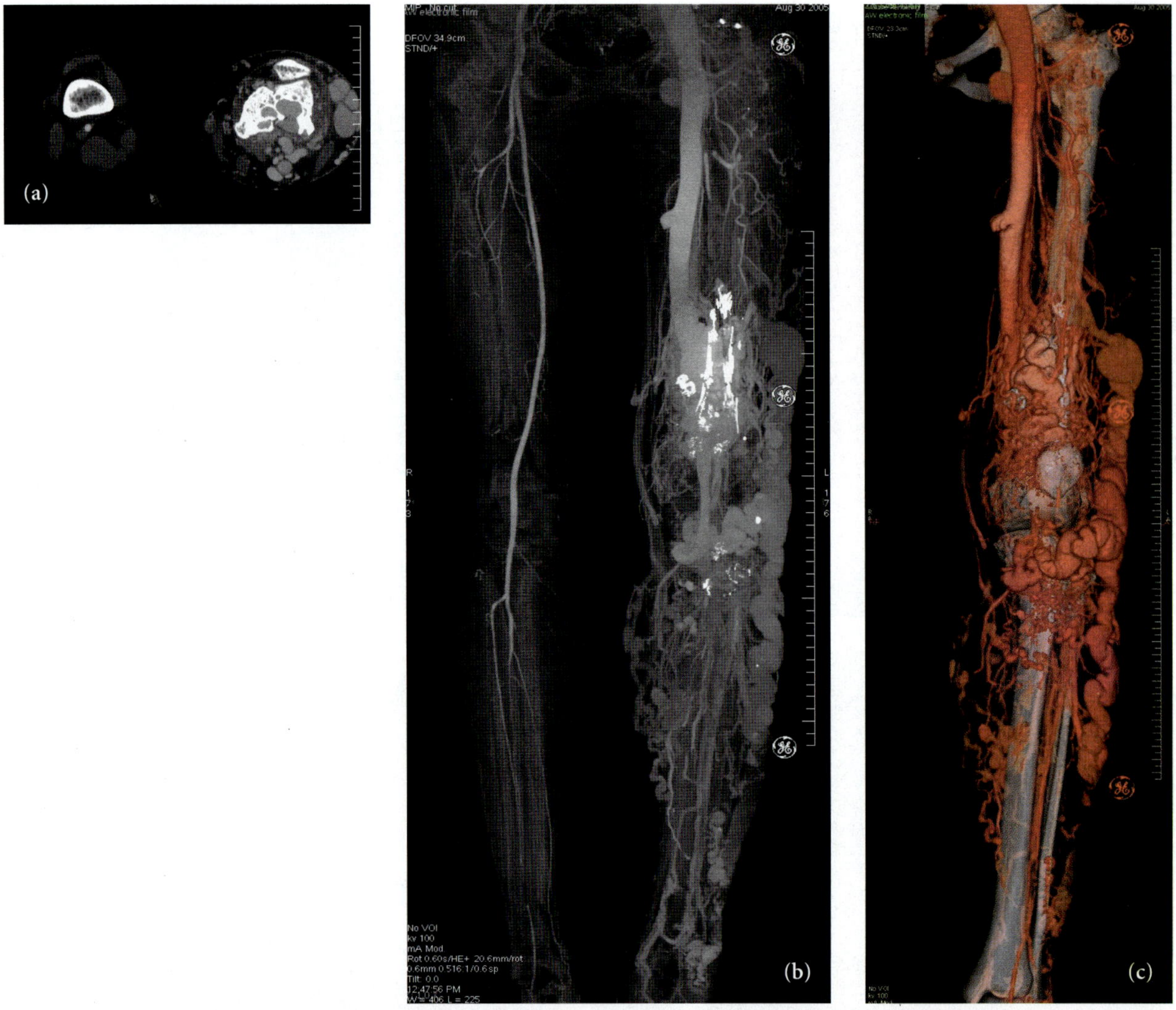

Arteriovenous malformation of the lower limb in Schobinger's stage III with bony lytic changes of the tibia evidenced by CT scan (a), corresponding to large draining veins permeating the bone, as shown on the angio-CT scan sequence (b) and its 3-D reconstruction (c). The patient avoids trauma as much as possible (no sport, no exercise, and thick protective elastic stockings) because of the risk of severe hemorrhage if a fracture occurs. Therapeutic discussion concerns the issue of treating the intraosseous vascular lesions, and injecting glue or cement to strengthen the bone, but with a risk of suppression of a possibly useful drainage after the AV shunting.

Specific Locations, Problems Created, Investigations, and Treatments

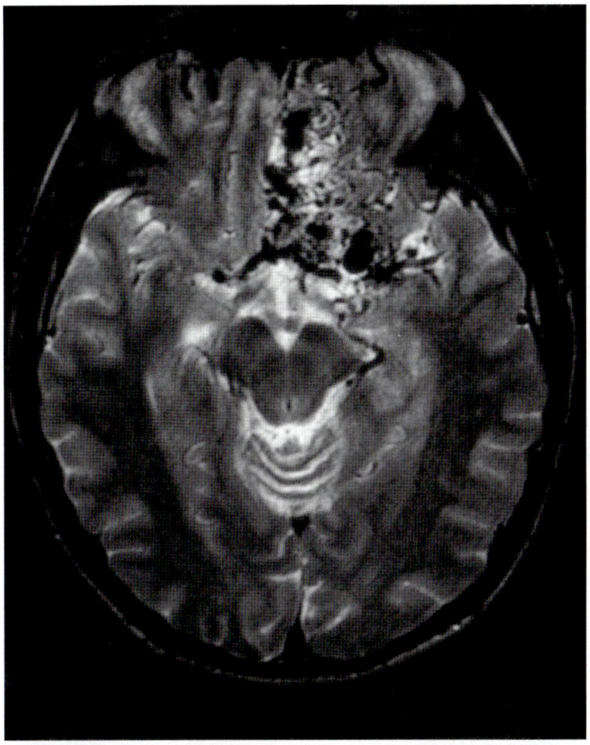

MRI of the brain involvement in a patient with Bonnet–Dechaume–Blanc syndrome. The Schobinger stage III skin AVM in the mid-forehead was resected after arterial embolization, and the long-term results were stable and good. As the cerebral lesion was not symptomatic and difficult to access, no treatment was offered.

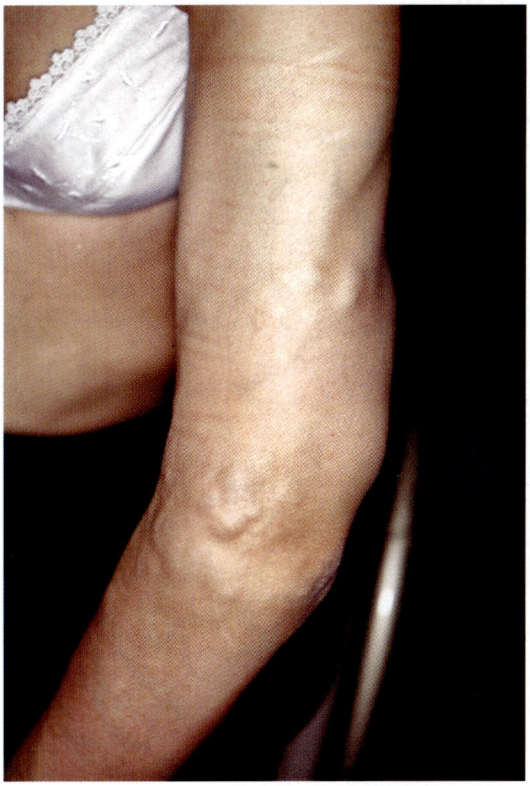

This woman has Cobb syndrome. She also has a diffuse extremity AVM with overgrowth of the affected arm, which constitutes Parkes Weber syndrome: a number of our patients with spinal lesions of Cobb syndrome also have such involvement of the extremity located in the same metamere. This young woman developed neurological signs from the spinal dorsal AVM; arterial embolization was not effective and she became paraplegic.

Specific Locations, Problems Created, Investigations, and Treatments

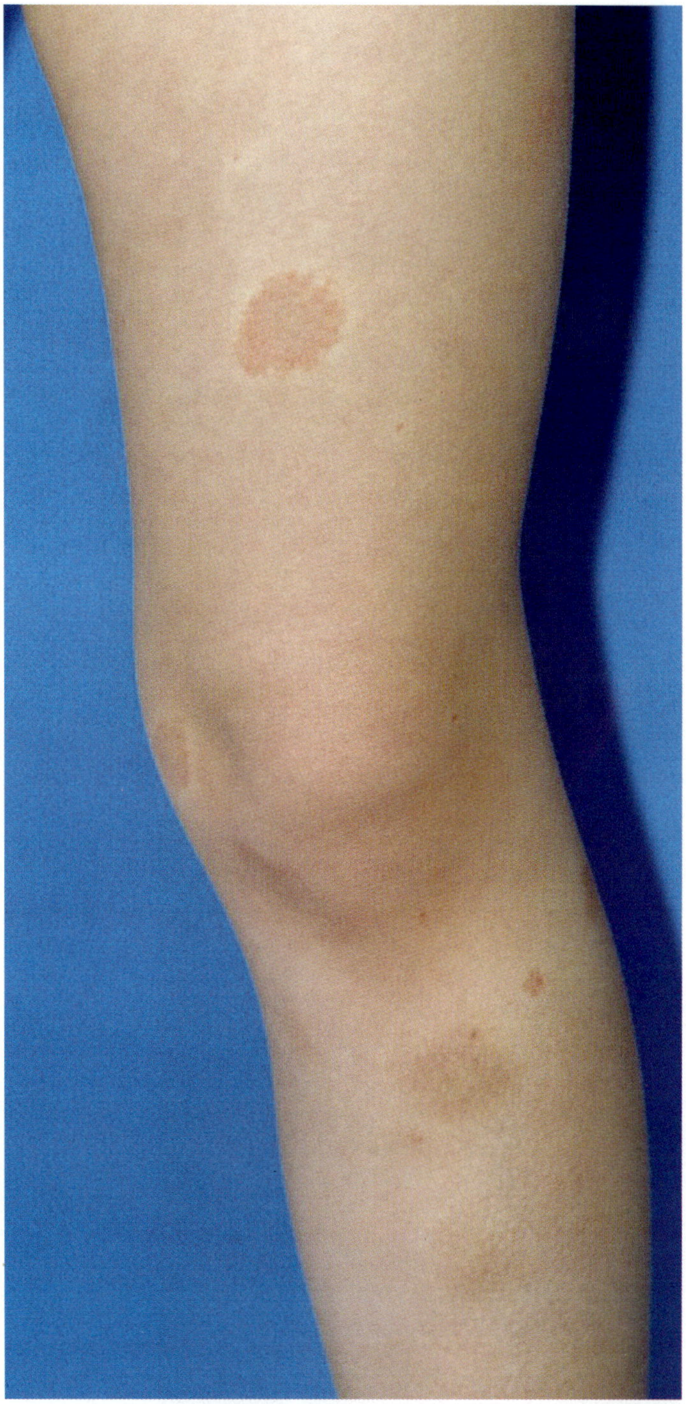

Like other members of her family, this girl has the typical small, multiple capillary stains with a thin pale halo, but in her case they are observed in association with a limb AVM, as part of the CM–AVM syndrome linked to *RASA1* mutation (7).

References

1 Bhattacharya JJ, Luo CB, Suh D. Wyburn-Mason or Bonnet–Dechaume–Blanc as cerebrofacial arteriovenous metameric syndromes (CAMS). *Intervent Neuroradiol* 2001; **7**: 5–17.

2 Bonnet P, Dechaume J, Blanc E. L'anévrisme cirsoide de la rétine (anévrisme racémeux). Ses relations avec l'anévrisme cirsoide du cerveau. *Le Journal Médical de Lyon* 1937; **18**: 165–78.

3 Burrows PB, Bisdorff A, Karian V, Mason K. Complications of ethanol embolization of arteriovenous malformations. Communication T21 in 15th ISSVA Workshop. Wellington, NZ. 22–25 February 2004.

4 Burrows PE, Laor T, Paltiel H, Robertson RL. Diagnostic imaging in the evaluation of vascular birthmarks. *Dermatol Clin* 1998; **16**: 455–88.

5 Do YS, Yakes WF, Shin SW, Lee BB, Kim DI, Liu WC et al. Ethanol embolization of arteriovenous malformations: interim results. *Radiology* 2005; **235**: 674–82.

6 Dubois J, Garel L, Grignon A, David M, Laberge L, Filiatrault D et al. Imaging of hemangiomas and vascular malformations in children. *Acad Radiol* 1998; **5**: 390–400.

7 Eerola I, Boon LM, Mulliken JB, Burrows PE, Dompmartin A, Watanabe S et al. Capillary malformation–arteriovenous malformation, a new clinical and genetic disorder caused by RASA1 mutations. *Am J Hum Genet* 2003; **73**: 1240–9.

8 Enjolras O, Chapot R, Merland JJ. Vascular anomalies and the growth of limbs: a review. *J Pediatr Orthop* B 2004; **13**: 349–57.

9 Enjolras O, Logeart I, Gelbert F, Lemarchand-Venencie F, Reizine D, Guichard JP et al. Arteriovenous malformations: a study of 200 cases. *Ann Dermatol Venereol* 2000; **127**: 17–22.

10 Enjolras O, Mulliken JB. Vascular tumors and vascular malformations (new issues). *Adv Dermatol* 1997; **13**: 375–423.

11 Gladbach B, Pfeil J, Heijens E. Percutaneous epiphyseodesis. Correction of leg length inequalities and frontal plane deformities. *Orthopade* 2000; **29**: 2–8.

12 Khong PL, Burrows PE, Kozakewich HP, Mulliken JB. Fast-flow lingual vascular anomalies in the young patient: is imaging diagnostic? *Pediatr Radiol* 2003; **33**: 118–22.

13 Kohout MP, Hansen M, Pribaz JJ, Mulliken JB. Arteriovenous malformations of the head and neck: natural history and management. *Plast Reconstr Surg* 1998; **102**: 643–54.

14 Larralde M, Gonzalez V, Marietti R, Nussembaum D, Peirano M, Schroh R. Pseudo-Kaposi sarcoma with arteriovenous malformation. *Pediatr Dermatol* 2001; **18**: 325–7.

15 Lee BB, Do YS, Yakes W, Kim DI, Mattassi R, Hyon WS. Management of arteriovenous malformations: a multidisciplinary approach. *J Vasc Surg* 2004; **39**: 590–600.

16 Park S, Tepper OM, Galiano RD, Capla JM, Baharestani S, Kleinman ME et al. Selective recruitment of endothelial progenitor cells to ischemic tissues with increased neo-vascularization. *Plast Reconstr Surg* 2004; **113**: 284–93.

17 Robertson RL, Robson CD, Barnes PD, Burrows PE. Head and neck vascular anomalies of childhood. *Neuroimaging Clin N Am* 1999; **9**: 115–32.

18 Rodesch G, Hurth M, Alvarez H, Tadie M, Lasjaunias P. Classification of spinal cord arteriovenous shunts: proposal for a reappraisal – the Bicetre experience with 155 consecutive patients treated between 1981 and 1999. *Neurosurgery* 2002; **51**: 374–9; discussion 379–80.

19 Sofocleous CT, Rosen RJ, Raskin K, Fioole B, Hofstee DJ. Congenital vascular malformations in the hand and forearm. *J Endovasc Ther* 2001; **8**: 484–94.

20 Takaya N, Iwase T, Maehara A, Nishiyama S, Nakanishi S, Yamana D et al. Transcatheter embolization of arteriovenous malformations in Cowden disease. *Jpn Circ J* 1999; **63**: 326–9.

21 Upton J, Coombs CJ, Mulliken JB, Burrows PE, Pap S. Vascular malformations of the upper limb: a review of 270 patients. *J Hand Surg Am* 1999; **24**: 1019–35.

22 Wu JK, Bisdorff A, Gelbert F, Enjolras O, Burrows PE, Mulliken JB. Auricular arteriovenous malformation: evaluation, management, and outcome. *Plast Reconstr Surg* 2005; **115**: 985–95.

23 Wyburn-Mason R. Arteriovenous aneurysm of midbrain and retina, facial nevi, and mental changes. *Brain* 1943; **66**: 163–203.

24 Yakes WF, Luethke JM, Merland JJ, Rak KM, Slater DD, Hollis HW et al. Ethanol embolization of arteriovenous fistulas: a primary mode of therapy. *J Vasc Interv Radiol* 1990; **1**: 89–96.

25 Yakes WF, Yee DC. Safety of ethanol embolization for the treatment of vascular malformations. Communication T20 in 15th ISSVA Workshop. Wellington, NZ. 22–25 February 2004.

Conclusion

This Color Atlas illustrates the most common aspects of the main vascular lesions, once identified as "angiomas" or "vascular birthmarks." It clarifies the problems of classification and we strongly recommend use of the ISSVA classification system. Our Atlas gives insight into the biological behavior and the differences between vascular tumors and vascular malformations. It focuses on the clinical aspects, the main pathological features, and radiological data, and it illustrates the various therapeutic approaches, their indications and their results.

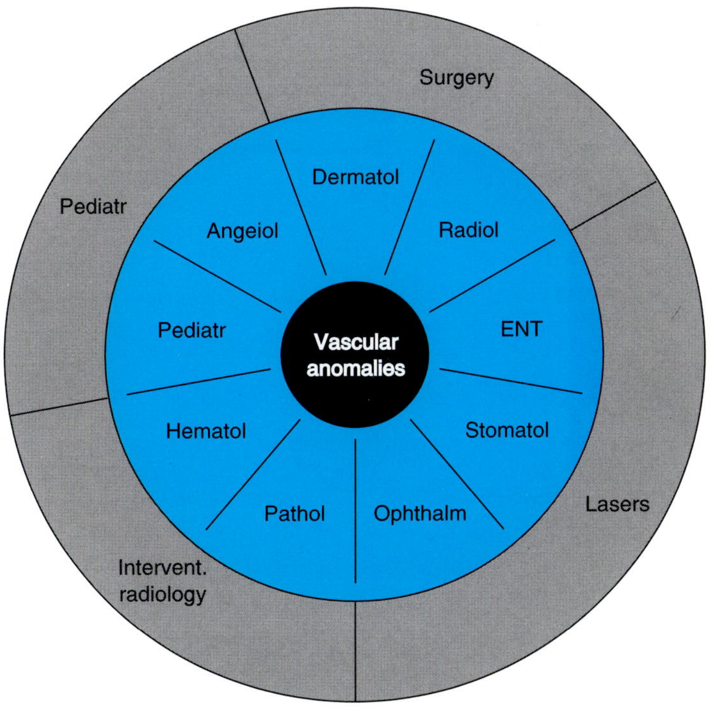

Figure 1 Specialists involved in a multidisciplinary team for diagnosis and treatment of vascular anomalies.

We do not attempt to offer an exhaustive book on the subject of vascular lesions. We only try to offer a comprehensive review of those previously called "angiomas" or "vascular birthmarks." Therefore this Atlas does not address in detail the many genetic syndromes that cause vascular anomalies, and does not display a dermatological pot-pourri of small uncommon dermatological vascular lesions that are clearly benign (such as pyogenic granuloma, hobnail hemangioma, epithelioid or histiocytoid hemangioma, etc.). Nor does it cover vascular tumors of possibly intermediate malignancy, such as the composite hemangioendothelioma. The vascular malignancies (angiosarcomas, lymphangiosarcomas) are beyond our scope (they were never considered "angiomas" or "birthmarks").

And finally, we want to stress the fact that identifying the diverse clinical, pathological, and radiological aspects of the various vascular tumors and malformations, as well as selecting their optimal therapeutic management, requires a multidisciplinary approach in the vast majority of cases.

Index